Controversies in Central Auditory Processing Disorder

Opening of Pandora's Box

The art work on the cover of this book portrays the famous painting of "Pandora" by John Williams Waterhouse. This neo-classical work-of-art (circa 1849–1917) depicts the beauty and allure of Pandora, as told in Greek mythology, and captures her intense curiosity for the unknown. Similarly, the domain of auditory processing and its disorders has elicited much interest and inquisitiveness among various professionals. But in contrast to warnings given to Pandora not to open the infamous box for what might be released, we encourage readers to open the covers of this book to unleash the unique intellectual gifts that lie within.

If the classical story about Pandora remains veridical, then lurking at the bottom of the opened box, we should expect to find hope. It is this same symbolism that we envision for this book; the hope that it will serve as a tool to educate, the expectation that it will spur new ideas, and the belief that these contemporary concepts will advance the field of auditory processing disorders to a new level.

Anthony T. Cacace
Dennis J. McFarland

Controversies in Central Auditory Processing Disorder

Edited by

Anthony T. Cacace, Ph.D.
Dennis J. McFarland, Ph.D.

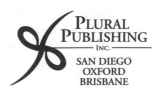

PLURAL
PUBLISHING
INC.

SAN DIEGO
OXFORD
BRISBANE

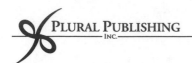

PLURAL PUBLISHING
INC.

5521 Ruffin Road
San Diego, CA 92123

e-mail: info@pluralpublishing.com
Web site: http://www.pluralpublishing.com

49 Bath Street
Abingdon, Oxfordshire OX14 1EA
United Kingdom

Library of Congress Cataloging-in-Publication Data

Controversies in central auditory processing disorder (CAPD) / [edited by] Anthony T.
Cacace and Dennis J. McFarland.
     p. ; cm.
  Includes bibliographical references and index.
  ISBN-13: 978-1-59756-260-7 (alk. paper)
  ISBN-10: 1-59756-260-2 (alk. paper)
  1. Word deafness. 2. Auditory perception. 3. Auditory pathways.
  [DNLM: 1. Language Development Disorders. 2. Auditory Cortex—physiopathology.
3. Auditory Pathways—physiopathology. 4. Auditory Perception—physiology. 5. Auditory
Perceptual Disorders. WL 340.2 C764 2008] I. Cacace, Anthony T. II. McFarland, Dennis J.
  RC394.W63C66 2008
  617.8—dc22

                                                                    2008009909

Contents

Foreword

If you are looking for a clinical cookbook on how to diagnose those suspected of having (central) auditory processing disorders (CAPD), and subsequently treat those so diagnosed, then you should not read this book. This book is much less than a clinical "cookbook," but much, much more. I will begin by telling the reader what this book does not do. This book does not offer any agreed upon definition of CAPD. It does not offer a clear underlying anatomic or physiologic basis for this clinical entity. It neither promises nor delivers a consensus statement about a test battery for diagnosing the disorder. It does not have separate chapters representing the various well-known groups who have their own unique and often idiosyncratic definitions, models, and tests of CAPD. No chapter focuses on treatment. Why, you might ask, did this book not include the above listed omissions? I believe that there are at least two good answers to this question. First, recently published books, or sections of books, have been dedicated to the above issues, and little would have been accomplished by producing yet another "cookbook." Second, there is currently great divisiveness in the field of audiology concerning CAPD. There is no broadly accepted definition of CAPD. No one really knows what causes CAPD. Despite lofty claims to the contrary, there is no clear consensus concerning the battery of tests that lead to a diagnosis of CAPD. Similarly, there is no widely accepted auditory (re)habilitation program that has been conclusively shown to help those with CAPD. The strength and value of this book is that it clearly points out that "the emperor has no clothes." We are hamstrung by the lack of agreement in definitions and test batteries in the area of CAPD.

This book does include several chapters that tell the reader what we currently know about the auditory nervous system from recent animal studies, as well as human studies using emerging functional-imaging modalities. Chapters are not limited to topics directly related to CAPD, but address multiple clinical entities, including auditory neuropathy, specific learning disabilities, and tinnitus. One chapter is dedicated to addressing age-related changes in auditory abilities. Lessons are offered about moving the field forward by those with expertise in epidemiology. It is clear that we must do a better job in designing studies to identify the incidence and prevalence of CAPD, with particular attention paid to the sensitivity and specificity of the test battery, as well as issues of validity and reliability. Arguments are made both for and against using linguistic stimuli in the CAPD battery. Tests that use language are potentially confounded by the linguistic competency of the patient. One chapter discusses the current generation of speech-discrimination tests. These tests are far from perfect in identifying subtle changes in speech-discrimination problems in those with peripheral hearing loss, and have limitations as tools to identify auditory processing problems. There is even a chapter on the processing of music in various clinical populations. Music is as complex spectrally and temporally as speech, but without the linguistic load of speech stimuli.

There are arguments made that, unless the problems in CAPD can be shown to be solely (or at least primarily) auditory in nature, then it should not be labeled an "auditory" processing problem. This is more than a semantic issue. It would mandate a multimodal evaluation process. If the test material were linguistic in nature, then the visual modality would need to be evaluated, as the auditory and visual modalities are the only two sensory systems that are commonly used to process linguistic stimuli. Designing tests in the auditory modality and visual modality that assess similar constructs is far from a straightforward problem. If multiple modalities are shown to be impaired in those with CAPD, then this would argue for a supramodal problem in CAPD. This would possibly move this disorder from the audiologic to the psychological domain, and possibly outside the scope of practice for audiologists.

The current divisiveness in the field is not a bad thing—it is simply the growing pains of an emerging area of study. You could read this book, and possibly walk away a little depressed about the lack of agreement. I, on the other hand, walked away feeling hopeful. Strong-willed, articulate, and intelligent clinicians/scientists have come together to offer new views and to kick sand in the face of convention. In their blatant identification of problems, they offer a path to salvation for the field in general: We must lose our ego involvement in old definitions, untestable theories, and mechanisms that are not borne out by experimental data. We must learn from our colleagues in other fields—we can and must design psychometrically sound test batteries. We must accept that cognitive, linguistic, and attentional factors can potentially influence our test results. We must be willing at least to consider the possibility that CAPD may not be solely or even predominantly auditory. We must continue to look for the underlying anatomic and/or physiologic basis for CAPD, as a better understanding of the underlying disorder should lead to better interventions. We must continue our functional-imaging and evoked-potential studies of those with CAPD, as these will likely shed light on the underlying cause of this disorder. Data are presented in this book suggesting that there may be no educational sequelae of CAPD. If this is the case, we must ask ourselves if it is worth the time and the financial resources to identify and treat this disorder. Longitudinal studies in a large group of those diagnosed with CAPD are needed to get a better handle on what happens to these children: Are they less likely to finish college, or hold a good job; will they make less money? Are they more likely to show processing problems in old age, have a lower perceived quality of life—do they become Republicans?

It is my most sincere hope that this book will lead to a better dialog among those involved in CAPD, both clinically and in the research arena. I hope that each author reads the book in its entirety. The value of this book is that it asks many more questions than it answers. It made me think—and I hope it makes you think too. I would like to see the issues raised debated at meetings, and argued about in the literature. Furthermore, I do hope to read a "clinical cookbook" on CAPD in the next decade or so, where there is consensus on the definition, test battery, underlying mechanism(s), and treatment of CAPD. It is only through discussion, debate, argument, and finally agreement that the muddy water of CAPD will become clear and palatable.

Robert F. Burkard

Preface

Our goal as editors was to highlight different viewpoints from individuals who have worked in the area of auditory processing; as clinicians, basic scientists, or both. In the clinical domain, the topic of auditory processing disorders has been a "lightning rod for controversy" that seems to have fostered ongoing debates for over 3 decades. In order to bring these issues to the forefront, we made a concerted effort to invite a representative sample of individuals to express a wide range of views on this topic to help resolve and/or better understand some of the relevant issues. However, not everyone accepted our invitation. Unfortunately, some individuals accepted initially but their commitment to put their thoughts in writing never materialized; one group formally withdrew.

However, the 17 chapters in this book represent a wide range of relevant viewpoints and topics ranging from modality specificity, innovative ways to define auditory cortex by magnetic resonance imaging, advanced concepts in anatomy and physiology, issues related to learning and plasticity, to topics dealing with musical perception and its disorders. Although some chapters express critical commentary with respect to the conceptualization and diagnosis of CAPD/APD, they are not intended to be offensive, nor should they be construed as acrimonious to any one person or group. Moreover, the editors made no attempt to shape or coerce any point of view and it was our underlying intention to allow the author(s) to express their personal opinions. The editorial review process focused primarily on issues related to conforming to style standards, although in some instances, clarification of certain points was needed.

We acknowledge the effort and due diligence put forth by the contributors in describing their work.

Additionally, we anticipate that the various chapters contained herein will clarify some issues, generate discussion and debate, and open up new vistas for research. The need to provide individuals entering the field with a full range of viewpoints is obvious and we endorse this approach as a healthy way to educate. At the same time, some of the novel ideas expressed in these chapters also may be of value to the experienced clinician and valued researcher. They may provide the impetus to reconsider certain points of view, help formulate novel hypotheses, and perform experiments needed to advance the field.

Lastly, we wish to thank Professor Robert F. Burkard for writing the Foreword to this book. Our selection of this individual was based on his editorial experience and scientific prowess. Indeed, we were interested in obtaining an independent overview from someone respected in the field of hearing science and known to be knowledgeable, always critical, but nonetheless fair.

We hope that readers enjoy the book and gain useful knowledge from it.

Anthony T. Cacace
Dennis J. McFarland

Contributors

Karen Banai, Ph.D.
Department of Communication Sciences
Northwestern University
Evanston, Illinois
Department of Communication Sciences
University of Haifa
Haifa, Israel
Chapter 15

Robert F. Burkard, Ph.D.
Professor and Chair
Department of Rehabilitation Science
University at Buffalo
Buffalo, New York
Chapter 17 and Foreword

Anthony T. Cacace, Ph.D.
Professor
Departments of Communication Sciences
    and Disorders and Otolaryngology
Wayne State University
Detroit, Michigan
Chapters 6, 12, and 17

Justin Cowan, Ph.D.
Postdoctoral Researcher
Department of Experimental Psychology
University of Oxford
Oxford, UK
Chapter 11

Karen J. Cruickshanks, Ph.D.
Professor
Departments of Ophthalmology and Visual
    Sciences
and Department of Population Health
    Sciences

University of Wisconsin School of
    Medicine and Public Health
Madison, Wisconsin
Chapter 7

Simone Dalla Bella, Ph.D.
Associate Professor
Department of Cognitive Psychology
University of Finance and Management
Warsaw, Poland
International Laboratory for Brain, Music,
    and Sound Research (BRAMS)
Montreal, Canada
Chapter 14

Dirk De Ridder, M.D., Ph.D.
Professor
Department of Neurosurgery
and Brain Research Center of Antwerp for
    Innovative Interdisciplinary
    Neuromodulation
University Hospital Antwerp
Edegem, Belgium
Chapter 16

Frank Eisner, Ph.D.
Institute of Cognitive Neuroscience
University College London
London, UK
Chapter 3

Troy A. Hackett, Ph.D.
Assistant Professor
Department of Hearing and Speech Sciences
Vanderbilt University School of Medicine
Nashville, Tennessee
Chapter 2

Larry E. Humes, Ph.D.
Professor
Department of Speech and Hearing
    Sciences
Indiana University
Bloomington, Indiana
Chapter 8

James F. Jerger, Ph.D.
Distinguished Scholar-in-Residence
School of Behavioral and Brain Sciences
The University of Texas at Dallas
Dallas, Texas
Chapter 1

Robert W. Keith, Ph.D.
Professor
Department of Communication Sciences
    and Disorders
College of Allied Health
Univerisity of Cincinnatti
Cincinnati, Ohio
Chapter 10

Gary R. Kidd, Ph.D.
Associate Scientist
Department of Speech and Hearing
    Sciences
Indiana University
Bloomington, Indiana
Chapter 13

Nina Kraus, Ph.D.
Hugh Knowles Professor
Department of Communication Sciences;
    Neurobiology; Otolaryngology
Northwestern University
Chicago, Illinois
Chapter 15

Rachel McArdle, Ph.D.
Chief
Audiology and Speech Pathology
    Service
Bay Pines VA Healthcare System
Bay Pines, Florida

and
Assistant Professor
Communication Sciences and Disorders
University of South Florida
Tampa, Florida
Chapter 9

Dennis J. McFarland, Ph.D.
Research Scientist
Laboratory of Nervous System Disorders
Wadsworth Laboratories
New York State Department of Health
Albany, New York
Chapters 6 and 12

Jennifer R. Melcher, Ph.D.
Assistant Professor
Department of Otology and Laryngology
Harvard Medical School
Eaton-Peabody Laboratory,
Massachusetts Eye and Ear Infirmary
Speech and Hearing Bioscience and
    Technology Program,
Harvard-MIT Division of Health Science
    and Technology
Boston, Massachusetts
Chapter 5

Tomas Menovsky, M.D., Ph.D.
Department of Neurosurgery
University Medical Center St. Radboud
Nijmegen, Belgium
Chapter 16

David R. Moore, Ph.D.
Director
MRC Institute of Hearing Research
University Park
Nottingham, U.K.
Chapter 11

Josef P. Rauschecker, Ph.D.
Professor of Physiology and Biophysics,
    Neurology and Psychology
Laboratory of Integrative Neuroscience
    and Cognition

Georgetown University
Washington, DC
Chapter 4

Stuart Rosen, Ph.D.
Professor of Speech and Hearing
    Science
Department of Phonetics and Linguistics
University College London
London, England
Chapter 11

Sophie K. Scott, Ph.D., B.Sc. (Hons)
Institute of Cognitive Neuroscience
University College London
London, England
Chapter 3

Paul H. Van de Heyning M.D., Ph.D.
Department of Otolaryngology
University Hospital Antwerp
Antwerp, Belgium
Chapter 16

Charles S. Watson, Ph.D.
Professor Emeritus
Department of Speech and Hearing
    Sciences and Psychology (Adj.)
Indiana University
and
President
Communication Disorders Technology,
    Inc.
Bloomington, Indiana
Chapter 13

Richard H. Wilson, Ph.D.
Senior Research Career Scientist
VA Medical Center
Mountain Home, Tennessee
and
Professor
Departments of Communication Disorders
    and Surgery
East Tennessee State University
Johnson City, Tennessee
Chapter 9

To my wife Lydia and children: Elizabeth, Cassandra, and Anthony, Jr.
A. T. Cacace

To my wife, Loretta
D. J. McFarland

CHAPTER 1

The Concept of Auditory Processing Disorder— A Brief History

JAMES F. JERGER

In order to understand current concepts of auditory processing disorder (APD), it may be instructive to trace the historical development of the idea. My first contact with the APD arena came as a graduate assistant in the clinic of Helmer Myklebust at Northwestern University in the early 1950s. Over the next half century I have observed the work of others, participated in some test development, and have thought a good deal about this enigmatic disorder. Any history must, necessarily, reflect a bit of the historian; colleagues may detect a personal bias here or there, but I have tried to tread a neutral path throughout. The story begins in the mid-19th century.

The Early Pioneers

The roots of APD lie in the seminal observations of the great 19th and early 20th century neurologists, especially Paul Broca, Carl Wernicke, John Hughlings Jackson, Henry Head, and Sigmund Freud. These pioneers firmly established the link between brain injury and disturbances of both receptive and expressive language processing, the disorders we now know as the various forms of aphasia. As they examined patients with symptoms of language disorder, however, they sometimes encountered individuals who seemed to have a qualitatively different sort of language processing problem. These individuals could hear words and see objects but appeared to have trouble understanding what they meant. Although Sigmund Freud introduced the term "Agnosia" to describe the general condition of inability to interpret received sensory stimuli, and S. E. Henschen introduced the term "Word Deafness" to describe a specifically auditory variant, nonetheless, Henry Head (1926) was the first to describe such disorders in detail. He had encountered many such patients in his studies of victims of head wounds during the First World War and concluded that such disorders were distinct from the aphasias. His description of the problem, more than 80 years ago, still resonates:

> *Word deafness ... is shown particularly by inability to understand spoken words. Like a person in a foreign country, the patient hears the sounds, distinguishes one from another, but they convey to him no meaning. ... Now it is obvious that such manifestations must represent a disturbance on a lower functional level than those of any form of aphasia or amnesia: They are primarily defects of perception.* (Head, 1926, p. 105)

Here, Head clearly elucidates the notion of a deficit in auditory perception as distinct from a higher order language processing disorder. This was the fundamental conceptual framework underlying the earliest view of APD. We shall see, however, that over the years it has become widely embellished.

Although this early work on aphasia and agnosia was based on the study of patients with demonstrable, usually severe, brain injury, it was only a short intuitive leap to the idea that milder manifestations of such perceptual disorders might be the result of less severe neurologic dysfunction, perhaps deriving from faulty development or childhood illness and lacking "hard" signs. One of the first to posit such a possibility was Helmer Myklebust, a psychologist with a strong background in the evaluation of deaf children.

Helmer Myklebust

When he came to Northwestern University's School of Speech in the late 1940s, Myklebust opened a diagnostic children's hearing clinic and encouraged parents, pediatricians, and other professionals to refer children suspected of possible hearing loss. This was, of course, a period that predated, by many years, the advent of tools like infant hearing screening, the auditory brainstem response (ABR) and otoacoustic emissions (OAEs), or even sophisticated play audiometry. Deciding whether a young child might have a hearing loss was based on a good deal of prior experience with hearing-impaired children, skillful observation, focused questioning, some controlled testing, and intuition.

The primary presenting symptom that brought children to the clinic, and indeed to most hearing-care professionals in that era, was "not talking" (i.e., failure to develop speech appropriate to the child's chronologic age), an inevitable sequela of moderate to severe hearing loss. And, indeed, Myklebust found such losses in many of the children referred to his clinic: but he also observed that a number of the children referred for lack of appropriate speech development had no apparent loss in auditory sensitivity. Something else seemed to be going on. They could "hear," but what they "heard" was apparently not sufficient for proper language development. Myklebust suggested that some of these children might have a form of mild auditory agnosia. In his words "... *A certain number of young children have disturbances of auditory perception without symbolic language disorders*" (Myklebust, 1952, p. 157). His descriptions of such children has a contemporary ring:

> *One of their fundamental difficulties is that they cannot listen; therefore, they cannot direct their attention selectively to an expected sound. To them the auditory environment does not consist of many individual sounds to be used as the immediate situation demands. Their auditory world is conglomerate; all sounds having equal importance and all being foreground sounds*

simultaneously. (Myklebust, 1952, pp. 256–257)

It is also noteworthy that Myklebust did not insist that such disorders must be "auditory-specific."

Inability to listen, to give sustained selected responses auditorially, is a characteristic of disturbed auditory perception. Such disturbances frequently are associated with analogous disorders in the area of vision. However, auditory perceptual disorders are not necessarily associated with visual perceptual disorders, either can occur as distinct from the other. (Myklebust, 1954, p. 159).

To fit Myklebust's contribution into the context of his times, it is important to remember that in those days the principal emphasis was on "deafness." If the problem was not clearly in the periphery, then it was called "central deafness." Myklebust introduced the term "auditory disorder" as a comprehensive descriptor covering not only peripheral hearing sensitivity loss but the consequences of problems at higher levels in the auditory system, especially as they affected language development. He then developed a systematic behavioral approach to the differential diagnosis of such disorders. It still serves as the model for many contemporary behavioral approaches to the diagnosis of APD.

The Italians

The years 1954 to 1955 saw the publication of two seminal papers by a group of Italian investigators led by Ettore Bocca. The conventional wisdom at this point in time was that lesions involving the auditory cortex were not likely to be revealed by conventional speech audiometric testing. Scores on monosyllabic word lists typically were well within normal limits (e.g., Goldstein, Goodman, & King, 1956). But Bocca and colleagues (Bocca, Calearo, & Cassinari, 1954; Bocca, Calearo, Cassinari, & Migliavacca, 1955) showed that, if you made the listening task sufficiently difficult, lesions affecting the auditory cortex in one hemisphere would be revealed as a depressed speech understanding score on the ear opposite the affected side of the brain. Initially they "sensitized" Italian word lists by low-pass filtering the speech, or by presenting the words at a very low sensation level. Later they employed "speeded" speech, by recording the words while speaking rapidly (Calearo & Lazzaroni, 1957), an early precursor to contemporary digital speech compression.

These findings had an electrifying effect on investigators throughout the world, but especially in the United States, where the implication for the diagnosis of central auditory disorders was apparent. The work of the Italians chiefly had been based on patients with tumors of the temporal lobe, but the intuitive leap to the investigation of persons with auditory complaints, but lacking "hard" neurologic signs, was irresistible. A number of investigators (Jerger, 1960; Keith, 1986; Lynn & Gilroy, 1977; Matzker, 1959; Musiek, 1983; Speaks & Jerger, 1965) set out to devise difficult or "sensitized" speech audiometric tasks in an attempt to capitalize on the lead provided by the pioneering Italian group.

The Dichotic Connection

Donald Broadbent was an English psychologist who became interested in the fact that airline flight traffic controllers were quite adept at handling communications from two or more aircraft at the same time. To answer the more general question of how many channels of auditory information could be processed simultaneously; he devised what we now know as the dichotic digits test (Broadbent, 1958). One, two, or three pairs of digits were presented to the listener sequentially. Each pair consisted of two different digits, one to the right ear and the other to the left ear. The listener was instructed to repeat back all digits heard in either ear. Broadbent was interested in the extent to which information presented in one channel interfered with information presented in the other channel.

Meanwhile, at the Montreal Neurological Institute, psychologists Brenda Milner and Doreen Kimura saw, in Broadbent's dichotic technique, an interesting possibility for studying patients with neurologic disorders, especially at the cortical level. An interesting byproduct of their research was destined to have a profound effect on the assessment of APD. While testing young-adult normal controls, they noted that there was a small but consistent difference between right-ear and left-ear scores (Kimura, 1967). The average right ear score seemed to be slightly, but significantly, higher than the left-ear score. This has come to be known as the "right-ear advantage (REA)" in dichotic listening, although subsequent experience suggests that "left-ear disadvantage (LED)" would be a more useful term.

This early work on the dichotic listening paradigm generated an interest in the development of dichotic listening tests that might prove useful in evaluating adults with brain lesions. There were two, almost mutually exclusive, rationales driving such development. One was a natural extension of the "sensitized test" idea. Here was a way to make speech processing really difficult, but with the advantage that the speech stimuli

need not be physically altered in any way. Difficult listening was inherent in the complex processing required rather than by modification of the stimuli, per se. In this approach both ears were expected to show deficits; there was no direct interest in interaural differences. The other rationale was related to research with commisurotomy patients (Milner, Taylor, & Sperry, 1968). When the corpus callosum was severed in cases of intractable epilepsy, these patients could understand speech well in either ear if it was presented monaurally, but under dichotic presentation the left-ear score was much worse than the right-ear score, indeed, often abolished entirely. These observations lent strong support to the structural or "hard-wired" theory of dichotic listening in which it is posited that, in most individuals; (a) the left hemisphere is specialized for language processing, (b) contralateral pathways suppress ipsilateral pathways, and, therefore, (c) the right ear input enjoys privileged access to the left hemisphere language processing center, whereas (d) left-ear input must take a less direct path via the right hemisphere and the interhemispheric connection to the left hemisphere via the corpus callosum.

Contemporary dichotic tests may be scored according to either rationale. The former, "sensitized test" rationale is based on no specific neurophysiologic deficit; the latter implicitly predicts either a unilateral hemispheric lesion, or delayed/faulty development of, or age-related decline in, interhemispheric connectivity (Musiek, Gollegly, & Baran, 1984).

Over the next two decades a number of dichotic tests or test batteries were developed for clinical use. In 1962, Katz developed the staggered spondee word (SSW) test. A pair of spondee words is presented dichotically, but the second syllable of one word overlaps the first syllable of the other. Scoring and interpretation are complex (Katz, 1968; Katz, Stecker, & Henderson, 1992).

During this same period, Willeford (1977) developed a dichotic sentence test using natural sentences. The procedure was used effectively by Lynn and Gilroy (1977) in their comprehensive study of adults with verified brain lesions. Shortly thereafter, Berlin, Lowe, Thompson, and Cullen (1968) developed a dichotic test procedure based on consonant-vowel nonsense syllables. Copies of the Berlin tapes were widely used worldwide for the next three decades. During the 1970s, Jerger and Jerger (1974, 1975) modified the synthetic sentence identification (SSI) paradigm by adding either an ipsilateral (SSI-ICM) or a contralateral (SSI-CCM) competing message. In 1983, a dichotic version of the SSI sentences, the dichotic sentence identification (DSI) test was developed (Fifer, Jerger, Berlin, Tobey, & Campbell, 1983).

It should be emphasized that virtually all of this early development of dichotic testing was focused on the study of adults, usually with *verified brain lesions*. Beginning in the late 1970s, however, interest turned toward children (e.g., Katz & Ivey, 1994, p. 242; Musiek, Gollegly, & Baran, 1984). Could "sensitized" speech testing and especially dichotic testing, be used to evaluate children suspected of auditory processing disorder?

Nondichotic Measures

Although dichotic tests have played a major role in APD assessment, other approaches have included low-pass filtering (Keith, 1986; Lynn & Gilroy, 1977), compressed or speeded speech (Beasley & Freeman, 1977; Kurdziel, Noffsinger, & Olsen, 1976), temporal and frequency patterning (Pinheiro & Musiek, 1985), and gap detection (Musiek, Shinn, et al. 2005).

The Psychoeducational Connection

The idea that some children might have particular problems with the processing of auditory input in spite of normal sensitivity spread rapidly during the 1980s. Although Myklebust had raised the issue three decades earlier, the burgeoning societal interest in reading problems, language delay, learning disability, and attention deficit disorder stimulated a widespread rebirth of the concept. Initial impetus came from a landmark publication, *The Psychopathology and Education of the Brain-Injured Child*, by psychoeducational consultants Alfred Strauss and Laura Lehtinen in 1947. The authors proposed a straightforward definition:

The brain-injured child is a child who, before, during, or after birth has received an injury to or suffered an infection of the brain. As a result of such organic impairment, defects of the neuromotor system may be present or absent; however, such a child may show disturbances in perception, thinking, and emotional behavior, either separately or in combination. These disturbances can be demonstrated by specific tests. These disturbances prevent or impede a normal learning process. Special educational methods have been devised to remedy these specific handicaps. (Strauss & Lehtinen, 1947, p. 4)

In these spare sentences, written almost 60 years ago, one can discern much of the current rationale for the diagnosis and treatment of children suspected of a broad variety of disorders including APD. The central theme of this approach was "learning disability." The child was targeted for evaluation because of an assumed learning problem, usually reflected in poor academic perform-ance. The first methodological approach to Strauss and Lehtinens' claim that *"These disturbances can be demonstrated by spe-cific tests"* was the development of the Illi-nois Test of Psycholinguistic Abilities (ITPA) by Sam Kirk (1968). Based on Osgood's model of communication, Kirk defined a number of theoretical constructs thought to underlie the communication skills neces-sary for adequate learning (Kavale & Forness, 1985), In the perceptual-motor domain the ITPA contained five auditory subtests:

- *Auditory Reception*
- *Auditory Association*
- *Auditory Sequential Memory*
- *Auditory Closure*
- *Sound Blending*

Poor performance on one or more these subtests was assumed to be consis-tent with an auditory perceptual problem. Here we can see the earliest stages of devel-opment of one popular contemporary view of auditory processing disorder shared by many audiologists and speech-language pathologists. Auditory perception is viewed as the summation of a number of discrete, measurable abilities. More recently, several additional hypothesized discrete abilities have been added to Kirk's original list.

Two Divergent Paths

At this point in our historical journey, we can already discern the development of two dissimilar approaches to the concept of auditory processing disorder: one might be called the "audiologic" approach; the other the "psychoeducational" approach.

The audiologic approach built on the earlier observations that persons with brain

injury affecting the auditory central nerv-ous system exhibited certain behaviors; *ergo*, if tests revealed these same behaviors, then a link to brain injury was established. Whereas some investigators noted the tau-tology inherent in this syllogism, others accepted the premise and set out to devise tests of the desired behavior appropriate for children. Based on the model of dichotic lis-tening, Keith (1986, 1994, 2000) developed two dichotic test procedures, one employ-ing competing words, the other competing sentences. His SCAN procedures for both adults and children have been widely used in pediatric evaluation. Willeford's battery (1977), including his competing sentences test and Katz' SSW procedure also have been widely applied to children with appar-ently poor listening skills (Arnst & Katz, 1982). In 1983, Jerger, Jerger, and Abrams (1983) developed the Pediatric Speech Intelligibility (PSI) test, a word and sentence-based test procedure, involving both ipsilat-eral and contralateral competing messages, for use with very young children.

The rationale for most of these proce-dures might be summarized as follows. If persons with known injury to the auditory nervous system perform in a characteristic way on these tests, then if a child performs in that same characteristic way, an injury to that same part of the auditory nervous sys-tem may be suspected. The validity of this rationale has only rarely been tested in chil-dren (e.g., Jerger, Johnson, & Loiselle, 1988; Jerger, 1987; Jerger & Zeller, 1989; Musiek, Baran, & Pinheiro, 1994).

The psychoeducational approach, on the other hand, is built on the premise of a set of primary auditory abilities that can be tested by appropriate techniques. The ques-tion of how this relates to brain function is not directly addressed. This approach is well exemplified by the auditory skills subtests of the Goldman-Fristoe-Woodcock Scale

(1974). This instrument posited four dimensions of auditory perceptual processing:

- Auditory Discrimination
- Auditory Memory
- Auditory Selective Attention
- Sound-Symbol Association

Other investigators have suggested additional dimensions (e.g., ASHA, 1996; Woodcock, McGrew, & Mather, 2001) but they were all variations on the same central theme of hypothesized discrete perceptual processes. Bellis (1996), uniquely combined an audiologic approach to testing within a framework of five discrete dimensions of processing.

The Plot Thickens

The idea that auditory processing ability underlies other basic abilities such as language development and reading was a natural outgrowth of the schema laid out so clearly by Strauss and Lehtinen. If learning is based on language, and if language is learned primarily through the auditory modality, then it is not unreasonable to suppose that problems in auditory perceptual processing could lead to problems in language acquisition and to subsequent learning disability. Christine Sloan was an early advocate of this position (Sloan, 1980, 1986, 1992). Paula Tallal and her colleagues (1973, 1980) were among the first to investigate the area systematically. Their early studies of children with language delay suggested that some showed "... *specific difficulty in responding to rapidly changing stimuli, regardless of whether stimuli are nonverbal or verbal"* (Tallal, 1980, p. 138).

Here is a suggestion that the number of primary auditory perceptual abilities underlying the auditory processing abilities which, in turn, underlie successful language development, may be fewer than many have thought. Tallal and colleagues have pursued this avenue vigorously, developing, in the process, techniques for evaluating and treating disorders of "rapid auditory processing" or RAP (e.g., Tallal et al., 1996).

Recently, a group of Australian investigators have suggested that a different unitary aspect of auditory perception, the ability to differentiate spatially dissimilar foreground and background sounds, might be present in a high proportion of children at risk for APD (Cameron, Dillon, & Newall, 2006). This is eerily reminiscent of Myklebust's original description quoted above.

The Language Processing Connection

Gradually, the initial emphasis on auditory processing has, in some circles, morphed into an emphasis on language processing (Richard, 2006). People whose primary interest is childhood language disorders, particularly their management, emphasize that auditory processing is only one component of the processing of language in hostile acoustic environments. This viewpoint is well illustrated by Medwetsky (2006).

If we recognize that the processing of spoken language involves an intertwining of auditory processing, cognition and language, ultimately we can construct an assessment battery that allows us to better understand the overall nature of an individual's difficulties. (Medwetsky, 2006, p. 6)

Inherent in this conceptualization is the idea that factors other than auditory perceptual disorder may contribute to what many have identified as symptoms of APD and that they may interact with auditory perceptual disorders to complicate language processing.

Three Divergent Paths

We have seen that a singular idea, auditory perceptual disorder, originally advanced as a hypothesized explanation for children who "didn't seem to hear well" but had normal auditory sensitivity, has morphed into at least three different paths; (1) an audiologic path, (2) a psychoeducational path, and (3) a language development path. A measure of the extent of the divergence is the fact that some professionals, especially in the language development arena, flatly deny the reality of auditory processing disorder as a distinct entity, insisting that all such children simply are reflecting receptive language dysfunction (Heine, Joffe, & Greaves, 2003; Heine, 2007).

How could this divergence have come about? I suggest that it has arisen from the differing models in which the various professionals, audiologists, speech pathologists, and language pathologists were trained and have subsequently operated. Two key models are the medical model and the educational model. Audiologists have tended to be strongly influenced by the medical model. When the patient, or his or her parents, complains that the child "does not seem to hear well," then the primary approach is to administer tests designed to reveal any problems in the auditory system. The idea is to employ tests that can be easily interpreted as normal or abnormal, and in which previous study has demonstrated that the result is abnormal when the problem lies in a particular part of the auditory nervous system: hence, the audiologists'

preoccupation with audiograms, ABRs, otoacoustic emissions, tests of speech understanding in noise, temporal and pitch pattern tests, and especially dichotic tests. The emphasis has been on differential diagnosis of neural dysfunction, first in adults, then in children. The audiologic test battery is used to exclude peripheral sensitivity loss, auditory neuropathy/dysynchrony, and nonauditory bases for the observed symptoms, then to identify deficits in auditory test performance known to be related to known brain dysfunction. Intervention strategies derive from the nature of these deficits.

The psychoeducational approach, in contrast, has been largely influenced by the educational model. In this model the observation that the child "does not seem to hear well" derives its significance from its impact on learning and academic performance. But learning can be subdivided; learning language, learning to read, learning to write, learning to spell, learning to do arithmetic, and so forth. In the psychoeducational approach each area of learning is further subdivided into hypothesized distinct abilities, and each hypothesized ability is tested with an appropriately norm'd instrument. Deficiency in a particular ability points the way to appropriate intervention. Within this conceptual framework, listening can easily be subdivided into distinct abilities; auditory discrimination, auditory memory, auditory closure, and so on. Here the emphasis is not on differential diagnosis of a neural dysfunction but on discovering which hypothesized ability or abilities need strengthening.

The primacy of language as fundamental to other learning leads, in the psycheducational approach, to emphasis on receptive and expressive language skills and to the notion that what is assumed to be an isolated auditory perceptual deficit may, in fact, be only one interactive component of a more basic receptive language disorder.

Voices of Dissent

Some have argued that we lack a clear framework for conceptualizing APD. Judging from the divergent strands traced above, however, it could as well be argued that we have too many conceptual frameworks. Norma Rees (1973) was an early critic of the movement to link language and learning disabilities to APD, arguing that, like Procrustes of Greek legend, who stretched or chopped off his victims limbs to fit a single iron bed, *"auditory processing disturbances have become the iron bed into which all sorts of language and learning deficits are made to fit"* (Rees, 1981, p. 94).

Other important issues have been raised relative to the auditory tests used in diagnostic batteries. The majority of procedures employ words and sentences as the test stimuli. But if auditory processing disorder affects language development, then the use of language-based test materials could be viewed as somewhat circular (cf., Jerger & Allen, 1998; Moore, 2006).

Another major criticism is the extent to which extra-auditory factors influence performance on language-based behavioral measures (Cacace & McFarland, 1998): how much of an apparent deficit may be attributable to flagging attention, cognitive deficit, motivation, and so forth. The significance of extra-auditory factors was well illustrated in a report by Silman, Silverman, and Ehmer (2000) highlighting the importance of just one such influence, motivation to cooperate in the testing activity. They report extremely interesting data on three children. Each had been diagnosed as CAPD on the basis of behavioral measures. In every case the child's performance was shifted into the normal range by the simple expedient of reinforcing correct responses with the child's favorite toy or treat.

The problem of extra-auditory influences is particularly acute in dichotic testing procedures, especially when attention must be divided between ears. It has been argued that many contemporary tests fail to control adequately for confounding by extra-auditory factors (Cacace & McFarland, 1998).

The notion of "sensitized" tests raises two important issues (Cacace & McFarland, 2006): first, it is never made clear just what perceptual processes are affected by the sensitization; second, sensitization opens the door to interaction with a host of nonauditory factors and processes.

Although the theme of "auditory-specific perceptual disorder" weaves through the last half century of APD conceptualization and diagnosis, McFarland and Cacace (2006) argue that the goal of demonstrating a genuine modality-specific disorder has seldom been achieved. Indeed, they argue, if only auditory tests are administered the outcome is forced. They have suggested that paired auditory and visual testing is necessary before it can be concluded that a deficit is, indeed, auditory-specific (but see Musiek, Bellis & Chermak, [2005] and the earlier quotation from Myklebust [1954], on the need for auditory specificity).

The concept of multiple discrete auditory perceptual abilities, so central in the psychoeducational approach, is, as Cacace and McFarland (2006) emphasize, strongly related to whatever specific tests are thought to measure. But *"Auditory processes that are operationally defined in terms of specific test performance do not provide theoretical constructs that can be related to . . . evolving concepts in auditory neuroscience"* (Cacace & McFarland, 2006, p. 48).

Finally, a number of investigators have pointed out the difficulty in differentiating APD from attention deficit disorders (e.g., Cook et al., 1993). When these authors administered a battery of APD tests to 15 children with ADHD, "all were found to have some degree of central auditory processing dysfunction . . . " (p. 135).

A principal concern associated with these various expressions of dissent is that the false-positive rate of identification of APD associated with current test procedures may be unacceptably high. Too many children, it is argued, may be labeled APD when the actual problem is something different.

Meanwhile, in the real world, multitudes of children are being "tested for APD" in the public schools every day, principally by dedicated educational specialists: they seek, but do not always find, clear guidance on how to do this. Many, under the press of time, rely on screening instruments to make diagnostic decisions. Although this practice is universally decried, a clear-cut, workable alternative is seldom offered.

Speech Versus Nonspeech

Over the past three decades conceptual frameworks of, and tests for, APD have become closely interwoven with speech, in the form of syllables, words, and sentences, as the stimulus of choice. On the audiologic path, words and sentences have been filtered, accelerated, masked, compressed, reverberated, and presented dichotically. On the psychoeducational path there has been a strong emphasis on phonological awareness, and the use of syllable and word stimuli to assess discrete auditory abilities. In the language development area the emphasis has been on nothing less than the comprehension of spoken language.

But within the past decade we have seen movements to define APD as a problem in the processing of nonspeech stimuli.

It is stated explicitly in the Working Definition of APD by the British Society of Audiology (2005) and implicitly in the position statement of the ASHA Working Group on Auditory Processing Disorder (2005). Movement in this direction could have substantial implications for future test materials and test construction. It might, moreover, cast into limbo much of the research data gathered in the last four decades using speech and speechlike stimuli. On the positive side, however, the use of nonspeech stimuli would, as Moore (2006) points out, facilitate the development of an animal model of APD.

Summary

In short, APD means different things to different people! It began as a fairly circumscribed perceptual concept—difficulty in separating auditory foreground from auditory background in children—but it has morphed along divergent paths. One path was developed by audiologists, initially studying brain-injured adults, then applying these findings to the testing of children. A second path was developed by psychoeducational specialists based on the concept of discrete auditory perceptual abilities, a paradigm subsequently adopted by many audiologists and speech-language pathologists as a model for diagnosing and treating disorders of auditory processing. A third path has been traced by persons primarily interested in the complex interactions among auditory processing disorder and other cognitive dimensions as they impact language acquisition and learning. It may be fair to say that none of these paths has yet solved, in totally satisfactory fashion, the diagnostic problem facing the clinician.

Only the future student of APD history will be able to record whether these paths continue to diverge, or whether they eventually begin to converge on a more unitary conceptualization of, and approach to, the problem.

Acknowledgment. I am grateful to Jeffrey Martin, Susan Jerger, and Christine Dollaghan for helpful suggestions.

References

Arnst, D., & Katz, J. (Eds.). (1982). *Central Auditory Assessment: The SSW Test*. San Diego, CA: College-Hill Press.

ASHA. (1996). Central auditory processing disorders: Current status of research and implications for clinical practice. *American Journal of Audiology, 5*, 41–54.

ASHA. (2005). *(Central) Auditory Processing Disorders—The role of the audiologist* [Position Statement]. From http://www.asha.org/members/deskref-journals/deskref/default

Beasley, D., & Freeman, B. (1977). Time-altered speech as a measure of central auditory processing. In R. Keith (Ed.), *Central auditory dysfunction* (pp. 129–176). New York: Grune & Stratton.

Bellis, T. (1996). *Assessment and management of central auditory processing disorders in the educational setting: From science to practice*. San Diego, CA: Singular.

Berlin, C., Lowe, S., Thompson, L., & Cullen, J. (1968). The construction and perception of simultaneous messages. *ASHA, 10*, 397.

Bocca, E., Calearo, C., & Cassinari, V. (1954). A new method for testing hearing in temporal lobe tumors. *Acta Otolaryngologica, 44*, 219–221.

Bocca, E., Calearo, C., Cassinari, V., & Migliavacca, F. (1955). Testing "cortical" hearing in temporal lobe tumors. *Acta Otolaryngologica, 45*, 289–304.

British Society of Audiology (2005). APD Steering Group: Working Definition of APD. From http://www.thebsa.org.uk/apd/Home.htm# working%20def

Broadbent, D. (1958). *Perception and communication*. New York: Macmillan.

Cacace, A., & McFarland, D. (1998). Central auditory processing disorder in school-aged children: A critical review. *Journal of Speech, Language, and Hearing Research, 41*, 355–373.

Cacace, A., & McFarland, D. (2006). Delineating auditory processing disorder (APD) and attention deficit hyperactivity disorder (ADHD): A conceptual, theoretical, and practical framework. In T. Parthasarathy (Ed.), *An introduction to auditory processing disorders in children* (pp. 39–61). Mahwah, NJ: Lawrence Erlbaum Associates.

Calearo, C., & Lazzaroni, A. (1957). Speech intelligibility in relation to the speed of the message. *Laryngoscope, 67*, 410–419.

Cameron, S., Dillon, H., & Newall, P. (2006). The listening in spatialized noise test: An auditory processing disorder study. *Journal of the American Academy of Audiology, 17*, 306–320.

Cook, J., Mausbach, T., Burd, L., Gascon, G., Slotnick, H., Patterson, B., et al. (1993). A preliminary study of the relationship between central auditory processing disorder and attention deficit disorder. *Journal of Psychiatric Neuroscience, 18*, 130–137.

Fifer, R., Jerger, J., Berlin, C., Tobey, E., & Campbell, J. (1983). Development of a dichotic sentence identification test for hearing-impaired adults. *Ear and Hearing, 4*, 300–305.

Goldman, R., Fristoe, M., & Woodcock, R. (1974). *Goldman-Fristoe-Woodcock Auditory Skills Test Battery*. Circle Pines, MN: American Guidance Service.

Goldstein, R., Goodman, A., & King, R. (1956). Hearing and speech in infantile hemiplegia before and after left hemispherectomy. *Neurology, 6*, 869–875.

Head, H. (1926). *Aphasia and kindred disorders of speech* (Vol. 1). Cambridge: Cambridge University Press.

Heine, C. (2007). Personal communication.

Heine, C., Joffe, B., & Greaves, E. (2003). *The dilemma of APD: Clinical decision-making.* Paper presented at the Nature Nurture Knowledge: Proceedings of the 2003 Speech Pathology Australia National Conference, Melbourne.

Jerger, J. (1960). Audiological manifestations of lesions in the auditory nervous system. *Laryngoscope, 70,* 417–425.

Jerger, J., & Jerger, S. (1974). Auditory findings in brainstem disorders. *Archives of Otolaryngology, 99,* 342–349.

Jerger, J., & Jerger, S. (1975). Clinical validity of central auditory tests. *Scandinavian Audiology, 4,* 147–163.

Jerger, S. (1987). Validation of the pediatric speech intelligibility test in children with central nervous system lesions. *Audiology, 26,* 298–311.

Jerger, S., & Allen, J. (1998). How global behavioral tests of central auditory processing may complicate management. In F. Bess (Ed.), *Children with hearing impairment. Contemporary trends* (pp. 163–177). Nashville, TN: Bill Wilkerson Center Press.

Jerger, S., Jerger, J., & Abrams, S. (1983). Speech audiometry in the young child. *Ear and Hearing, 4,* 56–66.

Jerger, S., Johnson, K., & Loiselle, L. (1988). Pediatric central auditory dysfunction: Comparison of children with confirmed lesions versus suspected processing disorders. *American Journal of Otology, 9,* 63–71.

Jerger, S., & Zeller, R. (1989). Dichotic listening in a child with a cerebral lesion: the "paradoxical" ipsilateral ear deficit. *Ear and Hearing, 10,* 167–172.

Katz, J. (1968). The SSW test: An interim report. *Journal of Speech and Hearing Disorders, 33,* 132–146.

Katz, J., & Ivey, R. (1994). Spondaic procedures in central testing. In J. Katz (Ed.), *Handbook of clinical audiology* (4th ed., pp. 239–255). Baltimore: Williams & Wilkins.

Katz, J., Stecker, N., & Henderson, D. (Eds.). (1992). *Central auditory processing: A transdisciplinary view.* St. Louis, MO: Mosby Yearbook.

Kavale, K., & Forness, S. (1985). *The science of learning disabilities.* San Diego, CA: College-Hill Press.

Keith, R. (1986). *SCAN: A screening test for auditory processing disorders.* San Antonio, TX: Psychological Corporation.

Keith, R. (1994). *SCAN-A: A test for auditory processing disorders in adolescents and adults.* San Antonio, TX: Psychological Corporation.

Keith, R. (2000). *SCAN-C: Test for auditory processing disorders in children-revised.* San Antonio, TX: Psychological Corporation.

Kimura, D. (1967). Functional asymmetry of the brain in dichotic listening. *Cortex, 3,* 163–178.

Kirk, S. (1968). Illinois Test of Psycholinguistic Abilities: Its origin and implications. In J. Helmuth (Ed.), *Learning disorders* (Vol. 3). Seattle, WA: Special Child Publications.

Kurdziel, S., Noffsinger, D., & Olsen, W. (1976). Performance by cortical lesion patients on 40 and 60% time-compressed material. *Journal of the American Auditory Society, 2,* 3–7.

Lynn, G., & Gilroy, J. (1977). Evaluation of central auditory dysfunction in patients with neurological disorders. In R. Keith (Ed.), *Central auditory dysfunction.* New York: Grune & Stratton.

Matzker, J. (1959). Two methods for the assessment of central auditory functions in cases of brain disease. *Annals of Otology, Rhinology, and Laryngology, 68,* 1185–1197.

McFarland, D., & Cacace, A. (2006). Current controversies in CAPD: From Procrustes bed to Pandora's box. In T. Parthasarathy (Ed.), *An introduction to auditory processing disorders in children* (pp. 247–263). Mahwah, NJ: Lawrence Erlbaum Associates.

Medwetsky, L. (2006). Spoken language processing: A convergent approach to conceptualizing (central) auditory processing. *ASHA Leader Online, 11,* 6–7, 30–31,33.

Milner, B., Taylor, L., & Sperry, R. (1968). Lateralized suppression of dichotically presented digits after commissural section in man. *Science, 161,* 184–186.

Moore, D. (2006). Auditory processing disorder (APD): Definition, diagnosis, neural basis, and intervention. *Audiological Medicine, 4,* 4–11.

Moore, D. (2007). Auditory processing disorder (APD)—Potential contribution of mouse research. *Brain Research, 1091*, 200-206.

Musiek, F. (1983). The results of three dichotic speech tests on subjects with intracranial lesions. *Ear and Hearing, 4*, 318-323.

Musiek, F., Baran, J., & Pinheiro, M. (1990). Duration pattern recognition in normal subjects and patients with cerebral and cochlear lesions. *Audiology, 29*, 304-313.

Musiek, F., Baran, J., & Pinheiro, M. (1994). *Neuroaudiology case studies.* San Diego, CA: Singular.

Musiek, F., Bellis, T., & Chermak, G. (2005). Non-modularity of the central auditory nervous system: Implications for (central) auditory processing disorder. *American Journal of Audiology, 14*, 128-138.

Musiek, F., Gollegly, K., & Baran, J. (1984). Myelination of the corpus callosum and auditory processing problems in children: theoretical and clinical correlates. *Seminars in Hearing, 5*, 231-240.

Musiek, F., Shinn, J., Jirsa, R., Bamiou, D., Baran, J., & Zaiden, E. (2005). The GIN (Gaps-in-Noise) test performance in subjects with confirmed central auditory nervous system involvement. *Ear and Hearing, 26*, 608-618.

Myklebust, H. (1954). *Auditory disorders in children.* New York: Grune & Stratton.

Pinheiro, M., & Musiek, F. (Eds.). (1985). *Assessment of central auditory dysfunction: foundations and correlates.* Baltimore: Williams & Wilkins.

Rees, N. (1973). Auditory processing factors in language disorders: the view from Procrustes' bed. *Journal of Speech and Hearing Research, 38*, 304-315.

Rees, N. (1981). Saying more than we know: Is auditory processing disorder a meaningful concept. In R. Keith (Ed.), *Central auditory and language disorders in children* (pp. 94-120). San Diego, CA: College-Hill Press.

Richard, G. (2006). Language-based assessment and intervention of APD. In T. Parthasarathy (Ed.), *An introduction to auditory processing disorders in children* (pp. 95-108). Mahwah, NJ: Lawrence Erlbaum Associates.

Silman, S., Silverman, C., & Emmer, M. (2000). Central auditory processing disorders and reduced motivation: three case studies. *Journal of the American Academy of Audiology, 11*, 57-63.

Sloan, C. (1980). Auditory processing disorders and language development. In P. Levinson & C. Sloan (Eds.), *Auditory processing and language: Clinical and research perspectives* (pp. 101-116). New York: Grune & Stratton.

Sloan, C. (1986). *Treating auditory processing difficulties in children.* San Diego, CA: College-Hill Press.

Sloan, C. (1992). Language, language learning, and language disorder: implications for central auditory processing. In J. Katz, N. Stecker, & D. Henderson (Eds.), *Central auditory processing: A transdisciplinary view.* St. Louis, MO: Mosby-Yearbook.

Speaks, C., & Jerger, J. (1965). Method for measurement of speech identification. *Journal of Speech and Hearing Research, 8*, 185-194.

Strauss, A., & Lehtinen, L. (1947). *Psychpathology and education of the brain-injured child.* New York: Grune & Stratton.

Tallal, P. (1980). Language disabilities in children: A perceptual or linguistic deficit? *Journal of Pediatric Psychology, 5*, 127-140.

Tallal, P., Miller, S., Bedi, G., Byma, G., Wang, X., Nagarajan, S., et al. (1996). Language comprehension in language-learning impaired children improved with acoustically modified speech. *Science, 271*, 81-84.

Tallal, P., & Piercy, M. (1973). Defects of nonverbal auditory perception in children with developmental aphasia. *Nature, 241*, 468-469.

Willeford, J. (1977). Assessing central auditory behavior in children: a test battery approach. In R. Keith (Ed.), *Central auditory dysfunction* (pp. 43-72). New York: Grune & Stratton.

Woodcock, R., McGrew, K., & Mather, N. (2001). *Woodcock-Johnson III Tests of Cognitive Abilities.* Itasca, IL: Riverside.

CHAPTER 2

Organization of the Central Auditory Pathways in Nonhuman Primates and Humans

TROY A. HACKETT

Introduction

The perception of sound depends on the extraction of meaningful information encoded in the activity of neurons in dozens of subcortical nuclei and cortical areas. Each of these fields has a distinct anatomical profile, defined by the morphology and connections of its neurons. The neurophysiologic profiles of each field depend on these features in ways that are gradually being revealed.

The major components of the mammalian auditory system are the outer ear, middle ear, inner ear, and central pathways. The central auditory pathways consist of an elaborate network of interconnected nuclear complexes in the brainstem and thalamus, and numerous areas, or fields, in the cerebral cortex. Each major stage of processing in the brainstem and thalamus initiates and integrates multiple segregated parallel pathways involving functionally distinct populations of neurons. These pathways are responsible for the distribution of specialized acoustic information to higher centers, including cortex, and to lower stages, including the cochlea. Thus, the modulation and integration of auditory input occurs in multiple pathways at all levels.

Comparative studies indicate that the fundamental organization of the central pathways is highly conserved between species, especially among the subcortical structures. Species differences are most apparent at the cortical level, where the number and arrangement of areas varies significantly. For example, rats have at least five areas (Polley, Read, Storace, & Merzenich, 2007; Rutkowski, Miasnikov, & Weinberger, 2003), ferrets and cats have at least seven (Bizley, Nodal, Nelken, & King, 2005; Lee, Imaizumi, Schreiner, & Winer, 2004; Winer, Miller, Lee, &

Schreiner, 2005), and nonhuman primates have about 12 (Hackett, Stepniewska, & Kaas, 1998a; Kaas & Hackett, 2000). The number of areas comprising the human auditory cortex is currently unknown, but it is likely that humans have more than other primates (Hackett, 2003, 2007a, 2007b). These anatomic differences are presumed to underlie species differences in the processing of auditory information, as well, but with the exception of species with unique auditory capabilities (e.g., echolocating bats); little is known about the functional roles of any auditory area. This chapter focuses on the organization of the thalamocortical system in nonhuman primates and humans. The organization of the brainstem pathways are reviewed briefly, but as few studies have addressed auditory brainstem organization in primates, this summary is mainly derived from other species. Detailed reviews of that literature are published elsewhere (Aitkin, 1986; Ehret & Romand, 1997; Malmierca, 2003; Oertel, Fay, & Popper, 2002; Popper & Fay, 1992).

The Subcortical Auditory Pathways

Compared to the somatosensory and visual systems, the organization of the subcortical auditory pathways is exceptionally complex (Figure 2–1). The pathways include five major nuclear groups, each of which contains several subdivisions that mediate ascending and descending projections of several parallel pathways. The outputs specific to each ear cross the midline shortly after entering the brainstem, and decussate several times thereafter; thus, input from both ears is available to both sides of the brain at nearly every level of processing. A complex network of connections between auditory nuclei at different levels provides

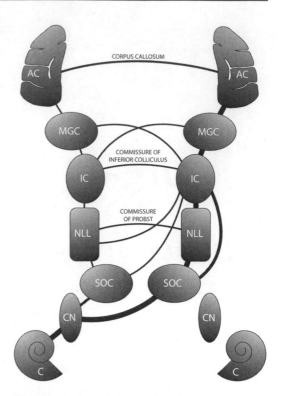

Figure 2–1. Schematic diagram of the ascending auditory pathway, showing the principal connections between auditory nuclei based on inputs from one cochlea. The subdivisions of each nuclear complex and the minor pathways are not shown. Stronger pathways are indicated by wider lines. C, cochlea; CN, cochlear nucleus; SOC, superior olivary complex; NLL, nuclei of the lateral lemniscus; IC, inferior colliculus; MGC, medial geniculate complex; AC, auditory cortex.

numerous opportunities for interaction between pathways. At present, most of what is known about subcortical auditory processing in mammals comes from studies of nonprimates, especially cats, bats, and rodents. Equivalent studies in primates are relatively few in number; therefore, it is common to generalize principles of auditory subcortical organization across taxonomic groups, including humans.

The Cochlear Nuclei

Although the cochlear nucleus represents only the first stage of subcortical auditory processing, the anatomic and physiologic diversity of this structure indicates that substantial auditory processing is mediated at this level. The cochlear nuclei contain a wide variety of cell types distributed among three major subdivisions. Each of the major cell types is associated with a unique response profile reflecting particular attributes of the original acoustic signal. Different populations of neurons appear to be specialized to extract particular aspects of the encoded auditory stimulus, and therefore give rise to a number of segregated pathways that are functionally distinct (Romand & Avan, 1997). The tonotopic organization of the cochlea and eighth nerve is maintained by an orderly pattern of projections to each subdivision of the cochlear nucleus, which bifurcate upon entering the brainstem. The ascending branches innervate the anteroventral division of the cochlear nucleus (AVCN). The posterior branches synapse in the posteroventral (PVCN) and/ or dorsal (DCN) divisions. Neurons in the cochlear nuclei project to nearly every auditory nucleus on both sides of the brainstem, including the reticular formation, and also receive modulatory (corticofugal) projections from higher auditory and nonauditory centers (Winer, 2005). Three major fiber bundles form the principal output connections of the cochlear nuclei. The largest band from the AVCN forms the *trapezoid body* with bilateral projections to the superior olivary complexes, and contralateral projections to the lateral lemniscus and inferior colliculus. Fibers from the PVCN form the *intermediate acoustic stria of Held* with projections to the contralateral lateral lemniscus and inferior colliculus. The *dorsal acoustic stria of von Monakow*

is formed by fibers of the DCN which also project primarily to the contralateral lateral lemniscus and inferior colliculus. The anatomic features of the cochlear nuclei generally are consistent across primate species (Bacsik & Strominger, 1973; Barnes, Magoun, & Ranson, 1943; Heiman-Patterson & Strominger, 1985; Hilbig, Nowack, Boeckler, Bidmon, & Zilles, 2007; Moskowitz & Liu, 1972; Strominger, 1973; Strominger, Nelson, & Dougherty, 1977; Strominger & Strominger, 1971; Sutton, Hathaway, Seib, & Spelman, 1991), and compare well with nonprimates, although minor structural variations have been found (Moore, 1980; Ryugo, Pongstaporn, Wright, & Sharp, 1995; Spatz, 1999).

The Superior Olivary Complex

The next major level of auditory brainstem processing is the superior olivary complex (SOC), which receives bilateral projections from the cochlear nuclei. The SOC consists of several nuclei that are known to exhibit substantial anatomic variation among species (Malmierca, 2003; Moore & Moore, 1971; Osen, Mugnaini, Dahl, & Christiansen, 1984; Schwartz, 1992). In mammals, the three main subnuclei are the lateral (LSO) and medial (MSO) superior olivary nuclei and the medial nucleus of the trapezoid body (MNTB). Each division is tonotopically organized and has variable patterns of projections to the lateral lemniscus and inferior colliculus (Oliver, 2000; Thompson & Schofield, 2000). These are bordered by several *periolivary* nuclei that have unique anatomical features and are an important component of the descending auditory pathway (Adams, 1983). Anatomic studies of primates and humans indicate that the LSO and MNTB are prominent, but relatively small in size, compared to other species, whereas the structural features of the periolivary nuclei appear to be the most variable (Barnes et al., 1943; Bazwinsky, Bidmon, Zilles, & Hilbig, 2005; Irving & Harrison, 1967; Kulesza & Randy, 2007; Moore, 2000; Moore, Guan, & Shi, 1998; Moore & Moore, 1971).

The SOC is the earliest stage of central auditory processing at which inputs from both ears converge. Accordingly, one of the primary functions associated with the SOC is the encoding of auditory cues pertaining to sound location (Moore, 1991; Pollak, Burger, Park, Klug, & Bauer, 2002; Tollin, 2003). Interaural differences in time and intensity associated with the location of a sound source can be resolved by the circuitry of the LSO and MSO (Jeffress, 1948; Smith, Joris, & Yin, 1993). Additional projections to the superior colliculus and motor nuclei in the brainstem contribute to the acoustic and startle reflexes, whereas modulation of cochlear function is achieved through direct bilateral projections from the MSO and LSO to inner and outer hair cells in the cochlea (Rasmussen, 1946, 1953).

The Lateral Lemniscus

The lateral lemniscus is the principal fiber tract connecting the SOC and IC. In most species, this pathway is associated with at least two major subnuclei (Covey & Casseday, 1995; Malmierca, 2003; Merchan, Malmierca, Bajo, & Bjaalie, 1997). The ventral nucleus (VNLL) receives monaural inputs primarily from the contralateral ventral cochlear nucleus, and mainly projects to the ipsilateral inferior colliculus. In contrast, the dorsal nucleus (DNLL) receives bilateral inputs from the CN and SOC and projects bilaterally to inferior colliculus and deep layers of the superior colliculus (Adams & Warr, 1976; Bajo, Merchan, Lopez, & Rouiller, 1993; Brunso-Bechtold, Thompson, & Masterton, 1981; Coleman & Clerici,

1987; Friauf & Ostwald, 1988; Glendenning, Brunso-Bechtold, Thompson, & Masterton, 1981; Henkel, 1997; Henkel & Spangler, 1983; Hutson, Glendenning, & Masterton, 1991; Kudo, 1981; Malmierca, Le Beau, & Rees, 1996; Malmierca, Leergaard, Bajo, Bjaalie, & Merchan, 1998; Merchan & Berbel, 1996; Merchan, Saldana, & Plaza, 1994; Shneiderman, Oliver, & Henkel, 1988). The bilateral projections of the DNLL to the IC are tonotopically organized, but the tonotopic organization of the VNLL to the ipsilateral IC is less clear. Although the precise roles of these nuclei remain unclear, they exhibit distinctive binaural and monaural response properties and have important influences on the activity of neurons in the IC (Aitkin, Anderson, & Brugge, 1970; Batra & Fitzpatrick, 2002; Brugge, Anderson, & Aitkin, 1970; Kelly & Li, 1997).

The Inferior Colliculus

The inferior colliculus (IC) is commonly divided into three major divisions: central (ICc), external cortex (EC), and the dorsal cortex (DC). Multiple ascending and descending auditory pathways converge in the IC from auditory nuclei on both sides of the brainstem, as well as descending inputs of from superior colliculus, thalamus, and cortex (Aitkin, 1986; Ehret & Romand, 1997; Malmierca, 2003; Pollak, Burger, & Klug, 2003; Winer, 2005; Winer, Chernock, Larue, & Cheung, 2002). The major ascending projections of the IC target the medial geniculate complex bilaterally. Other outputs target the superior colliculi, reticular formation, periaqueductal gray, contralateral IC, and lower auditory nuclei. As the connection patterns indicate, the IC is responsible for the integration of monaural and binaural information processed by lower and higher auditory centers, including cortex. This is reflected in the wide variety of response patterns among different subdivisions of the structure.

The primary ascending pathway in the brainstem proceeds through the ICc and maintains the tonotopic organization of the cochlea. Within the ICc, neurons are narrowly tuned and topographically arranged by characteristic frequency (Aitkin, Webster, Veale, & Crosby, 1975; Hind, Goldberg, Greenwood, & Rose, 1963; Merzenich & Reid, 1974; Serviere, Webster, & Calford, 1984; Webster, Serviere, Crewther, & Crewther, 1984). In addition to stimulus frequency, other features (e.g., latency, response threshold, tuning bandwidth, and best azimuth) may be arranged topographically in distinct maps in the ICc (Aitkin, Pettigrew, Calford, Phillips, & Wise, 1985; Schreiner & Langner, 1988; Stiebler, 1986). Recent studies in macaque monkeys reveal that neurons in the ICc are modulated by eye position (Groh, Trause, Underhill, Clark, & Inati, 2001) and behavioral context (Metzger, Greene, Porter, & Groh, 2006), suggesting that connections with higher stages of processing within and outside of the auditory pathways influence activity in the primary ascending pathway. Although there is no clear map of auditory space in the ICc of primates, its neurons are tuned to spatial location (Groh, Kelly, & Underhill, 2003; Zwiers, Versnel, & Van Opstal, 2004), indicating that information about location is encoded by activity in the primary pathway (Sterbing, Hartung, & Hoffmann, 2003).

The Medial Geniculate Complex

The medial geniculate complex (MGC) is the final stage of subcortical processing of ascending auditory information (Jones, 2007; Sherman & Guillery, 2001). Ascending inputs arise bilaterally from all divisions of the IC, although the ipsilateral set of projections is considerably stronger. Outputs target primary and nonprimary fields of auditory cortex, all of which project back to the MGC, forming a feedback loop. The MGC is commonly divided into three divisions: ventral (MGv), dorsal (MGd), and magnocellular or medial (MGm). In primates the MGd is further subdivided into anterodorsal, (MGad) and posterodorsal (MGpd) (Burton & Jones, 1976; de la Mothe, Blumell, Kajikawa, & Hackett, 2006b; FitzPatrick & Imig, 1978; Hackett et al., 2007). As in other mammals (Rouiller & de Ribaupierre, 1985; Winer, 1984, 1985; Winer, Kelly, & Larue, 1999), these divisions are distinguished on the bases of their unique architecture, patterns of cortical and subcortical connections, and physiology. In addition to the MGC, adjoining nuclei in the thalamus (e.g., suprageniculate, limitans, posterior], and medial pulvinar) also appear to play a role in auditory and multisensory processing via their connections with cortical and subcortical auditory fields.

The inputs and outputs of the MGC suggest that each division is primarily associated with one of perhaps several parallel pathways reaching the auditory cortex (Andersen, Knight, & Merzenich, 1980; Andersen, Roth, Aitkin, & Merzenich, 1980; Calford & Aitkin, 1983; Evans, 1974; Jones, 2007; Poljak, 1926; Rouiller & de Ribaupierre, 1985; Rouiller, Simm, Villa, de Ribaupierre, & de Ribaupierre, 1991; Winer & Lee, 2007; Winer et al., 2005). The primary ascending pathway, also known as the tonotopic or lemniscal pathway, continues from the ICc to the MGv. Neurons in the MGv are arranged in laminae corresponding to the tonotopic organization of the cochlca, presumably inherited from the ICc (Calford, 1983; Morest, 1965). The primary pathway extends from the MGv through the posterior limb of the internal capsule, targeting primary (core) auditory cortex (Calford & Aitkin, 1983; de la Mothe et al., 2006b; Morel, Garraghty, & Kaas, 1993; Morel & Kaas,

1992; Rouiller, 1997; Winer & Lee, 2007). The nonprimary, or extralemniscal, ascending pathways involve the MGd and MGm. The MGd receives inputs from the DC and EC divisions of the inferior colliculus (Andersen, Knight, Merzenich, 1980; Calford & Aitkin, 1983; Kudo & Niimi, 1980) and projects primarily to areas of auditory cortex outside of A1. In primates, the MGd projection targets areas that comprise the belt and parabelt regions surrounding the core (Burton & Jones, 1976; de la Mothe et al., 2006b; Hackett et al., 2007; Hackett, Stepniewska, & Kaas, 1998b; Molinari et al., 1995; Morel et al., 1993; Morel & Kaas, 1992). The MGd appears to lack tonotopic organization and neurons tend to be broadly tuned to frequency (Calford, 1983; Calford & Aitkin, 1983; He, 2002). For this reason, the MGd is often considered part of the nontonotopic, or diffuse, auditory pathway (de Ribaupierre, 1997; Rouiller, 1997). Finally, the MGm, which receives projections from the ICc and EC, contributes to a third pathway passing through the MGC (Calford & Aitkin, 1983; Kudo & Niimi, 1980). In contrast to the ventral and dorsal divisions of the MGC, the MGm projects diffusely to all areas of auditory cortex (Jones, 2007; Winer & Lee, 2007). Neurons in the MGm are dominated by responses to auditory stimuli, but some units also respond to vestibular and somatic stimulation (Blum, Abraham, & Gilman, 1979; Curry, 1972; Love & Scott, 1969; Wepsic, 1966), possibly reflecting connections with the nuclei of other sensory systems (de la Mothe et al., 2006b; Jones, 2007). Therefore, the MGm is often considered part of a multisensory pathway (de Ribaupierre, 1997), although some aspects of this conclusion remain uncertain (Jones, 2007). Overall, then, the organization of the MGC and surrounding nuclei reflects the presence of multiple parallel pathways in which distinct aspects of auditory and multisensory processing appear to be mediated.

Summary

The picture of auditory processing that emerges from the foregoing is that each major stage of hierarchical processing in the brainstem and thalamus initiates and integrates *multiple parallel pathways* involving functionally distinct populations of neurons. These pathways are responsible for the distribution of specialized acoustic information to higher centers, including cortex, and to lower stages, including the cochlea. Thus, the modulation and integration of auditory input occurs in multiple pathways at all levels. Although the unique anatomic and physiologic features of these pathways support their segregation into functionally distinct subsystems, these details are still being elucidated. Some clarification has come from studying the organization of auditory cortex, as described below.

Auditory Cortical Organization in Nonhuman Primates

Our working model of the primate auditory cortex represents the collective findings of the field, compiled from studies of New World and Old World primates over several decades (for reviews, see Aitkin, 1990; Hackett, 2007a; Hackett & Kaas, 2004; Kaas & Hackett, 2000; Woolsey & Walzl, 1982). The model incorporates the anatomic and physiologic features reported in studies of several species into a schematic diagram that illustrates the flow of information into and out of the cortical auditory system (Figure 2–2). As such, the model provides a useful structural framework for the interpretation of data collected from studies of central auditory processing. However, as noted throughout this chapter, several aspects of the model remain incomplete.

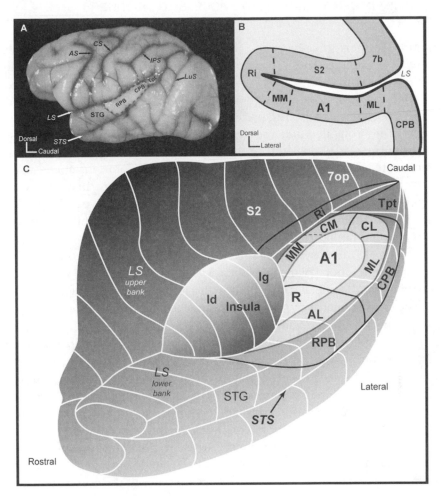

Figure 2–2. Schematic diagrams of macaque monkey auditory cortex.
A. Lateral view of left hemisphere. The dashed ovoid on the superior
temporal gyrus (STG) circumscribes the location of rostral (RPB) and
caudal (CPB) parabelt areas. The temporal parietotemporal area (Tpt)
adjoins the CPB caudally. **B.** Coronal section through the lateral sulcus
(LS) showing locations of areas 7b, somatosensory area 2 (S2),
retroinsular area (Ri), primary (core) area (A1), middle lateral (ML) and
middle medial (MM) belt areas, and CPB. **C.** The lateral sulcus (LS) of
the left hemisphere was graphically opened to reveal the locations of
caudal and lateral auditory cortical areas on its lower bank. Two of the
three core areas are visible on the lower bank (A1 and R, rostral). The
most rostral area of the core (RT) and medial belt (RM, RTM) are hid-
den from view within the circular sulcus that borders the ventral insula.
A1 is surrounded by several belt areas (CM, caudomedial; CL, caudolateral; ML, middle lateral; AL, anterolateral). The upper bank of the LS is
retracted to show the locations of S2, Ri, area 7 opercular (7op), gran-
ular insula (Ig), and dysgranular insula (Id). The superior temporal sulcus (STS), containing the temporal parietal occipital area (TPO) was
not graphically opened.

Refinements are periodically made as required by new findings, and substantial revisions are still possible.

We define *auditory cortex* as those areas of cerebral cortex that are the preferential targets of neurons in either the ventral (MGv) or dorsal (MGd) divisions of the medial geniculate complex (MGC) in the thalamus. By this definition, a large portion of the superior half of the temporal lobe is occupied by the auditory cortex (see Figure 2–2). Its medial boundaries lie within the lateral sulcus (LS) (i.e., sylvian fissure) where the superior temporal plane joins the insula (rostrally) and parietal operculum (caudally). The lateral boundary varies somewhat between species, but generally extends to edge of the superior temporal sulcus (STS) or slightly onto its dorsal bank. The caudal boundary is located near the junction of the lateral and superior temporal sulci at the border of the temporoparietal temporal area (Tpt). Rostrally, auditory cortex occupies most of the superior temporal gyrus (STG) excluding the temporal pole.

Numerous cortical fields outside the boundaries of auditory cortex also process auditory information. As these areas receive inputs from some portion of auditory cortex, and generally do not receive significant inputs from the MGC, they are referred to as *auditory-related*. These areas are located in the temporal pole, portions of the superior temporal sulcus, intraparietal sulcus, and prefrontal cortex. Auditory-related areas tend to be sites of multisensory convergence where neurons integrate inputs from auditory, visual, and somatosensory modalities.

Subdivisions of Auditory Cortex

A major feature of our working model is that the auditory cortex is divided into three regions: *core*, *belt*, and *parabelt*. Each region is further subdivided into a variable number of individual areas, or subdivisions, on the basis of anatomic or physiologic features. Generally, the anatomic features of an area are fairly uniform, permitting the formulation of a structural profile unique to that area. In some instances, a key neurophysiologic feature may also characterize an area, adding to its overall profile. At present, however, anatomic features comprise the profiles of most auditory areas.

The core region contains three subdivisions (A1, R, RT), and is considered to be the initial (primary) stage of auditory processing in cortex. This assumption is largely based on two observations. First, the thalamic inputs to the core are dominated by the MGv, which is part of the primary subcortical auditory pathway. Second, the output projections of neurons in the core tend to be limited to areas within the surrounding belt region, whereas the belt and parabelt areas are broadly connected with auditory-related fields elsewhere in the brain. The architecture of the core region is characterized by dense myelination from layers III to VI, accompanied by dense expression of several protein markers in a band involving layers III and IV (i.e., cytochrome oxidase, acetylcholinesterase, parvalbumin). Although the functional significance of these features is not clear, this pattern is typical of the primary cortex of other sensory modalities. Neurons in each subdivision of the core are arranged in a manner that preserves the tonotopic (frequency) organization of the cochlea. In A1, neurons that are most sensitive to high frequencies are located caudally, whereas neurons tuned to low frequencies are located rostrally; thus, the basilar membrane is represented by a gradient that proceeds from high to low frequencies along the caudal-rostral axis in A1. The gradient is reversed in R, and once again in RT, indicating that there are three distinct representations of the basilar membrane in the core region.

In the belt region surrounding the core (see Figure 2–2), seven subdivisions have been tentatively identified (CM, CL, ML, AL, RM, RTL, RTM). Thalamic inputs to the belt areas mainly arise from one of the nonprimary dorsal divisions (MGd) of the MGC: anterodorsal (MGad), and posterodorsal (MGpd). The cortical connections of the belt areas include both the core and parabelt regions, which places the belt region at an intermediate (secondary) stage of processing. With respect to cellular architecture, the expression of myelin and other protein markers is significantly reduced in most of the belt areas, but typically higher than the parabelt region. Although less robust, tonotopic organization has been observed in several of the belt areas, suggesting that basilar membrane organization remains a functionally significant aspect of auditory processing at this stage (Petkov, Kayser, Augath, & Logothetis, 2006; Rauschecker & Tian, 2004; Rauschecker, Tian, & Hauser, 1995).

The parabelt region adjoining the lateral belt areas appears to contain two subdivisions (CPB, RPB) (Hackett et al., 1998a; Morel et al., 1993; Morel & Kaas, 1992). Thalamic inputs to the parabelt favor MGpd and MGad (Hackett et al., 1998b). Cortical inputs arise from the belt areas, but not the core. This pattern of connections places the parabelt at a higher stage than the belt in the auditory processing hierarchy. However, as the belt and parabelt regions both receive inputs from the MGd, some of these inputs may be processed in parallel by neurons in both regions (see below). The expression of myelin and the other protein markers are low in the parabelt. It is not known whether neurons are tonotopically organized.

Serial and Parallel Organization of Auditory Cortex

A second major feature of the model is that auditory cortical processing involves both serial and parallel components. Anatomically, the main evidence for serial transmission of information comes from the observation that neurons in the core project to the belt region, but not the parabelt. This pattern of connections suggests that information processing in primate auditory cortex proceeds in a hierarchy beginning in the core and moving sequentially through the belt and parabelt regions (Kaas & Hackett, 1998). Physiologic support for this hypothesis rests on two principal observations. First, Rauschecker, Tian, Pons, and Mishkin (1997) found that after ablation of the core area A1, neurons in the adjacent belt area, CM, no longer responded to tones, whereas neurons in the adjacent core area, R, were unaffected. These results implied that responsiveness to tones in CM was dependent on serial relay of information from A1. Second, neurons in the belt areas tend to have longer response latencies and broader frequency tuning compared to neurons in the core (Kajikawa, de la Mothe, Blumell, & Hackett, 2005; Lakatos et al., 2005; Tian, Reser, Durham, Kustov, & Rauschecker, 2001; Woods, Lopez, Long, Rahman, & Recanzone, 2006). Taken together, these findings suggest that neuronal activity in the belt areas reflects the integration of activity from the core.

Evidence of parallel processing also has anatomic and physiologic support. Anatomically, all three core areas receive their principal thalamic input from the MGv, whereas thalamic input to most of the belt and parabelt areas arises from either the MGad or MGpd. This implies that areas within the same region may be processing identical, or at least similar, inputs in parallel.

In addition, each area of auditory cortex projects to more than one auditory cortical field. For example, A1 projects to all of the adjoining belt areas (i.e., CM, CL, ML), suggesting that all three receive the same or similar information from A1. However, even tonotopically matched portions of the belt areas receive only a small percentage of inputs from the same neurons in A1. Thus, the processing is not strictly parallel. Physiologically, perhaps the best evidence of parallel processing was found in the study by Rauschecker et al. (1997), reviewed above. Recall that after ablation of A1, responses in R were unaffected. This indicates that MGv inputs to R remained intact, whereas parallel inputs from MGv to A1 were destroyed.

In summary, the core, belt, and parabelt regions represent different levels of processing in the auditory cortex of primates. The subcortical projections target each region via at least two parallel pathways, whereas inputs to areas within each region, or level of processing, arise from the same subcortical pathway. Therefore, information processing with a region is largely parallel, but information exchange between regions is roughly hierarchical.

Topographic Connections and Processing Streams

A third feature of auditory cortical organization is that the connections between areas are topographically organized (see Figure 2–2). Within auditory cortex, the caudal areas of the core, belt, and parabelt are densely interconnected, whereas connections between the rostral and caudal areas are generally less dense (Hackett & Kaas, 2004; Kaas & Hackett, 1998). Between the rostral and caudal poles of auditory cortex overlap is greater, suggesting that there is a gradient of

interconnectivity in which the most widely separated areas have the weakest connections. The rostrocaudal topography extends to connections with auditory-related areas, as well (Figure 2–3). Rostral areas of the belt and parabelt have stronger connections with the temporal pole and rostral and orbital prefrontal cortex. Caudal areas have few connections with those areas, but robust connections with caudal prefrontal cortex and posterior parietal areas (Hackett, Stepniewska, & Kaas, 1999; Kaas & Hackett, 2000; Romanski, Bates, & Goldman-Rakic, 1999; Romanski, Tian, et al., 1999).

These topographic relationships lend anatomical support to the dual streams hypothesis, in which rostral areas of auditory cortex are considered more specialized for the processing of nonspatial (what) information, whereas the caudal areas contributed to the processing of spatial (where) relationships (Kaas & Hackett, 1999; Rauschecker & Tian, 2000; Romanski, Tian, et al., 1999). There may also be differences between the caudal and rostral areas with respect to multisensory integration, as discussed in the next section. The functional significance of the dual streams hypothesis has been controversial since its inception, and remains in flux, although it is rather clear that the caudal and rostral streams contribute uniquely to auditory and perhaps nonauditory sensory processing in primate cerebral cortex (Poremba et al., 2004; Romanski, Averbeck, & Diltz, 2005; Woods et al., 2006).

Multisensory Integration in Auditory Cortex

Until recently, it was assumed that processing in auditory and other sensory cortices was unimodal, and that their outputs subsequently converged downstream, in regions

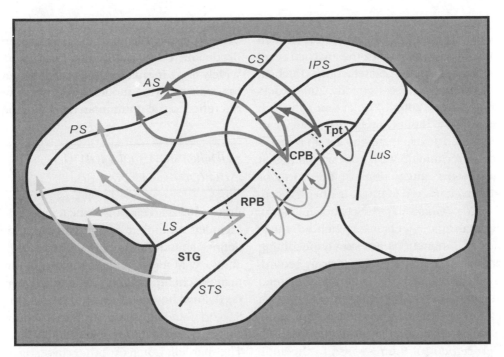

Figure 2–3. Auditory-related connections in the primate cerebral cortex. Darker arrows indicate connections with caudal belt and caudal parabelt areas of auditory cortex, and the adjoining temporal parietotemporal area (Tpt). Lighter arrows depict connections of rostral belt and parabelt areas of auditory cortex, and the rostral STG. Core and belt regions of auditory cortex not shown. Refer to Figure 2–2 for other abbreviations.

such as the superior temporal sulcus, prefrontal cortex, or posterior parietal cortex. Therefore, in the case of auditory cortex, nonauditory influences on auditory cortical activity were attributed to feedback projections from higher order multisensory fields. That perspective is now changing to accommodate the discovery of robust multisensory activity in some areas of auditory cortex. A series of recent studies in the macaque monkey demonstrated that neurons in at least one of the auditory belt areas (area CM) were responsive to both auditory and somatosensory stimulation (Fu et al., 2003; Kayser, Petkov, Augath, & Logothetis, 2005; Schroeder & Foxe, 2005; Schroeder, Lakatos, Smiley, & Hackett, 2007; Schroeder et al., 2001). Moreover, the robust sensitivity to tactile stimulation appears to be driven by feedforward inputs from secondary somatosensory areas (e.g., retroinsular area, Ri), rather than modulation of activity by downstream feedback projections (see Figure 2–2) (Cappe & Barone, 2005; de la Mothe, Blumell, Kajikawa, & Hackett, 2006a; Hackett, Smiley, Ulbert, Karmos, Lakatos, de la Mothe, Schroeder, 2007). Visual stimuli have also been found to activate auditory cortex of macaque monkeys in both visual and audiovisual modes of stimulation (Ghazanfar, Maier, Hoffman, & Logothetis, 2005; Kayser, Petkov, Augath, & Logothetis, 2007; Schroeder

& Foxe, 2002). Connections between auditory and visual cortex have been identified that appear to be part of the anatomic network underlying these interactions (Falchier, Clavagnier, Barone, & Kennedy, 2002; Rockland & Ojima, 2003). The extent to which nonauditory inputs target other areas of auditory cortex (e.g., rostral areas) remains to be determined, but it appears likely that multisensory interactions of one form or another characterize most, if not all, cortical fields (Ghazanfar & Schroeder, 2006). The neuronal mechanisms behind these kinds of interactions are slowly becoming clearer. For example, laminar array recordings in A1 revealed that when contralateral somatosensory stimulation was paired with an auditory stimulus, the phase of ongoing neural oscillations was reset, resulting in *enhancement* of the response to the auditory stimulus, in the apparent absence of a response to tactile stimulation (Lakatos, Chen, O'Connell M, Mills, & Schroeder, 2007). The effect was greatest in the high-δ (2.3–4 Hz), β (10–24 Hz), and high-γ (52–100 Hz) frequency bands. In contrast, ipsilateral somatosensory stimulation reset the phase associated with low excitability, suggesting that *suppression* of the auditory response may result in certain conditions. Thus, one effect of multisensory integration at early stages of auditory cortical processing may be to modulate stimulus salience by the synchronization of ongoing activity (Schroeder & Foxe, 2005). The functional significance of these interactions is discussed further below.

Auditory Cortical Organization in Humans

The establishment of a working model of human auditory cortex has lagged behind that of the nonhuman primate model. Numerous schemes have been proposed over the last century, but the parcellation of Brodmann (1909) still remains the most widely used. In this section, recent progress toward a working model is reviewed, with reference to the nonhuman primate model.

Subdivisions of Human Auditory Cortex

Brodmann's parcellation of the temporal lobe included a number of areas that could be defined as auditory, auditory-related, or nonauditory. Modern interpretations of Brodmann's scheme suggest that auditory cortex (as defined herein) is largely confined to the STG/STP and includes all or part of areas 41, 42, 52, and 22 (Hackett, 2003, 2007a). The parcellations of other investigators include as many as 50 additional subdivisions (Beck, 1928; Campbell, 1905; Flechsig, 1920; Galaburda & Sanides, 1980; Hopf, 1954; Morosan et al., 2001; Morosan, Schleicher, Amunts, & Zilles, 2005; Rademacher, Caviness, Steinmetz, & Galaburda, 1993; Rivier & Clarke, 1997; Vogt & Vogt, 1919; von Economo & Horn, 1930; von Economo & Koskinas, 1925; Wallace, Johnston, & Palmer, 2002). In comparing these studies, two observations stand out. First, there is rather poor agreement with respect to the number and arrangement of subdivisions. Extensive anatomic and physiologic studies (in progress) will be needed for validation, and so it may be quite some time before an accurate map is obtained. Second, though distinct in their details, the various conceptions reflect a general coherence to the less detailed parcellation of Brodmann (Figure 2-4). That is, there is a central core region with an unknown number of subdivisions that corresponds to area 41 on the first transverse temporal gyrus (TTG). The core is flanked by a beltlike arrangement

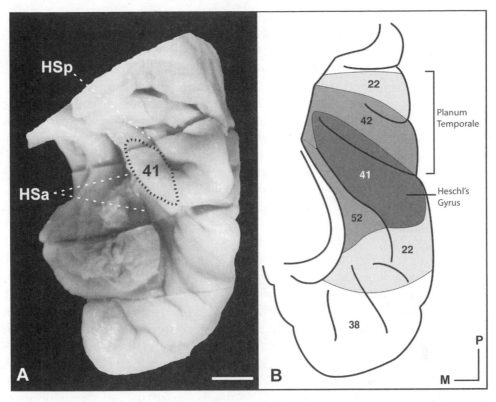

Figure 2–4. Dorsal views of the human left superior temporal plane. **A.** Black dashed ovoid indicates the boundaries of the core region (Brodmann's area 41) on Heschl's gyrus. Dashed white lines designate sulci flanking Heschl's gyrus: HSa, anterior Heschl's sulcus; HSp, posterior Heschl's sulcus. Scale bar = 5 mm. **B.** Schematic diagram of the human superior temporal plane. Area 41 occupies a large portion of the transverse temporal gyrus of Heschl, and corresponds to the core region. Area 42 flanks area 41 on the posterolateral side of Heschl's gyrus, and appears to correspond to the lateral belt and parts of the parabelt region on the planum temporale. Area 52 occupies the anteriomedial side of area 41 and corresponds to the medial belt region. Area 22 flank all three regions and extends onto the superior temporal gyrus (not shown).

of areas that correspond to the territory covered by areas 42, 52, and 22 (Galaburda & Sanides, 1980; Hackett, 2007a; Sweet, Dorph-Petersen, & Lewis, 2005). Comparative anatomical studies suggest that the architectonic profiles of *areas* 41, 42, 52, and 22 resemble profiles of the core, lateral belt, medial belt, and parabelt *regions* identified in monkeys (Hackett, Preuss, & Kaas,

2001; Sweet et al., 2005). In that case, a large portion of the belt and parabelt regions may be contained within the PT. As the human temporal lobe is greatly expanded compared to monkeys, a one-to-one correspondence of areas is unlikely. However, the similarities in organization are enough to support the establishment of a working model based on this arrangement.

Tonotopic organization is an expected organizational feature of the human core region; however, it has been surprisingly difficult to establish this feature due to methodological limitations of functional imaging or electrophysiology. Tonotopic organization is best observed at near-threshold intensities, as employed in single or multiunit studies, whereas higher intensities are generally needed to detect signal change using noninvasive methods. Nevertheless, a number of studies have produced evidence of tonotopic gradients and reversals along the TTG axis, comparable to studies of the core region in nonhuman primates (Cansino, Ducorps, & Ragot, 2003; Formisano et al., 2003; Fujioka et al., 2003; Howard et al., 1996; Langers, Backes, & van Dijk, 2007; Talavage, Ledden, Benson, Rosen, & Melcher, 2000; Talavage et al., 2004; Yetkin, Roland, Christensen, & Purdy, 2004). Those findings suggest that at least two areas comprise the core region of human auditory cortex, whereas there is little evidence of tonotopic gradients outside of the core.

Serial and Parallel Organization

Functional studies of the human cerebral cortex (fMRI, EEG, MEG, PET) indicate that auditory stimulation activates an extensive network of auditory and auditory-related areas in the temporal, parietal, and frontal lobes (Binder et al., 2000; Friederici, 2002; Griffiths, Warren, Scott, Nelken, & King, 2004; Hall, Hart, & Johnsrude, 2003; Scott, 2005; Scott & Johnsrude, 2003; Wise et al., 2001; Zatorre, 2007). Within this network, it is reasonably clear that auditory information ascends a hierarchy of areas proceeding through auditory cortex and terminating in auditory-related areas downstream which may process some of those

inputs in parallel (Davis & Johnsrude, 2003; Griffiths, 2001; Griffiths et al., 2007; Langers, Backes, & Dijk, 2003; Schonwiesner et al., 2007; Uppenkamp, Johnsrude, Norris, Marslen-Wilson, & Patterson, 2006). The PT, for example, has long been thought to operate at a higher level than the core region on HG, and is itself a region comprised of functionally distinct subregions specialized for the processing particular attributes of sound (Binder, Frost, Hammeke, Rao, & Cox, 1996; Griffiths & Warren, 2002; Warren & Griffiths, 2003). Functional connections have also been established between HG and an area located on the posterior STG, referred to as PLST (Brugge, Volkov, Garell, Reale, & Howard, 2003; Howard et al., 2000; Oya et al., 2006). In these studies, evoked potentials were directly recorded from human auditory cortex using a combination of surface and penetrating electrode arrays. Activation of PLST was observed after electrical stimulation of the HG, with progressive shifts in latency and amplitude that varied topographically along the medial to lateral axis of the gyrus. Stimulation of PLST generated complementary activity in HG. These findings indicate that the connections between HG and PLST are reciprocal and provide direct evidence of a serial flow of information from core to lateral belt or parabelt areas on the PT and STG. Several studies have demonstrated that activation between regions (i.e., core–belt) can be dissociated (Hall, Barrett, Akeroyd, & Summerfield, 2005; Hall et al., 2003; Hall et al., 2002; Harms, Guinan, Sigalovsky, & Melcher, 2005; Hart, Palmer, & Hall, 2002; Langers et al., 2007; Patterson, Uppenkamp, Johnsrude, & Griffiths, 2002; Seifritz et al., 2006; Seifritz et al., 2002; Tramo, Cariani, Koh, Makris, & Braida, 2005; Wessinger et al., 2001; Zatorre & Belin, 2001). For example, Seifritz et al. (2002) reported that the core region on the TTG exhibited a sustained BOLD response to auditory stimulation, whereas activation of the surrounding belt areas in the PT and anterior to TTG was characterized by a transient (phasic) response to the same stimulus. Similar results were obtained by Harms et al. (2005). Wessinger et al. (2001) and Seifritz et al. (2006) demonstrated greater activation in the core to narrow-band sounds, whereas sounds with broader bandwidth were preferred in the surrounding belt regions. In addition to being consistent with a model in which the core and belt regions represent different levels of processing, the relatively homogeneous activation within regions is consistent with parallel processing within each of those regions. These predictions were tested in a recent modeling study designed to examine the analysis of auditory objects by regions of auditory and auditory-related cortex (Griffiths et al., 2007). Serial and parallel models were tested to determine whether the analysis of spectral envelope proceeds in a serial fashion from HG to PT to the STS, or whether the PT and STS receive the information from the HG in parallel. The results strongly supported a serial model of auditory object processing (Griffiths & Warren, 2004), consistent with the connectional relationships observed in nonhuman primates and other network models (Husain & Horwitz, 2006). Within that hierarchy, there is evidence that earlier stages of processing in auditory cortex respond to different classes of sound (e.g., speech and nonspeech) with less specificity, whereas later stages show greater selectivity for speech (Uppenkamp et al., 2006). This may reflect the successive abstraction of perceptual features at later stages of processing in auditory cortex, and perhaps a transition from feature-based to object-based representation of auditory inputs (Schnupp, 2006).

Topographic Connections and Processing Streams

The topographic connections of the rostral and caudal areas of the macaque monkey auditory to auditory-related regions elsewhere in the brain were discussed above. These findings suggested that rostral auditory areas were preferentially linked to regions in the temporal and frontal lobes primarily concerned with the nonspatial attributes of sensory stimuli, whereas the caudal auditory areas were linked to posterior areas in parietal and frontal cortex that contribute to multimodal spatial processing. Perhaps the strongest evidence for the segregation of auditory activity into processing streams comes from functional studies of humans. Excellent reviews and commentaries of this rapidly growing literature are available (Arnott, Binns, Grady, & Alain, 2004; Belin & Zatorre, 2000; Boatman, 2006; Friederici, 2002; Griffiths et al., 2004; Hall, 2003; Hickok & Poeppel, 2004; Scott, 2005; Scott & Johnsrude, 2003; Warren, Wise, & Warren, 2005) The majority of these studies identify topographic differences in the processing of spatial (where) information by a dorsal stream, and nonspatial (what) information by a ventral stream. Topographic segregation of auditory processing is evident at two levels: (1) within the network of fields that comprise auditory cortex, and (2) within the network of auditory-related areas throughout the brain. At the level of auditory cortex, activation of the anterior and lateral portions of HG, PT, and STG tends to favor nonspatial features (e.g., speech sounds, pitch, sound patterns), whereas their posterior and medial domains are broadly responsive to sounds of all kinds, and tend to be more strongly activated by spatial features including moving auditory stimuli (Ahveninen et al., 2006; Altmann, Bledowski, Wibral, & Kaiser, 2007; Barrett & Hall, 2006; Binder, Liebenthal, Possing, Medler, & Ward, 2004; Hart, Palmer, & Hall, 2004; Hewson-Stoate, Schonwiesner, & Krumbholz, 2006; Krumbholz et al., 2005; Pavani, Macaluso, Warren, Driver, & Griffiths, 2002; Warren & Griffiths, 2003; Zatorre & Belin, 2001). The divergence of these two streams becomes more apparent in their downstream projections to auditory-related fields. The dorsal stream targets areas in posterior parietal and superior frontal regions, which tend to be activated by auditory spatial processing. The ventral stream is characterized by increased activity in anterior/ventral temporal and inferior frontal areas during nonspatial tasks (Alain, Arnott, Hevenor, Graham, & Grady, 2001; Belin, Zatorre, & Ahad, 2002; Belin, Zatorre, Lafaille, Ahad, & Pike, 2000; De Santis, Clarke, & Murray, 2007; Griffiths et al., 1996; Griffiths et al., 1998; Krumbholz et al., 2005; Maeder et al., 2001; Scott, Blank, Rosen, & Wise, 2000; Warren, Green, Rauschecker, & Griffiths, 2002).

Other studies have revealed other topographic differences that are less directly related to spatial and nonspatial processing. An alternative, or amplified view of the spatial and nonspatial theme links the dorsal stream to the sensory-motor aspects of speech production and the ventral stream to the meaning of sound (for a review, see Hickok & Poeppel, 2004). These authors review evidence that the dorsal stream contributes to auditory-motor integration by mapping sound onto its articulatory-based representation, whereas the ventral stream maps sound onto its meaning (Hickok & Poeppel, 2000; Wise et al., 2001). Similarly, Scott (2005) noted that the medial posterior fields are activated during speech production, regardless of whether the articulation is overt or specific to speech. Thus,

the posteromedial portion of human auditory cortex appears to contribute to a sensory motor interface that links perception and production.

It is important to note here that segregation of the dorsal and ventral streams is not complete, as there is anatomic evidence of interactions between streams (Kaas & Hackett, 1999), which can be revealed by adjusting task demands (Zatorre, Bouffard, Ahad, & Belin, 2002). Thus, the delineation of two streams in which spatial and nonspatial processing is completely segregated is clearly overly simplistic.

Multisensory Integration

The integration of information captured by multiple sensory modalities underlies the formation of unified percepts of our environment. An important benefit of that kind of perceptual synchrony is enhanced detection and identification of sensory events (King, 2005; Spence & Squire, 2003). Multisensory interactions are well documented in the classic multisensory regions of frontal, parietal, and temporal cortex where the outputs of the sensory cortices converge, but it has recently become clear that multisensory interactions also occur in areas of sensory cortex previously thought to be unimodal (Ghazanfar & Schroeder, 2006). In auditory cortex, both tactile and visual modes of stimulation modulate activity in auditory and auditory-related areas, contributing to a wide variety of observations (Schroeder & Foxe, 2005; Schroeder et al., 2007).

One class of interactions impacts the detection and discrimination of stationary and moving objects. For example, electrophysiologic activity and reaction times associated with combined auditory and visual stimuli are typically enhanced compared to stimulation of either modality alone (Molholm et al., 2002; Senkowski, Molholm, Gomez-Ramirez, & Foxe, 2006). Similarly, subjects more rapidly detected an audiotactile stimulus compared to their unimodal presentations, irrespective of the spatial alignment of the auditory and tactile stimuli (Murray et al., 2005; Zampini, Torresan, Spence, & Murray, 2007). With respect to multisensory influences on motion perception, numerous psychophysical studies have documented the effects of combining auditory, tactile, or visual stimulation (Soto-Faraco, Kingstone, & Spence, 2003). Generally, performance is best when stimuli are spatially or temporally congruent. Imaging and electrophysiologic recordings indicate that these effects correlate positively with enhanced activation of auditory and auditory-related areas. In one recent study, subjects were best at judging motion when the auditory and visual sources were in phase (Baumann & Greenlee, 2007). Compared to static noise, activation in the in-phase and antiphase conditions was enhanced in the belt and parabelt regions of the right hemisphere, among others. Thus, multisensory contributions to motion perception appear to modulate activity in early stages of cortical sensory processing.

A second class of interactions occurs when perception of an event in one modality is altered by an event in another modality. The best known examples include the ventriloquist or McGurk effects, in which the visual representation of an event alters perception of the acoustic properties associated with that event (Alais & Burr, 2004; McGurk & MacDonald, 1976; Recanzone, 1998). These effects appear to involve modulation of activity in auditory areas, where even lip movements alone can activate primary auditory cortex (Calvert et al., 1997; Sams et al., 1991). Pairing a visual stimulus with auditory imagery can generate activation of secondary auditory areas in the PT

and STG (Jancke & Shah, 2004). Alternatively, temporal features, such as a repetitive flutter or flicker sound, in the auditory domain can alter the perception of flicker rates in the visual domain (Recanzone, 2003; Welch, DuttonHurt, & Warren, 1986), supporting psychophysical evidence that audition dominates vision in temporal processing, whereas vision is dominant in spatial tasks (Guttman, Gilroy, & Blake, 2005; Wada, Kitagawa, & Noguchi, 2003). As for audiotactile interactions, it has been shown that tactile sensations can be predictably altered by concurrent acoustic stimulation, as in the parchment skin illusion (Guest, Catmur, Lloyd, & Spence, 2002; Jousmaki & Hari, 1998). Tactile perception is also affected by the acoustic properties of solids and liquids while eating or drinking (Kitagawa & Spence, 2006; Spence & Zampini, 2006). Related studies indicate that tinnitus can be evoked in some patients by tactile stimulation after complete and acute unilateral deafferentation of the periphery following neurosurgery (Cacace, Cousins, Parnes, McFarland, et al., 1999; Cacace, Cousins, Parnes, Semenoff, et al., 1999), suggesting that cross-modal plasticity may enhance activity in the circuits linking the auditory and somatosensory modalities (Levanen, Jousmaki, & Hari, 1998). The anatomic substrates of these interactions are not entirely clear, but there is evidence that parts of auditory cortex are involved (Cacace, Cousins, Parnes, Semenoff, et al., 1999; Lockwood et al., 1998).

Within human auditory cortex, multisensory interactions appear to exhibit some degree of topographic specificity. The clearest examples involve the posterior-medial portion of the planum temporale, which is frequently activated by audiotactile stimulation (Caetano & Jousmaki, 2006; Foxe et al., 2000; Foxe et al., 2002; Gobbele et al., 2003; Lehmann et al., 2006; Murray et al., 2005;

Schurmann, Caetano, Hlushchuk, Jousmaki, & Hari, 2006). Audiotactile convergence in this region may be related to evidence of sensory-motor interactions in the temporal-parietal region during speech production (discussed above). Audiovisual interactions also modulate activity in the core and belt areas of HG, PT, and STG (Buchsbaum et al., 2005; Johanna Pekkola, 2006; Laurienti et al., 2002; Martuzzi et al., 2006; Meyer, Baumann, Marchina, & Jancke, 2007; Ojanen et al., 2005; Pekkola et al., 2006; Pekkola et al., 2005; Reale et al., 2007; Rinne et al., 2005), but topographic specificity is less clear and the results have been more variable compared to audiotactile studies. More specifically, the areas of auditory and auditory-related cortex involved vary with methodological and task demands, and therefore the precise network underlying audiovisual integration remains uncertain (Bushara, Grafman, & Hallett, 2001; Calvert, 2001; Calvert, Hansen, Iversen, & Brammer, 2001).

Summary

The central auditory pathways of humans and nonhuman primates are fundamentally similar in their organization. As in all mammals, the auditory areas of the primate cerebral cortex receive inputs from auditory nuclei in the medial geniculate complex of the thalamus after extensive processing by brainstem nuclei, including the cochlear nuclei, superior olivary complex, lateral lemniscus, and inferior colliculus. In contrast to the subcortical nuclei, which are highly conserved across mammals, the organization of auditory cortex appears to vary significantly. Compared to nonprimates, the greatest number of auditory cortical areas has been identified in monkeys. In humans, where auditory cortex is greatly expanded in size, it is possible that additional areas may be present. Although the generation of maps of auditory cortex is ongoing and expected to continue for quite some time, comparative analyses of human and nonhuman primates indicate that the principles of auditory cortex organization are comparable.

A primary, or core region, is flanked medially and laterally by belt and parabelt regions that cover much of the superior temporal gyrus. The regions are hierarchically arranged, and each contains multiple subdivisions, or areas. The belt and parabelt regions are connected with a number of auditory-related fields elsewhere in the brain. These fields are typically sites of multisensory integration where the outputs of auditory, visual, and somatosensory cortices converge. Within this system of connections, the rostral and caudal areas of auditory cortex project topographically to functionally distinct auditory-related areas. These two pathways are generally thought to represent segregated streams for the processing of nonspatial and spatial information, analogous to the dual streams of the visual system. Although the auditory-related areas are considered the principal sites of multisensory convergence in the brain, it has recently become clear that even the auditory cortex receives inputs from other sensory modalities. These inputs appear to contribute to a range of psychophysical observations which demonstrate the interactive effects of combined auditory, visual, and somatosensory stimulation.

References

Adams, J. C. (1983). Cytology of periolivary cells and the organization of their projections in the cat. *Journal of Comparative Neurology*, *215*, 275–289.

Adams, J. C., & Warr, W. B. (1976). Origins of axons in the cat's acoustic striae determined by injection of horseradish peroxidase into severed tracts. *Journal of Comparative Neurology, 170,* 107–121.

Ahveninen, J., Jaaskelainen, I. P., Raij, T., Bonmassar, G., Devore, S., Hamalainen, M., et al. (2006). Task-modulated "what" and "where" pathways in human auditory cortex. *Proceedings of the National Academy of Sciences, 103,* 14608–14613.

Aitkin, L. (1986). *The auditory midbrain: Structure and function in the central auditory pathway.* Clifton, NJ: Humana Press.

Aitkin, L. M. (1990). *The auditory cortex, structural and functional bases of auditory perception.* London: Chapman and Hall.

Aitkin, L. M., Anderson, D. J., & Brugge, J. F. (1970). Tonotopic organization and discharge characteristics of single neurons in nuclei of the lateral lemniscus of the cat. *Journal of Neurophysiology, 33,* 421–440.

Aitkin, L. M., Pettigrew, J. D., Calford, M. B., Phillips, S. C., & Wise, L. Z. (1985). Representation of stimulus azimuth by low-frequency neurons in inferior colliculus of the cat. *Journal of Neurophysiology, 53,* 43–59.

Aitkin, L. M., Webster, W. R., Veale, J. L., & Crosby, D. C. (1975). Inferior colliculus. I. Comparison of response properties of neurons in central, pericentral, and external nuclei of adult cat. *Journal of Neurophysiology, 38,* 1196–1207.

Alain, C., Arnott, S. R., Hevenor, S., Graham, S., & Grady, C. L. (2001). "What" and "where" in the human auditory system. *Proceeding of the National Academy of Science, 98,* 12301–12306.

Alais, D., & Burr, D. (2004). The ventriloquist effect results from near-optimal bimodal integration. *Current Biology, 14,* 257–262.

Altmann, C. F., Bledowski, C., Wibral, M., & Kaiser, J. (2007). Processing of location and pattern changes of natural sounds in the human auditory cortex. *NeuroImage, 35,* 1192–1200.

Andersen, R. A., Knight, P. L., & Merzenich, M. M. (1980). The thalamocortical and corticothalamic connections of AI, AII, and the anterior auditory field (AAF) in the cat: evidence for two largely segregated systems of connections. *Journal of Comparative Neurology, 194,* 663–701.

Andersen, R. A., Roth, G. L., Aitkin, L. M., & Merzenich, M. M. (1980). The efferent projections of the central nucleus and the pericentral nucleus of the inferior colliculus in the cat. *Journal of Comparative Neurology, 194,* 649–662.

Arnott, S. R., Binns, M. A., Grady, C. L., & Alain, C. (2004). Assessing the auditory dual-pathway model in humans. *NeuroImage, 22,* 401–408.

Bacsik, R. D., & Strominger, N. L. (1973). The cytoarchitecture of the human anteroventral cochlear nucleus. *Journal of Comparative Neurology, 147,* 281–289.

Bajo, V. M., Merchan, M. A., Lopez, D. E., & Rouiller, E. M. (1993). Neuronal morphology and efferent projections of the dorsal nucleus of the lateral lemniscus in the rat. *Journal of Comparative Neurology, 334,* 241–262.

Barnes, W. T., Magoun, H. W., & Ranson, S. W. (1943). The ascending auditory pathway in the brain stem of the monkey. *Journal of Comparative Neurology, 79,* 129–152.

Barrett, D. J. K., & Hall, D. A. (2006). Response preferences for "what" and "where" in human non-primary auditory cortex. *NeuroImage, 32,* 968–977.

Batra, R., & Fitzpatrick, D. C. (2002). Monaural and binaural processing in the ventral nucleus of the lateral lemniscus: A major source of inhibition to the inferior colliculus. *Hearing Research, 168,* 90–97.

Baumann, O., & Greenlee, M. W. (2007). Neural correlates of coherent audiovisual motion perception. *Cerebral Cortex, 17,* 1433–1443.

Bazwinsky, I., Bidmon, H.-J., Zilles, K., & Hilbig, H. (2005). Characterization of the rhesus monkey superior olivary complex by calcium binding proteins and synaptophysin. *Journal of Anatomy, 207,* 745–761.

Beck, E. (1928). Die myeloarchitektonische Felderung es in der Sylvischen Furche gelegenen Teiles des menschlichen Schläfenlappens. *Journal of Psychology and Neurology, 36,* 1–21.

Belin, P., & Zatorre, R. J. (2000). "What," "where" and "how" in auditory cortex. *Nature Neuroscience, 3,* 965–966.

Belin, P., Zatorre, R. J., & Ahad, P. (2002). Human temporal-lobe response to vocal sounds. *Cognitive Brain Research, 13*, 17–26.

Belin, P., Zatorre, R. J., Lafaille, P., Ahad, P., & Pike, B. (2000). Voice-selective areas in human auditory cortex. *Nature, 403*, 309–312.

Binder, J. R., Frost, J. A., Hammeke, T. A., Bellgowan, P. S. F., Springer, J. A., Kaufman, J. N., et al. (2000). Human temporal lobe activation by speech and nonspeech sounds. *Cerebral Cortex, 10*, 512–528.

Binder, J. R., Frost, J. A., Hammeke, T. A., Rao, S. M., & Cox, R. W. (1996). Function of the left planum temporale in auditory and linguistic processing. *Brain, 119*, 1239–1247.

Binder, J. R., Liebenthal, E., Possing, E. T., Medler, D. A., & Ward, B. D. (2004). Neural correlates of sensory and decision processes in auditory object identification. *Nature Neuroscience, 7*, 295–301.

Bizley, J. K., Nodal, F. R., Nelken, I., & King, A. J. (2005). Functional organization of ferret auditory cortex. *Cerebral Cortex, 15*, 1637–1653.

Blum, P. S., Abraham, L. D., & Gilman, S. (1979). Vestibular, auditory, and somatic input to the posterior thalamus of the cat. *Experimental Brain Research, 34*, 1–9.

Boatman, D. F. (2006). Cortical auditory systems: Speech and other complex sounds. *Epilepsy and Behavior, 8*, 494–503.

Brodmann, K. 1909. *Vergleichende Lokalisationslehre der Grosshirnrinde*. Barth, Leipzig.

Brugge, J. F., Anderson, D. J., & Aitkin, L. M. (1970). Responses of neurons in the dorsal nucleus of the lateral lemniscus of cat to binaural tonal stimulation. *Journal of Neurophysiology, 33*, 441–458.

Brugge, J. F., Volkov, I. O., Garell, P. C., Reale, R. A., & Howard, M. A., 3rd. (2003). Functional connections between auditory cortex on Heschl's gyrus and on the lateral superior temporal gyrus in humans. *Journal of Neurophysiology, 90*, 3750–3763.

Brunso-Bechtold, J. K., Thompson, G. C., & Masterton, R. B. (1981). HRP study of the organization of auditory afferents ascending to central nucleus of inferior colliculus in cat. *Journal of Comparative Neurology, 197*, 705–722.

Buchsbaum, B. R., Olsen, R. K., Koch, P. F., Kohn, P., Kippenhan, J. S., & Berman, K. F. (2005). Reading, hearing, and the planum temporale. *NeuroImage, 24*, 444–454.

Burton, H., & Jones, E. G. (1976). The posterior thalamic region and its cortical projection in New World and Old World monkeys. *Journal of Comparative Neurology, 168*, 249–301.

Bushara, K. O., Grafman, J., & Hallett, M. (2001). Neural correlates of auditory-visual stimulus onset asynchrony detection. *Journal of Neuroscience, 21*, 300–304.

Cacace, A. T., Cousins, J. P., Parnes, S. M., McFarland, D. J., Semenoff, D., Holmes, T., et al. (1999). Cutaneous-evoked tinnitus. II. Review Of neuroanatomical, physiological and functional imaging studies. *Audiology and Neuro-otology, 4*, 258–268.

Cacace, A. T., Cousins, J. P., Parnes, S. M., Semenoff, D., Holmes, T., McFarland, D. J., et al. (1999). Cutaneous-evoked tinnitus. I. Phenomenology, psychophysics and functional imaging. *Audiology and Neuro-otology, 4*, 247–257.

Caetano, G., & Jousmaki, V. (2006). Evidence of vibrotactile input to human auditory cortex. *NeuroImage, 29*, 15–28.

Calford, M. B. (1983). The parcellation of the medial geniculate body of the cat defined by the auditory response properties of single units. *Journal of Neuroscience, 3*, 2350–2364.

Calford, M. B., & Aitkin, L. M. (1983). Ascending projections to the medial geniculate body of the cat: Evidence for multiple, parallel auditory pathways through thalamus. *Journal of Neuroscience, 3*, 2365–2380.

Calvert, G. A. (2001). Crossmodal processing in the human brain: Insights from functional neuroimaging studies. *Cerebral Cortex, 11*, 1110–1123.

Calvert, G. A., Bullmore, E. T., Brammer, M. J., Campbell, R., Williams, S. C., McGuire, P. K., et al. (1997). Activation of auditory cortex during silent lipreading. *Science, 276*, 593–596.

Calvert, G. A., Hansen, P. C., Iversen, S. D., & Brammer, M. J. (2001). Detection of audiovisual integration sites in humans by application of electrophysiological criteria to the BOLD effect. *NeuroImage, 14*, 427–438.

Campbell, H. W. (1905). In *Histological studies on the localization of cerebral function.* Cambridge, UK: Cambridge University Press.

Cansino, S., Ducorps, A., & Ragot, R. (2003). Tonotopic cortical representation of periodic complex sounds. *Human Brain Mapping, 20*, 71-81.

Cappe, C., & Barone, P. (2005). Heteromodal connections supporting multisensory integration at low levels of cortical processing in the monkey. *European Journal of Neuroscience, 22*, 2886-2902.

Coleman, J. R., & Clerici, W. J. (1987). Sources of projections to subdivisions of the inferior colliculus in the rat. *Journal of Comparative Neurology, 262*, 215-226.

Covey, E., & Casseday, H. J. (1995). The lower brainstem auditory pathways. In A. Popper & R. Fay (Eds.), *Hearing in bats* (pp. 146-190). New York: Springer-Verlag.

Curry, M. J. (1972). The exteroceptive properties of neurones in the somatic part of the posterior group (PO). *Brain Research, 44*, 439-462.

Davis, M. H., & Johnsrude, I. S. (2003). Hierarchical processing in spoken language comprehension. *Journal of Neuroscience, 23*(8), 3423-3431.

de la Mothe, L. A., Blumell, S., Kajikawa, Y., & Hackett, T. A. (2006a). Cortical connections of auditory cortex in marmoset monkeys: core and medial belt regions. *Journal of Comparative Neurology, 496*, 27-71.

de la Mothe, L. A., Blumell, S., Kajikawa, Y., & Hackett, T. A. (2006b). Thalamic connections of auditory cortex in marmoset monkeys: core and medial belt regions. *Journal of Comparative Neurology, 496*, 72-96.

de Ribaupierre, F. (1997). *Acoustical information processing in the auditory thalamus and cortex.* New York: Oxford Press.

De Santis, L., Clarke, S., & Murray, M. M. (2007). Automatic and intrinsic auditory "What" and "Where" processing in humans revealed by electrical neuroimaging. *Cerebral Cortex, 17*, 9-17.

Ehret, G., & Romand, R. (1997). *The central auditory system.* New York: Oxford University Press.

Evans, E. (1974). *Neural processes for the detection of acoustic patterns and for sound localization.* Cambridge, MA: MIT Press.

Falchier, A., Clavagnier, S., Barone, P., & Kennedy, H. (2002). Anatomical evidence of multimodal integration in primate striate cortex. *Journal of Neuroscience, 22*, 5749-5759.

FitzPatrick, K. A., & Imig, T. J. (1978). Projections of auditory cortex upon the thalamus and midbrain in the owl monkey. *Journal of Comparative Neurology, 177*, 537-555.

Flechsig, P. (1920). In *Anatomie des Menschlichen Gehirns und Ruckenmarks auf Myelogenetischer Grundlage.* Leipzig, Germany: Thieme.

Formisano, E., Kim, D. S., Di Salle, F., van de Moortele, P. F., Ugurbil, K., & Goebel, R. (2003). Mirror-symmetric tonotopic maps in human primary auditory cortex. *Neuron, 40*, 859-869.

Foxe, J. J., Morocz, I. A., Murray, M. M., Higgins, B. A., Javitt, D. C., & Schroeder, C. E. (2000). Multisensory auditory-somatosensory interactions in early cortical processing revealed by high-density electrical mapping. *Brain Research and Cognitive Brain Research, 10*, 77-83.

Foxe, J. J., Wylie, G. R., Martinez, A., Schroeder, C. E., Javitt, D. C., Guilfoyle, D., et al. (2002). Auditory-somatosensory multisensory processing in auditory association cortex: an fMRI study. *Journal of Neurophysiology, 88*, 540-543.

Friauf, E., & Ostwald, J. (1988). Divergent projections of physiologically characterized rat ventral cochlear nucleus neurons as shown by intra-axonal injection of horseradish peroxidase. *Experimental Brain Research, 73*, 263-284.

Friederici, A. D. (2002). Towards a neural basis of auditory sentence processing. *Trends in Cognitive Science, 6*, 78-84.

Fu, K. M., Johnston, T. A., Shah, A. S., Arnold, L., Smiley, J., Hackett, T. A., et al. (2003). Auditory cortical neurons respond to somatosensory stimulation. *Journal of Neuroscience, 23*, 7510-7515.

Fujioka, T., Ross, B., Okamoto, H., Takeshima, Y., Kakigi, R., & Pantev, C. (2003). Tonotopic representation of missing fundamental complex sounds in the human auditory cortex. *European Journal of Neuroscience, 18*, 432-440.

Galaburda, A., & Sanides, F. (1980). Cytoarchitectonic organization of the human auditory cortex. *Journal of Comparative Neurology, 190*, 597-610.

Ghazanfar, A. A., Maier, J. X., Hoffman, K. L., & Logothetis, N. K. (2005). Multisensory integration of dynamic faces and voices in rhesus monkey auditory cortex. *Journal of Neuroscience, 25*, 5004-5012.

Ghazanfar, A. A., & Schroeder, C. E. (2006). Is neocortex essentially multisensory? *Trends in Cognitive Science, 10*, 278-285.

Glendenning, K. K., Brunso-Bechtold, J. K., Thompson, G. C., & Masterton, R. B. (1981). Ascending auditory afferents to the nuclei of the lateral lemniscus. *Journal of Comparative Neurology, 197*, 673-703.

Gobbele, R., Schurmann, M., Forss, N., Juottonen, K., Buchner, H., & Hari, R. (2003). Activation of the human posterior parietal and temporoparietal cortices during audiotactile interaction. *NeuroImage, 20*, 503-511.

Griffiths, T. D. (2001). The neural processing of complex sounds. *Annals of the New York Academy of Sciences, 930*, 133-142.

Griffiths, T. D., Kumar, S., Warren, J. D., Stewart, L., Stephan, K. E., & Friston, K. J. (2007). Approaches to the cortical analysis of auditory objects. *Hearing Research, 229*, 46-53.

Griffiths, T. D., Rees, A., Witton, C., Shakir, R. A., Henning, G. B., & Green, G. G. (1996). Evidence for a sound movement area in the human cerebral cortex. *Nature, 383*, 425-427.

Griffiths, T. D., Rees, G., Rees, A., Green, G. G., Witton, C., Rowe, D., et al. (1998). Right parietal cortex is involved in the perception of sound movement in humans. *Nature Neuroscience, 1*, 74-79.

Griffiths, T. D., & Warren, J. D. (2002). The planum temporale as a computational hub. *Trends in Neuroscience, 25*, 348-353.

Griffiths, T. D., & Warren, J. D. (2004). What is an auditory object? *Nature Reviews Neuroscience, 5*, 887-892.

Griffiths, T. D., Warren, J. D., Scott, S. K., Nelken, I., & King, A. J. (2004). Cortical processing of complex sound: A way forward? *Trends in Neuroscience, 27*, 181-185.

Groh, J. M., Kelly, K. A., & Underhill, A. M. (2003). A monotonic code for sound azimuth in primate inferior colliculus. *Journal of Cognitive Neuroscience, 15*, 1217-1231.

Groh, J. M., Trause, A. S., Underhill, A. M., Clark, K. R., & Inati, S. (2001). Eye position influences auditory responses in primate inferior colliculus. *Neuron, 29*, 509-518.

Guest, S., Catmur, C., Lloyd, D., & Spence, C. (2002). Audiotactile interaction in roughness perception. *Experimental Brain Research, 146*, 161-171.

Guttman, S. E., Gilroy, L. A., & Blake, R. (2005). Hearing what the eyes see. Auditory encoding of visual temporal sequences. *Psychological Science, 16*, 228-235.

Hackett, T. (2003). The comparative anatomy of the primate auditory cortex. In A. Ghazanfar (Ed.), *Primate audition: Behavior and neurobiology* (pp. 199-226). Boca Raton, FL: CRC Press.

Hackett, T. A. (2007a). Organization and correspondence of the auditory cortex of humans and nonhuman primates. In J. Kaas (Ed.), *Evolution of the nervous system* (pp. 109-119). Oxford, UK: Elsevier.

Hackett, T. A. (2007b). Organization of the thalamocortical auditory pathways in primates. In R. F. Burkard, M. Don, & J. J. Eggermont (Eds.), *Auditory evoked potentials: Basic principles and clinical application* (pp. 428-440). Baltimore: Lippincott Williams & Wilkins.

Hackett, T. A., De La Mothe, L. A., Ulbert, I., Karmos, G., Smiley, J., & Schroeder, C. E. (2007). Multisensory convergence in auditory cortex, II. Thalamocortical connections of the caudal superior temporal plane. *Journal of Comparative Neurology, 502*, 924-952.

Hackett, T. A., & Kaas, J. H. (2004). Auditory cortex in primates: functional subdivisions and processing streams. In M. Gazzaniga (Ed.), *The cognitive neurosciences III* (pp. 215-232). Cambridge, MA: MIT Press.

Hackett, T. A., Preuss, T. M., & Kaas, J. H. (2001). Architectonic identification of the core region in auditory cortex of macaques, chimpanzees, and humans. *Journal of Comparative Neurology, 441,* 197–222.

Hackett, T. A., Smiley, J.F., Ulbert, I., Karmos, G., Lakatos, P., de la Mothe, L.A., Schroeder, C.E. (2007). Sources of somatosensory input to the caudal belt areas of auditory cortex. *Perception, 36,* 1419–1430.

Hackett, T. A., Stepniewska, I., & Kaas, J. H. (1998a). Subdivisions of auditory cortex and ipsilateral cortical connections of the parabelt auditory cortex in macaque monkeys. *Journal of Comparative Neurology, 394,* 475–495.

Hackett, T. A., Stepniewska, I., & Kaas, J. H. (1998b). Thalamocortical connections of the parabelt auditory cortex in macaque monkeys. *Journal of Comparative Neurology, 400,* 271–286.

Hackett, T. A., Stepniewska, I., & Kaas, J. H. (1999). Prefrontal connections of the parabelt auditory cortex in macaque monkeys. *Brain Research, 817,* 45–58.

Hall, D. A. (2003). Auditory pathways: Are 'what' and 'where' appropriate? *Current Biology, 13,* R406–R408.

Hall, D. A., Barrett, D. J. K., Akeroyd, M. A., & Summerfield, A. Q. (2005). Cortical representations of temporal structure in sound. *Journal of Neurophysiology, 94,* 3181–3191.

Hall, D. A., Hart, H. C., & Johnsrude, I. S. (2003). Relationships between human auditory cortical structure and function. *Audiology and Neuro-Otology, 8,* 1–18.

Hall, D. A., Johnsrude, I. S., Haggard, M. P., Palmer, A. R., Akeroyd, M. A., & Summerfield, A. Q. (2002). Spectral and temporal processing in human auditory cortex. *Cerebral Cortex, 12,* 140–149.

Harms, M. P., Guinan, J. J., Jr., Sigalovsky, I. S., & Melcher, J. R. (2005). Short-term sound temporal envelope characteristics determine multisecond time patterns of activity in human auditory cortex as shown by fMRI. *Journal of Neurophysiology, 93,* 210–222.

Hart, H. C., Palmer, A. R., & Hall, D. A. (2002). Heschl's gyrus is more sensitive to tone level than non-primary auditory cortex. *Hearing Research, 171,* 177–190.

Hart, H. C., Palmer, A. R., & Hall, D. A. (2004). Different areas of human non-primary auditory cortex are activated by sounds with spatial and nonspatial properties. *Human Brain Mapping, 21,* 178–190.

He, J. (2002). OFF responses in the auditory thalamus of the guinea pig. *Journal of Neurophysiology, 88,* 2377–2386.

Heiman-Patterson, T. D., & Strominger, N. L. (1985). Morphological changes in the cochlear nuclear complex in primate phylogeny and development. *Journal of Morphology, 186,* 289–306.

Henkel, C. K. (1997). Axonal morphology in fibrodendritic laminae of the dorsal nucleus of the lateral lemniscus: afferent projections from the medial superior olivary nucleus. *Journal of Comparative Neurology, 380,* 136–144.

Henkel, C. K., & Spangler, K. M. (1983). Organization of the efferent projections of the medial superior olivary nucleus in the cat as revealed by HRP and autoradiographic tracing methods. *Journal of Comparative Neurology, 221,* 416–428.

Hewson-Stoate, N., Schonwiesner, M., & Krumbholz, K. (2006). Vowel processing evokes a large sustained response anterior to primary auditory cortex. *European Journal of Neuroscience, 24,* 2661–2671.

Hickok, G., & Poeppel, D. (2000). Towards a functional neuroanatomy of speech perception. *Trends in Cognitive Science, 4,* 131–138.

Hickok, G., & Poeppel, D. (2004). Dorsal and ventral streams: a framework for understanding aspects of the functional anatomy of language. *Cognition, 92,* 67–99.

Hilbig, H., Nowack, S., Boeckler, K., Bidmon, H.-J., & Zilles, K. (2007). Characterization of neuronal subsets surrounded by perineuronal nets in the rhesus auditory brainstem. *Journal of Anatomy, 210,* 507–517.

Hind, J. E., Goldberg, J. M., Greenwood, D. D., & Rose, J. E. (1963). Some discharge characteristics of single neurons in the inferior colliculus of the cat. II. Timing of the discharges and observations on binaural stimulation. *Journal of Neurophysiology, 26,* 321–341.

Hopf, P. (1954). Die myeloarchitektonic des isocortex temporalis beim menschen. *Journal of Hirnforsch, 1*, 208-279.

Howard, M. A., 3rd, Volkov, I. O., Abbas, P. J., Damasio, H., Ollendieck, M. C., & Granner, M. A. (1996). A chronic microelectrode investigation of the tonotopic organization of human auditory cortex. *Brain Research, 724*, 260-264.

Howard, M. A., Volkov, I. O., Mirsky, R., Garell, P. C., Noh, M. D., Granner, M., et al. (2000). Auditory cortex on the human posterior superior temporal gyrus. *Journal of Comparative Neurology, 416*, 79-92.

Husain, F. T., & Horwitz, B. (2006). Experimental-neuromodeling framework for understanding auditory object processing: integrating data across multiple scales. *Journal of Physiology, 100*, 133-141.

Hutson, K. A., Glendenning, K. K., & Masterton, R. B. (1991). Acoustic chiasm. IV: Eight midbrain decussations of the auditory system in the cat. *Journal of Comparative Neurology, 312*, 105-131.

Irving, R., & Harrison, J. M. (1967). The superior olivary complex and audition: a comparative study. *Journal of Comparative Neurology, 130*, 77-86.

Jancke, L., & Shah, N. J. (2004). 'Hearing' syllables by 'seeing' visual stimuli. *European Journal of Neuroscience, 19*, 2603-2608.

Jeffress, L. A. (1948). A place theory of sound localization. *Journal of Comparative Physiology and Psychology, 41*, 35-39.

Jones, E. G. (2003). Chemically defined parallel pathways in the monkey auditory system. *Annals of the New York Academy of Sciences, 999*, 218-233.

Jones, E. G. (2007). *The thalamus* (2nd ed., Vol. II). Cambridge, UK: Cambridge University Press.

Jousmaki, V., & Hari, R. (1998). Parchment-skin illusion: Sound-biased touch. *Current Biology, 8*, R190.

Kaas, J. H., & Hackett, T. A. (1998). Subdivisions of auditory cortex and levels of processing in primates. *Audiology and Neuro-Otology, 3*, 73-85.

Kaas, J. H., & Hackett, T. A. (1999). "What" and "where" processing in auditory cortex. *Nature Neuroscience, 2*, 1045-1047.

Kaas, J. H., & Hackett, T. A. (2000). Subdivisions of auditory cortex and processing streams in primates. *Proceedings of the National Academy of Sciences, 97*, 11793-11799.

Kajikawa, Y., de la Mothe, L. A., Blumell, S., & Hackett, T. A. (2005). A comparison of neuron response properties in areas A1 and CM of the marmoset monkey auditory cortex: tones and broad band noise. *Journal of Neurophysiology, 93*, 22-34.

Kayser, C., Petkov, C. I., Augath, M., & Logothetis, N. K. (2005). Integration of touch and sound in auditory cortex. *Neuron, 48*, 373-384.

Kayser, C., Petkov, C. I., Augath, M., & Logothetis, N. K. (2007). Functional imaging reveals visual modulation of specific fields in auditory cortex. *Journal of Neuroscience, 27*, 1824-1835.

Kelly, J. B., & Li, L. (1997). Two sources of inhibition affecting binaural evoked responses in the rat's inferior colliculus: The dorsal nucleus of the lateral lemniscus and the superior olivary complex. *Hearing Research, 104*, 112-126.

King, A. J. (2005). Multisensory integration: Strategies for synchronization. *Current Biology, 15*, R339-R341.

Kitagawa, N., & Spence, C. (2006). Audiotactile multisensory interactions in human information processing. *Japanese Psychological Research, 48*, 158-173.

Krumbholz, K., Schonwiesner, M., von Cramon, D. Y., Rubsamen, R., Shah, N. J., Zilles, K., et al. (2005). Representation of interaural temporal information from left and right auditory space in the human planum temporale and inferior parietal lobe. *Cerebral Cortex, 15*, 317-324.

Kudo, M. (1981). Projections of the nuclei of the lateral lemniscus in the cat: an autoradiographic study. *Brain Research, 221*, 57-69.

Kudo, M., & Niimi, K. (1980). Ascending projections of the inferior colliculus in the cat: an autoradiographic study. *Journal of Comparative Neurology, 191*, 545-556.

Kulesza, J., & Randy J. (2007). Cytoarchitecture of the human superior olivary complex: Medial and lateral superior olive. *Hearing Research*, *225*, 80-90.

Lakatos, P., Chen, C. M., O'Connell M, N., Mills, A., & Schroeder, C. E. (2007). Neuronal oscillations and multisensory interaction in primary auditory cortex. *Neuron*, *53*, 279-292.

Lakatos, P., Pincze, Z., Fu, K. G., Javitt, D. C., Karmos, G., & Schroeder, C. E. (2005). Timing of pure tone and noise-evoked responses in macaque auditory cortex. *NeuroReport*, *16*, 933-937.

Langers, D. R. M., Backes, W. H., & Dijk, P. v. (2003). Spectrotemporal features of the auditory cortex: The activation in response to dynamic ripples. *NeuroImage*, *20*, 265-275.

Langers, D. R. M., Backes, W. H., & van Dijk, P. (2007). Representation of lateralization and tonotopy in primary versus secondary human auditory cortex. *NeuroImage*, *34*, 264-273.

Laurienti, P. J., Burdette, J. H., Wallace, M. T., Yen, Y.-F., Field, A. S., & Stein, B. E. (2002). Deactivation of sensory-specific cortex by cross-modal stimuli. *Journal of Cognitive Neuroscience*, *14*, 420-429.

Lee, C. C., Imaizumi, K., Schreiner, C. E., & Winer, J. A. (2004). Concurrent tonotopic processing streams in auditory cortex. *Cerebral Cortex*, *14*, 441-451.

Lehmann, C., Herdener, M., Esposito, F., Hubl, D., di Salle, F., Scheffler, K., et al. (2006). Differential patterns of multisensory interactions in core and belt areas of human auditory cortex. *NeuroImage*, *31*, 294-300.

Levanen, S., Jousmaki, V., & Hari, R. (1998). Vibration-induced auditory-cortex activation in a congenitally deaf adult. *Current Biology*, *8*, 869-872.

Lockwood, A. H., Salvi, R. J., Coad, M. L., Towsley, M. L., Wack, D. S., & Murphy, B. W. (1998). The functional neuroanatomy of tinnitus: evidence for limbic system links and neural plasticity. *Neurology*, *50*, 114-120.

Love, J. A., & Scott, J. W. (1969). Some response characteristics of cells of the magnocellular division of the medial geniculate body of the cat. *Canadian Journal of Physiology and Pharmacology*, *47*, 881-888.

Maeder, P. P., Meuli, R. A., Adriani, M., Bellmann, A., Fornari, E., Thiran, J. P., et al. (2001). Distinct pathways involved in sound recognition and localization: A human fMRI study. *NeuroImage*, *14*, 802-816.

Malmierca, M. S. (2003). The structure and physiology of the rat auditory system: an overview. *International Review of Neurobiology*, *56*, 147-211.

Malmierca, M. S., Le Beau, F. E., & Rees, A. (1996). The topographical organization of descending projections from the central nucleus of the inferior colliculus in guinea pig. *Hearing Research*, *93*, 167-180.

Malmierca, M. S., Leergaard, T. B., Bajo, V. M., Bjaalie, J. G., & Merchan, M. A. (1998). Anatomic evidence of a three-dimensional mosaic pattern of tonotopic organization in the ventral complex of the lateral lemniscus in cat. *Journal of Neuroscience*, *18*, 10603-10618.

Martuzzi, R., Murray, M. M., Michel, C. M., Thiran, J. P., Maeder, P. P., Clarke, S., et al. (2006). Multisensory Interactions within human primary cortices revealed by BOLD dynamics. *Cerebral Cortex*, *17*, 1672-1679.

McGurk, H., & MacDonald, J. (1976). Hearing lips and seeing voices. *Nature*, *264*, 746-748.

Merchan, M. A., & Berbel, P. (1996). Anatomy of the ventral nucleus of the lateral lemniscus in rats: A nucleus with a concentric laminar organization. *Journal of Comparative Neurology*, *372*, 245-263.

Merchan, M. A., Malmierca, M. S., Bajo, V. M., & Bjaalie, J. G. (1997). The nuclei of the lateral lemniscus, old views and new perspectives. In J. Syka (Ed.), *Acoustical signal processing in the central auditory system* (pp. 211-226). London: Plenum Press.

Merchan, M. A., Saldana, E., & Plaza, I. (1994). Dorsal nucleus of the lateral lemniscus in the rat: concentric organization and tonotopic projection to the inferior colliculus. *Journal of Comparative Neurology*, *342*, 259-278.

Merzenich, M. M., & Reid, M. D. (1974). Representation of the cochlea within the inferior colliculus of the cat. *Brain Research*, *77*, 397-415.

Metzger, R. R., Greene, N. T., Porter, K. K., & Groh, J. M. (2006). Effects of reward and behavioral context on neural activity in the primate inferior colliculus. *Journal of Neuroscience, 26,* 7468-7476.

Meyer, M., Baumann, S., Marchina, S., & Jancke, L. (2007). Hemodynamic responses in human multisensory and auditory association cortex to purely visual stimulation. *BMC Neuroscience, 8,* 14.

Molholm, S., Ritter, W., Murray, M. M., Javitt, D. C., Schroeder, C. E., & Foxe, J. J. (2002). Multisensory auditory-visual interactions during early sensory processing in humans: A high-density electrical mapping study. *Brain Research and Cognitive Brain Research, 14,* 115-128.

Molinari, M., Dell'Anna, M. E., Rausell, E., Leggio, M. G., Hashikawa, T., & Jones, E. G. (1995). Auditory thalamocortical pathways defined in monkeys by calcium-binding protein immunoreactivity. *Journal of Comparative Neurology, 362,* 171-194.

Moore, D. R. (1991). Anatomy and physiology of binaural hearing. *Audiology, 30,* 125-134.

Moore, J. K. (1980). The primate cochlear nuclei: loss of lamination as a phylogenetic process. *Journal of Comparative Neurology, 193,* 609-629.

Moore, J. K. (2000). Organization of the human superior olivary complex. *Microscopy Research and Technique, 51,* 403-412.

Moore, J. K., Guan, Y.-L., & Shi, S.-R. (1998). MAP2 expression in developing dendrites of human brainstem auditory neurons. *Journal of Chemical Neuroanatomy, 16,* 1-15.

Moore, J. K., & Moore, R. Y. (1971). A comparative study of the superior olivary complex in the primate brain. *Folia Primatologica, 16,* 35-51.

Morel, A., Garraghty, P. E., & Kaas, J. H. (1993). Tonotopic organization, architectonic fields, and connections of auditory cortex in macaque monkeys. *Journal of Comparative Neurology, 335,* 437-459.

Morel, A., & Kaas, J. H. (1992). Subdivisions and connections of auditory cortex in owl monkeys. *Journal of Comparative Neurology, 318,* 27-63.

Morest, D. K. (1965). The laminar structure of the medial geniculate body of the cat. *Journal of Anatomy, 99,* 143-160.

Morosan, P., Rademacher, J., Schleicher, A., Amunts, K., Schormann, T., & Zilles, K. (2001). Human primary auditory cortex: Cytoarchitectonic subdivisions and mapping into a spatial reference system. *NeuroImage, 13,* 684-701.

Morosan, P., Schleicher, A., Amunts, K., & Zilles, K. (2005). Multimodal architectonic mapping of human superior temporal gyrus. *Anatomy and Embryology, 210,* 401-406.

Moskowitz, N., & Liu, J. C. (1972). Central projections of the spiral ganglion of the squirrel monkey. *Journal of Comparative Neurology, 144,* 335-344.

Murray, M. M., Molholm, S., Michel, C. M., Heslenfeld, D. J., Ritter, W., Javitt, D. C., et al. (2005). Grabbing your ear: Rapid auditory-somatosensory multisensory interactions in low-level sensory cortices are not constrained by stimulus alignment. *Cerebral Cortex, 15,* 963-974.

Oertel, D., Fay, R., & Popper, A. (2002). *Integrative functions in the mammalian auditory pathway.* New York: Spring-Verlag.

Ojanen, V., Mottonen, R., Pekkola, J., Jaaskelainen, I. P., Joensuu, R., Autti, T., et al. (2005). Processing of audiovisual speech in Broca's area. *NeuroImage, 25,* 333-338.

Oliver, D. L. (2000). Ascending efferent projections of the superior olivary complex. *Microscopy Research and Technique, 51,* 355-363.

Osen, K. K., Mugnaini, E., Dahl, A. L., & Christiansen, A. H. (1984). Histochemical localization of acetylcholinesterase in the cochlear and superior olivary nuclei. A reappraisal with emphasis on the cohlear granule cell system. *Archives of Italian Biology, 122,* 169-212.

Oya, H., Poon, P. W. F., Brugge, J. F., Reale, R. A., Kawasaki, H., Volkov, I. O., et al. (2007). Functional connections between auditory cortical fields in humans revealed by Granger causality analysis of intra-cranial evoked potentials to sounds: Comparison of two methods. *Biosystems., 89,* 198-207.

Patterson, R. D., Uppenkamp, S., Johnsrude, I. S., & Griffiths, T. D. (2002). The processing of temporal pitch and melody information in auditory cortex. *Neuron, 36,* 767-776.

Pavani, F., Macaluso, E., Warren, J. D., Driver, J., & Griffiths, T. D. (2002). A common cortical substrate activated by horizontal and vertical sound movement in the human brain. *Current Biology*, *12*, 1584-1590.

Pekkola, J., Laasonen, M., Ojanen, V., Autti, T., Jaaskelainen, I. P., Kujala, T., et al. (2006). Perception of matching and conflicting audiovisual speech in dyslexic and fluent readers: an fMRI study at 3 T. *NeuroImage*, *29*, 797-807.

Pekkola, J., Ojanen, V., Autti, T., Jääskeläinen, I. P., Möttönen, R., & Sams, M. (2006). Attention to visual speech gestures enhances hemodynamic activity in the left planum temporale. *Human Brain Mapping*, *27*, 471-477.

Pekkola, J., Ojanen, V., Autti, T., Jaaskelainen, I. P., Mottonen, R., Tarkiainen, A., et al. (2005). Primary auditory cortex activation by visual speech: an fMRI study at 3 T. *NeuroReport*, *16*, 125-128.

Petkov, C. I., Kayser, C., Augath, M., & Logothetis, N. K. (2006). Functional imaging reveals numerous fields in the monkey auditory cortex. *PLoS Biology*, *4*, 1-14.

Poljak, S. (1926). The connections of the acoustic nerve. *Journal of Anatomy*, *60*, 465-469.

Pollak, G. D., Burger, R. M., & Klug, A. (2003). Dissecting the circuitry of the auditory system. *Trends in Neuroscience*, *26*, 33-39.

Pollak, G. D., Burger, R. M., Park, T. J., Klug, A., & Bauer, E. E. (2002). Roles of inhibition for transforming binaural properties in the brainstem auditory system. *Hearing Research*, *168*, 60-78.

Polley, D. B., Read, H. L., Storace, D. A., & Merzenich, M. M. (2007). Multiparametric auditory receptive field organization across five cortical fields in the albino rat. *Journal of Neurophysiology*, *97*, 3621-3638.

Popper, A., & Fay, R. (1992). *The mammalian auditory pathway: Neurophysiology*. New York: Springer-Verlag.

Poremba, A., Malloy, M., Saunders, R. C., Carson, R. E., Herscovitch, P., & Mishkin, M. (2004). Species-specific calls evoke asymmetric activity in the monkey's temporal poles. *Nature*, *427*, 448-451.

Rademacher, J., Caviness, V. J., Steinmetz, H., & Galaburda, A. (1993). Topographical variation of the human primary cortices: implications for neuroimaging, brain mapping, and neurobiology. *Cerebral Cortex*, *3*, 313-329.

Rasmussen, G. L. (1946). The olivary peduncle and other fiber connections of the superior olivary complex. *Journal of Comparative Neurology*, *84*, 141-219.

Rasmussen, G. L. (1953). Further observations on the efferent cochlear bundle. *Journal of Comparative Neurology*, *99*, 61-74.

Rauschecker, J. P., & Tian, B. (2000). Mechanisms and streams for processing of "what" and "where" in auditory cortex. *Proceedings of the National Academy of Sciences*, *97*, 11800-11806.

Rauschecker, J. P., & Tian, B. (2004). Processing of band-passed noise in the lateral auditory belt cortex of the rhesus monkey. *Journal of Neurophysiology*, *91*, 2578-2589.

Rauschecker, J. P., Tian, B., & Hauser, M. (1995). Processing of complex sounds in the macaque nonprimary auditory cortex. *Science*, *268*, 111-114.

Rauschecker, J. P., Tian, B., Pons, T., & Mishkin, M. (1997). Serial and parallel processing in rhesus monkey auditory cortex. *Journal of Comparative Neurology*, *382*, 89-103.

Reale, R. A., Calvert, G. A., Thesen, T., Jenison, R. L., Kawasaki, H., Oya, H., et al. (2007). Auditory-visual processing represented in the human superior temporal gyrus. *Neuroscience*, *145*, 162-184.

Recanzone, G. H. (1998). Rapidly induced auditory plasticity: the ventriloquism aftereffect. *Proceedings on the National Academy of Sciences*, *95*, 869-875.

Recanzone, G. H. (2003). Auditory influences on visual temporal rate perception. *Journal of Neurophysiology*, *89*, 1078-1093.

Rinne, T., Pekkola, J., Degerman, A., Autti, T., Jaaskelainen, I. P., Sams, M., et al. (2005). Modulation of auditory cortex activation by sound presentation rate and attention. *Human Brain Mapping*, *26*, 94-99.

Rivier, F., & Clarke, S. (1997). Cytochrome oxidase, acetylcholinesterase, and NADPH-diaphorase staining in human supratemporal and insular cortex: Evidence for multiple auditory areas. *NeuroImage*, *6*, 288-304.

Rockland, K. S., & Ojima, H. (2003). Multisensory convergence in calcarine visual areas in macaque monkey. *International Journal of Psychophysiology, 50*, 19-26.

Romand, R., & Avan, P. (1997). Anatomical and functional aspects of the cochlear nucleus. In G. Ehret & R. Romand (Eds.), *The central auditory system* (pp. 97-191). New York: Oxford Press.

Romanski, L. M., Averbeck, B. B., & Diltz, M. (2005). Neural representation of vocalizations in the primate ventrolateral prefrontal cortex. *Journal of Neurophysiology, 93*, 734-747.

Romanski, L. M., Bates, J. F., & Goldman-Rakic, P. S. (1999). Auditory belt and parabelt projections to the prefrontal cortex in the rhesus monkey. *Journal of Comparative Neurology, 403*, 141-157.

Romanski, L. M., Tian, B., Fritz, J., Mishkin, M., Goldman-Rakic, P. S., & Rauschecker, J. P. (1999). Dual streams of auditory afferents target multiple domains in the primate prefrontal cortex. *Nature Neuroscience, 2*, 1131-1136.

Rouiller, E. (1997). *Functional organization of the auditory pathways*. New York: Oxford Press.

Rouiller, E. M., & de Ribaupierre, F. (1985). Origin of afferents to physiologically defined regions of the medial geniculate body of the cat: Ventral and dorsal divisions. *Hearing Research, 19*, 97-114.

Rouiller, E. M., Simm, G. M., Villa, A. E., de Ribaupierre, Y., & de Ribaupierre, F. (1991). Auditory corticocortical interconnections in the cat: evidence for parallel and hierarchical arrangement of the auditory cortical areas. *Experimental Brain Research, 86*, 483-505.

Rutkowski, R. G., Miasnikov, A. A., & Weinberger, N. M. (2003). Characterisation of multiple physiological fields within the anatomical core of rat auditory cortex. *Hearing Research, 181*, 116-130.

Ryugo, D. K., Pongstaporn, T., Wright, D. D., & Sharp, A. H. (1995). Inositol 1,4,5-trisphosphate receptors: immunocytochemical localization in the dorsal cochlear nucleus. *Journal of Comparative Neurology, 358*, 102-118.

Sams, M., Aulanko, R., Hamalainen, M., Hari, R., Lounasmaa, O. V., Lu, S. T., et al. (1991). Seeing speech: Visual information from lip movements modifies activity in the human auditory cortex. *Neuroscience Letters, 127*, 141-145.

Schnupp, J. (2006). Auditory filters, features, and redundant representations. *Neuron, 51*, 278-280.

Schonwiesner, M., Novitski, N., Pakarinen, S., Carlson, S., Tervaniemi, M., & Naatanen, R. (2007). Heschl's gyrus, posterior superior temporal gyrus, and mid-ventrolateral prefrontal cortex have different roles in the detection of acoustic changes. *Journal of Neurophysiology, 97*, 2075-2082.

Schreiner, C. E., & Langner, G. (1988). Periodicity coding in the inferior colliculus of the cat. II. Topographical organization. *Journal of Neurophysiology, 60*, 1823-1840.

Schroeder, C. E., & Foxe, J. J. (2002). The timing and laminar profile of converging inputs to multisensory areas of the macaque neocortex. *Brain Research and Cognitive Brain Research, 14*, 187-198.

Schroeder, C. E., & Foxe, J. J. (2005). Multisensory contributions to low-level, "unisensory" processing. *Current Opinion in Neurobiology, 15*, 454-458.

Schroeder, C. E., Lakatos, P., Smiley, J., & Hackett, T. A. (2007). How and why is auditory processing shaped by multisensory convergence? In R. F. Burkard, M. Don, & J. J. Eggermont (Eds.), *Auditory evoked potentials: basic principles and clinical application* (pp. 651-670). Baltimore: Lippincott Williams and Wilkins.

Schroeder, C. E., Lindsley, R. W., Specht, C., Marcovici, A., Smiley, J. F., & Javitt, D. C. (2001). Somatosensory input to auditory association cortex in the macaque monkey. *Journal of Neurophysiology, 85*, 1322-1327.

Schurmann, M., Caetano, G., Hlushchuk, Y., Jousmaki, V., & Hari, R. (2006). Touch activates human auditory cortex. *NeuroImage, 30*, 1325-1331.

Schwartz, I. R. (1992). The superior olivary complex and lateral lemniscal nuclei. In D. Webster, A. Popper, & R. Fay (Eds.), *The mammalian auditory pathway: Neuroanatomy* (pp. 117-167). New York: Springer-Verlag.

Scott, S. K. (2005). Auditory processing—speech, space and auditory objects. *Current Opinion in Neurobiology, 15*, 197–201.

Scott, S. K., Blank, C. C., Rosen, S., & Wise, R. J. (2000). Identification of a pathway for intelligible speech in the left temporal lobe. *Brain, 123*, 2400–2406.

Scott, S. K., & Johnsrude, I. S. (2003). The neuroanatomical and functional organization of speech perception. *Trends in Neuroscience, 26*, 100–107.

Seifritz, E., Di Salle, F., Esposito, F., Herdener, M., Neuhoff, J. G., & Scheffler, K. (2006). Enhancing BOLD response in the auditory system by neurophysiologically tuned fMRI sequence. *NeuroImage, 29*, 1013–1022.

Seifritz, E., Esposito, F., Hennel, F., Mustovic, H., Neuhoff, J. G., Bilecen, D., et al. (2002). Spatiotemporal pattern of neural processing in the human auditory cortex. *Science, 297*, 1706–1708.

Senkowski, D., Molholm, S., Gomez-Ramirez, M., & Foxe, J. J. (2006). Oscillatory beta activity predicts response speed during a multisensory audiovisual reaction time task: A high-density electrical mapping study. *Cerebral Cortex, 16*, 1556–1565.

Serviere, J., Webster, W. R., & Calford, M. B. (1984). Isofrequency labelling revealed by a combined [14C]-2-deoxyglucose, electrophysiological, and horseradish peroxidase study of the inferior colliculus of the cat. *Journal of Comparative Neurology, 228*, 463–477.

Sherman, G. F., & Guillery, R. W. (2001). *Exploring the thalamus*. San Diego, CA: Academic Press.

Shneiderman, A., Oliver, D. L., & Henkel, C. K. (1988). Connections of the dorsal nucleus of the lateral lemniscus: an inhibitory parallel pathway in the ascending auditory system? *Journal of Comparative Neurology, 276*, 188–208.

Smith, P. H., Joris, P. X., & Yin, T. C. (1993). Projections of physiologically characterized spherical bushy cell axons from the cochlear nucleus of the cat: Evidence for delay lines to the medial superior olive. *Journal of Comparative Neurology, 331*, 245–260.

Soto-Faraco, S., Kingstone, A., & Spence, C. (2003). Multisensory contributions to the perception of motion. *Neuropsychologia, 41*, 1847–1862.

Spatz, W. B. (1999). Unipolar brush cells in the cochlear nuclei of a primate (Callithrix jacchus). *Neuroscience Letters, 270*, 141–144.

Spence, C., & Squire, S. (2003). Multisensory integration: maintaining the perception of synchrony. *Current Biology, 13*, R519–R521.

Spence, C., & Zampini, M. (2006). Auditory contributions to multisensory product perception. *Acta Acustica, 92*, 1–17.

Sterbing, S. J., Hartung, K., & Hoffmann, K.-P. (2003). Spatial tuning to virtual sounds in the inferior colliculus of the guinea pig. *Journal of Neurophysiology, 90*, 2648–2659.

Stiebler, I. (1986). Tone-threshold mapping in the inferior colliculus of the house mouse. *Neuroscience Letters, 65*, 336–340.

Strominger, N. L. (1973). The origins, course and distribution of the dorsal and intermediate acoustic striae in the rhesus monkey. *Journal of Comparative Neurology, 147*, 209–233.

Strominger, N. L., Nelson, L. R., & Dougherty, W. J. (1977). Second order auditory pathways in the chimpanzee. *Journal of Comparative Neurology, 172*, 349–366.

Strominger, N. L., & Strominger, A. I. (1971). Ascending brainstem projections of the anteroventral cochlear nucleus in the rhesus monkey. *Journal of Comparative Neurology, 252*, 353–365.

Sutton, D., Hathaway, O. Y., Seib, T., & Spelman, F. A. (1991). Macaque anteroventral cochlear nucleus: developmental anatomy. *Developmental Brain Research, 58*, 59–65.

Sweet, R. A., Dorph-Petersen, K. A., & Lewis, D. A. (2005). Mapping auditory core, lateral belt, and parabelt cortices in the human superior temporal gyrus. *Journal of Comparative Neurology, 491*, 270–289.

Talavage, T. M., Ledden, P. J., Benson, R. R., Rosen, B. R., & Melcher, J. R. (2000). Frequency-dependent responses exhibited by multiple regions in human auditory cortex. *Hearing Research, 150*, 225–244.

Talavage, T. M., Sereno, M. I., Melcher, J. R., Ledden, P. J., Rosen, B. R., & Dale, A. M. (2004). Tonotopic organization in human auditory cortex revealed by progressions of frequency sensitivity. *Journal of Neurophysiology, 91,* 1282–1296.

Thompson, A. M., & Schofield, B. R. (2000). Afferent projections of the superior olivary complex. *Microscopy Research and Technique, 51,* 330–354.

Tian, B., Reser, D., Durham, A., Kustov, A., & Rauschecker, J. P. (2001). Functional specialization in rhesus monkey auditory cortex. *Science, 292,* 290–293.

Tollin, D. J. (2003). The lateral superior olive: A functional role in sound source localization. *Neuroscientist, 9,* 127–143.

Tramo, M. J., Cariani, P. A., Koh, C. K., Makris, N., & Braida, L. D. (2005). Neurophysiology and neuroanatomy of pitch perception: auditory cortex. *Annals of the New York Academy of Sciences, 1060,* 148–174.

Uppenkamp, S., Johnsrude, I. S., Norris, D., Marslen-Wilson, W., & Patterson, R. D. (2006). Locating the initial stages of speech-sound processing in human temporal cortex. *Neuro-Image, 31,* 1284–1296.

Vogt, C., & Vogt, O. (1919). Allgemeinere Ergebnisse unserer Hirnforschung. *Journal of Psychological Neurology, 24,* 279–462.

von Economo, C., & Horn, L. (1930). Uber Windungsrelief, Masse und Rindenarchitektonik der Supratemporalflache, ihre individuellen und ihre Seitenunterschiede. *Zeitschrift fur die gesamte Neurologic Psychiatrie, 130,* 678–757.

von Economo, C., & Koskinas, G. (1925). *Die Cytoarchitectonik der Hirnrinde des erwachsenen menschen.* Berlin: Julius-Springer.

Wada, Y., Kitagawa, N., & Noguchi, K. (2003). Audio-visual integration in temporal perception. *International Journal of Psychophysiology, 50,* 117–124.

Wallace, M. N., Johnston, P. W., & Palmer, A. R. (2002). Histochemical identification of cortical areas in the auditory region of the human brain. *Experimental Brain Research, 143,* 499–508.

Warren, J. D., Zielinski, B.A., Green, G., Rauschecker, J. P., & Griffiths, T. D. (2002). Perception of sound source motion by the human brain. *Neuron, 34,* 139–148.

Warren, J. D., & Griffiths, T. D. (2003). Distinct mechanisms for processing spatial sequences and pitch sequences in the human auditory brain. *Journal of Neuroscience, 23,* 5799–5804.

Warren, J. E., Wise, R. J. S., & Warren, J. D. (2005). Sounds do-able: auditory-motor transformations and the posterior temporal plane. *Trends in Neurosciences, 28,* 636–643.

Webster, W. R., Serviere, J., Crewther, D., & Crewther, S. (1984). Iso-frequency 2–DG contours in the inferior colliculus of the awake monkey. *Experimental Brain Research, 56,* 425–437.

Welch, R. B., DuttonHurt, L. D., & Warren, D. H. (1986). Contributions of audition and vision to temporal rate perception. *Perception and Psychophysics, 39,* 294–300.

Wepsic, J. G. (1966). Multimodal sensory activation of cells in the magnocellular medial geniculate nucleus. *Experimental Neurology, 15,* 299–318.

Wessinger, C. M., VanMeter, J., Tian, B., Van Lare, J., Pekar, J., & Rauschecker, J. P. (2001). Hierarchical organization of the human auditory cortex revealed by functional magnetic resonance imaging. *Journal of Cognitive Neuroscience, 13,* 1–7.

Winer, J. A. (1984). The human medial geniculate body. *Hearing Research, 15,* 225–247.

Winer, J. A. (1985). The medial geniculate body of the cat. *Advanced Anatomy and Embryology Cell Biology, 86,* 1–97.

Winer, J. A. (2005). Decoding the auditory corticofugal systems. *Hearing Research, 207,* 1–9.

Winer, J. A., Chernock, M. L., Larue, D. T., & Cheung, S. W. (2002). Descending projections to the inferior colliculus from the posterior thalamus and the auditory cortex in rat, cat, and monkey. *Hearing Research, 168,* 181–195.

Winer, J. A., Kelly, J. B., & Larue, D. T. (1999). Neural architecture of the rat medial geniculate body. *Hearing Reseach, 130,* 19–41.

Winer, J. A., & Lee, C. C. (2007). The distributed auditory cortex. *Hearing Research, 229,* 3–13.

Winer, J. A., Miller, L. M., Lee, C. C., & Schreiner, C. E. (2005). Auditory thalamocortical transformation: structure and function. *Trends in Neuroscience, 28,* 255–263.

Wise, R. J., Scott, S. K., Blank, S. C., Mummery, C. J., Murphy, K., & Warburton, E. A. (2001). Separate neural subsystems within "Wernicke's area." *Brain, 124*, 83–95.

Woods, T. M., Lopez, S. E., Long, J. H., Rahman, J. E., & Recanzone, G. H. (2006). Effects of stimulus azimuth and intensity on the single-neuron activity in the auditory cortex of the alert macaque monkey. *Journal of Neurophysiology, 96*, 3323–3337.

Woolsey, C. N., & Walzl, E. M. (1982). Cortical auditory area of Macaca mulatta and its relation to the second somatic sensory area (Sm II). In C. N. Woolsey (Ed.), *Cortical sensory organization multiple auditory areas* (pp. 231–256). Cliffton, NJ: Humana.

Yetkin, F. Z., Roland, P. S., Christensen, W. F., & Purdy, P. D. (2004). Silent functional magnetic resonance imaging (fMRI) of tonotopicity and stimulus intensity coding in human primary auditory cortex. *Laryngoscope, 114*, 512–518.

Zampini, M., Torresan, D., Spence, C., & Murray, M. M. (2007). Auditory-somatosensory multisensory interactions in front and rear space. *Neuropsychologia. 45*, 1869–1877.

Zatorre, R. J. (2007). There's more to auditory cortex than meets the ear. *Hearing Research, 229*, 24–30.

Zatorre, R. J., & Belin, P. (2001). Spectral and temporal processing in human auditory cortex. *Cerebral Cortex, 11*, 946–953.

Zatorre, R. J., Bouffard, M., Ahad, P., & Belin, P. (2002). Where is 'where' in the human auditory cortex? *Nature Neuroscience, 5*, 905–909.

Zwiers, M. P., Versnel, H., & Van Opstal, A. J. (2004). Involvement of monkey inferior colliculus in spatial hearing. *Journal of Neuroscience, 24*, 4145–4156.

CHAPTER 3

Speech and Auditory Processing in the Cortex: Evidence from Functional Neuroimaging

FRANK EISNER AND SOPHIE K. SCOTT

Introduction

Much of the current discussion on central auditory processing disorder (CAPD) revolves around the question of which aspects of the auditory perceptual system are affected, and to what extent there is interaction of these systems with other cognitive domains. In this chapter, we outline a neuroanatomic framework for this discussion by drawing on evidence from functional neuroimaging in humans.

Recent advances in imaging methodology have made it possible to extend investigations on the functional anatomy of the auditory system from nonhuman primates to humans. We focus mostly on imaging techniques that measure cortical blood flow to allow for a relatively precise localization of the underlying neural activity. The most widely used techniques for anatomic in vivo brain imaging in human subjects are positron emission tomography (PET) and functional magnetic resonance imaging (fMRI). Both of these methods take advantage of the fact that an increase in synaptic activity in a given part of the brain is accompanied by an increase in demand for oxygen, which, in turn, triggers an increase in local blood supply. PET and fMRI are capable of tracing the concentration of oxygenated blood over space and time under different experimental conditions. Because of this capability, they have proven to be extremely useful in the investigation of structure–function relationships in the brain.

CAPD is described as a deficit in speech perception, or sometimes auditory perception in general (Moore, 2006). It can be clinically delineated from other conditions that may exhibit similar symptoms, such as specific language disorder, autism spectrum disorder, attention deficit hyperactivity disorder, or hearing impairment. Part of the recent debate on defining CAPD concerns whether the disorder should be defined as modality-specific, that is, whether it should only be diagnosed in the absence of a deficit in other perceptual domains (Cacace & McFarland, 2005; Rosen, 2005). Our aim in this chapter is not to contribute to a definition of CAPD, but to provide a functional neuroanatomic context in which patterns of deficits can be further investigated and classified. We argue that there is clear evidence from neuroimaging for functional hierarchies in the cortical processing of sound, which are particularly striking in the speech perception system. From what is now known about structure–function relationships in auditory processing, it is hoped that more specific predictions can be generated regarding the cortical localization of deficits in CAPD.

A Hierarchical Functional Architecture of Speech Processing

Deriving meaning from spoken utterances requires the evaluation of basic acoustic cues in the speech signal. These cues are used to access relatively stable, stored representational units of linguistic meaning such as syllables or words. The process of getting from the acoustics to word recognition takes place most of the time without any conscious effort by the listener, which may indicate that the human perceptual system engages highly specialized processes to handle numerous sources of variability and noise in the signal.

Many current psycholinguistic models of spoken word recognition include a pre-lexical level of processing where the speech signal is mapped onto abstract phonetic categories, which in turn pass their activation on to a lexical level of processing (Gaskell & Marslen-Wilson, 1997; McClelland & Elman, 1986; Norris, 1994; Stevens, 2002). Furthermore, models of speech comprehension often are hierarchically organized: Increasingly abstract information flows from early acoustic analysis and prelexical mapping to some kind of perceptual unit (e.g., phonemes, features, diphones), from there to a lexical level of processing, and finally to higher order syntactic and semantic analysis (McQueen, 2005). This view from cognitive psychology has been supported by several recent functional neuroimaging studies which have presented evidence for a hierarchical organization in the neural systems that are engaged in the processing of spoken language (Davis & Johnsrude, 2003; Kaas & Hackett, 1999; Rauschecker, 1998; Scott & Johnsrude, 2003; Wise et al., 2001).

Cortical processing of a sound starts at the primary auditory cortex (PAC), which occupies roughly the medial two-thirds of the transverse temporal gyri, and receives projections primarily from subcortical, ascending auditory pathways. Secondary auditory cortex expands lateral, anterior, and posterior to PAC, and, in humans, comprises the superior temporal gyrus and the superior temporal sulcus, insular cortex, and the planum temporale (Color Plate 3–1; Kaas, Hackett, & Tramo, 1999; Kaas & Hackett, 2000; Rauschecker, 1998; Rauschecker & Tian, 2000). More distant and multimodal regions, including the inferior frontal gyrus, supramarginal gyrus, middle temporal gyrus, and the precentral gyrus, also are frequently seen to be involved in the processing of speech in functional imaging studies. Regions more removed from PAC are often activated in experiments involving higher level language processing (such as lexical, syntactic, and semantic integration), and include the inferior frontal and inferior temporal gyri as well as the anterior superior temporal sulcus (Color Plate 3–2; Davis & Johnsrude, 2003; Hagoort, Hald, Bastiaansen, & Petersson, 2004; Rodd, Davis, & Johnsrude, 2005; Scott, Blank, Rosen, & Wise, 2000; Sharp, Scott, & Wise, 2003). Functional imaging experiments that employ active tasks (e.g., tasks that require metalinguistic judgments and behavioral responses) often find activation in brain regions that typically are not considered to be receptive language areas (Hickok & Poeppel, 2000; Norris & Wise, 2000; Zatorre, 1997).

Although auditory information passes through multiple processing stages in the subcortical auditory pathways and the core regions of PAC (Eggermont, 2001), it is unlikely that any speech-specific processing occurs in these systems. Functional imaging studies have shown that core regions of the auditory cortex are tonotopically organized (Engelien et al., 2002; Formisano et al., 2003; Yang et al., 2000) and respond to pure tones and complex sounds alike. The surrounding cortex, in contrast, is selective for sounds with a more complex spectrotemporal structure. Integration of input from the core areas therefore may take place in these secondary auditory areas (Wessinger et al., 2001). Speech-specific responses begin to emerge on the superior temporal gyrus both anteriorly and posteriorly to primary auditory areas. Selective activations for speech in the superior temporal cortex are often left-lateralized in adults (Binder et al., 1997, 2000; Narain et al., 2003; Scott et al., 2000; Wise et al., 1991) and infants (Dehaene-Lambertz, Dehaene, & Hertz-Pannier, 2002; Dehaene-Lambertz et al., 2006; Peña et al., 2003).

In the following sections, we discuss the hierarchical organization of auditory processing in more detail. We begin by reviewing studies that have investigated the perception of simple acoustic cues in the ascending auditory pathway. We then turn to prelexical and lexical processing of speech, and conclude with a brief discussion of other cognitive systems that interact with audition and speech comprehension.

Temporal Dynamics: Effects of Rate

Increasing the rate of distinct acoustic events can cause those events to be perceived as a single auditory object or "stream." In a typical demonstration of this phenomenon, the interstimulus interval (ISI) between noise bursts is shortened until, at a certain point, one continuous buzzing sound is perceived. Harms and colleagues have investigated where in the auditory pathway this type of perceptual integration occurs (Harms & Melcher, 2002). Using fMRI, it could be shown that there is a systematic progression from midbrain to thalamus to auditory cortex in the characteristic shape and amplitude of the hemodynamic response while listening to trains of noise bursts with varying ISIs (1, 2, 10, 20, or 35 bursts per second). Increasing the rate of acoustic events had a strong effect on amplitude in the inferior colliculus, a moderate effect in the medial geniculate body, and a weak effect in auditory cortex. Interestingly, the shape of the hemodynamic response also changed as a function of increased rate along this pathway. The auditory cortex showed a phasic response at shorter ISIs, such that there were distinct peaks after onset and offset of the train of noise bursts. The inferior colliculus showed a sustained response at all ISIs, and in the thalamus there was a moderate peak only after onset at short ISIs.

These results suggest that the perceptual integration of auditory stimuli emerges at the level of the thalamus and is stable at the level of the auditory cortex. In a further investigation, Harms, Guinan, Sigalovsky, and Melcher (2005) found that amplitude envelope is the primary acoustic cue that elicits a phasic response at cortical levels (as compared to frequency spectrum or overall intensity).

Temporal Dynamics: Amplitude and Frequency Modulation

Amplitude modulation (AM) has been shown to be critically important for speech perception, especially at lower rates (approximately relating to syllable duration). Giraud, Lorenzi and colleagues (2000) investigated the neural processing of AM across a range of AM rates (from 4-256 Hz) using fMRI. This study showed responses to AM in the ascending auditory pathway (brainstem, inferior colliculus, medial geniculate body) and cortex (Heschl's gyrus [HG], superior temporal gyrus [STG], superior temporal sulcus [STS], and inferior parietal lobe). All AM rates showed similar brain responses, though the responses were stronger to the low (4-16 Hz) rates. Although there were peaks in HG (regions corresponding to primary auditory cortex (PAC), there were greater responses in STG and STS. The greatest responses were in STS, and all the responses were bilateral. As in the Harms and Melcher (2002) study, this study also revealed a difference in the shape of the neural response to the different rates, with slow AM rates showing a sustained response and fast AM rates showing a transient response. The results of this study are again consistent with a hierarchical response to sound structure in the auditory cortex. Although there was no cortical selectivity for specific AM rates, the peak responses were stronger to low AM rates, and all responses were greater in auditory association cortex (STS and STG) than in PAC.

Frequency modulation was investigated in a study by Hall, Johnsrude, and colleagues (2002). Contrasting a modulated with an unmodulated signal revealed responses in HG, areas lateral to HG on the supratemporal plane, and the STG and STS bilaterally. A direct comparison of AM and FM (Hart et al., 2003) indicated that both modulation types lead to overlapping auditory responses when compared to unmodulated signals. Of course, frequency modulation entails AM modulation, but this heterogeneous response might also reflect a more basic property of auditory processing, where properties of sounds are not processed in discrete auditory areas (Brechmann & Scheich, 2005; Eggermont, 1998).

Spectral modulation has been studied by Thivard and colleagues. By contrasting fast and slow spectrally changing sounds with unchanging stimuli, selective responses to spectral change were seen in peaks lateral and anterior to PAC in both the left and right superior temporal gyrus (Thivard et al., 2000).

Prelexical Processing of Speech

Consistent with the view of a hierarchical organization of cortical auditory systems, evidence for prelexical processing in brain activation studies often is found in regions that lie anterior and lateral to PAC in the superior temporal gyrus and superior temporal sulcus (Indefrey & Cutler, 2004; Scott & Wise, 2004). Magnetoencephalography studies have shown that, in this region, different phonemes elicit discernible patterns in source localization and latency in the N100m component (Obleser, Elbert, Lahiri,

& Eulitz, 2003; Obleser, Lahiri, & Eulitz, 2004). Studies that have attempted to map activations to natural speech sounds with fMRI or PET have typically used acoustically based subtraction designs (e.g., speech vs. Gaussian noise, speech vs. pure tones; Jäncke, Wüstenberg, Scheich, & Heinze, 2002). The conclusions that can be drawn from these types of baseline comparison are limited as they are confounded along other dimensions, such as acoustic complexity, and therefore often cannot differentiate between simple acoustic, and speech-specialized processing (Norris & Wise, 2000; Scott & Wise, 2004). This problem has been approached by designing baseline stimuli that are acoustically similar to speech in terms of spectrotemporal complexity, are based on natural speech, and yet are not intelligible utterances. When the acoustic complexity of speech is controlled for in the baseline condition, regions in the anterior and posterior superior temporal sulcus have been demonstrated to selectively respond to intelligible speech (Narain et al., 2003; Scott et al., 2000). These studies used a conjunction design (Price & Friston, 1997), where brain regions that responded to both speech and noise vocoded speech (over spectrally rotated equivalents) were identified.

Other experimental designs address this problem by avoiding a "static" acoustic baseline subtraction design altogether and instead hold the acoustic signal constant while inducing a change in the phonemic percept. Dehaene-Lambertz et al. (2005) used fMRI to measure cortical activity elicited by sine-wave analogues of spoken syllables-sounds with extremely reduced spectral detail (see Remez, Fellowes, & Rubin, 1997). Their study took advantage of the phenomenon that sine-wave replicas are spectrally so impoverished that they are not perceived as speech by naïve listeners, but can be understood when listeners are told to switch to a "speech mode." Perceiving the sine-wave replicas as speech compared to perceiving the same sounds as nonspeech produced a left-lateralized activation of the posterior superior temporal gyrus, and the left supramarginal gyrus showed differential activity for different types of speech sounds when listening in "speech mode." Using sine-wave analogues of spoken words, Liebenthal, Binder, Piorkowski, and Remez (2003) found a similar, differential fMRI response slightly more ventrally in the left anterolateral transverse temporal gyrus and in the superior temporal gyrus.

Several studies have attempted to pin down phonological processes against early, nonspecific acoustic analysis by using training paradigms. The rationale in these experiments is that inducing a change along a dimension of interest will show a corresponding change in the fMRI signal relative to a control condition. For example, an initially nonphonemic acoustic pattern, such as an unfamiliar speech sound, can become a perceptual unit after listeners have learned to recognize this sound as belonging to a novel phonemic category. Golestani and Zatorre (2004) trained native English monolingual listeners on a nonnative place contrast (retroflex vs. alveolar stops). They found that only after training did the nonnative sounds elicit similar activations to native sounds in areas including both left and right superior temporal gyri, the right middle frontal gyrus and frontal operculum, and the left caudate. Another study addressing acquisition of a nonnative phoneme contrast (the [r]/[l] distinction in Japanese listeners; Callan, Tajima, Callan, Kubo, & Akahane-Yamada, 2003), in contrast, found activation of extensive cortical networks to be associated with increased discrimination performance after training. Both the native and nonnative contrasts activated superior temporal cortex, but the trained nonnative sounds additionally activated frontal, prefrontal, and subcortical areas.

Native-language phonological processing has been investigated with fMRI in an elegant study by Jacquemot, Pallier, LeBihan, Dehaene, and Dupoux (2003). Instead of a relatively short-term training procedure, this study examined phonotactics, that is, phonological restrictions that are learned as a result of long-term experience (on the order of years) with a native language. A crossed design was used, with two language groups (French and Japanese) and two phonological contrasts: presence or absence of an epenthetic vowel in a consonant cluster (CVC vs. CC), which is phonologically distinctive in French but illegal in Japanese; and presence of a long vowel (CV:C) versus a short vowel (CVC), which is a phonological contrast in Japanese but not in French. For Japanese listeners, a CVC sequence is difficult to discriminate from a CC sequence, where they tend to perceive an epenthetic vowel that is not physically there; French listeners, in contrast, find it diffcult to distinguish the long and short vowels (Dupoux, Kakehi, Hirose, Pallier, & Mehler, 1999). Listeners performed an AAX discrimination task in the scanner. The critical comparison was between trials where a "different" final item constituted a phonological change (i.e., epenthetic vowel for the French, vowel length for the Japanese listeners) and trials where the difference was acoustical (i.e., vowel length for the French, epenthetic vowel for the Japanese; note that the comparison therefore is based on physically identical stimuli). Jacquemot et al. found increased activity for phonological change relative to acoustic change in the left superior temporal and supramarginal gyri, and no activation for the reverse comparison.

Verbal Working Memory

Auditory cortex posterior and medial to primary auditory cortex has been shown to be sensitive to the articulation of speech, regardless to whether the speech is spoken or silently mouthed (Hickok et al., 2000; Wise et al., 2001). This has been proposed to form a sensorimotor link between speech production and speech perception (Scott & Johnsrude, 2003), which may be mediated by the possibilities of "feasible" articulations (Warren, Wise, & Warren, 2005). Apart from the known importance of speech production and perception links in language development, there is an important role for articulation in verbal aspects of short-term memory (Jacquemot & Scott, 2006). Left posterior auditory cortical fields have been activated in verbal and musical rehearsal tasks, with time courses of activation consistent with a role in working memory (Buchsbaum, Hickok, & Humphries, 2001; Hickok, Buchsbaum, Humphries, & Muftuler, 2003). The left posterior superior temporal gyrus has been implicated in both repetition (Wise et al., 2001) and a buffering role in speech perception (Scott et al., 2006). The supramarginal gyrus also has been specifically linked to the articulatory loop in working memory tasks. Verbal working memory thus may rely on a network of areas connecting temporal lobe areas with parietal and prefrontal networks (Jacquemot & Scott, 2006).

Attentional Influences on Speech Comprehension

The role of attention in the perception of speech and sound has been studied using a variety of techniques. Studies in which stimuli were held constant, but the task was altered, have demonstrated that task-dependent patterns of activation can be seen to identical stimuli. This variation in activation must mean that attentional processing is driving the results, rather than purely bottom-up perceptual processing of the stimuli. For example, variation in auditory processing has been demonstrated by asking subjects to attend to frequency modulated tones, and asking them to attend to the direction of modulation (rising vs. falling) or the duration (short vs. long; Brechmann & Scheich, 2005). As well as demonstrating the heterogeneity of neural responses in early auditory cortex, this study also reveals that attentional modulation can affect responses in early auditory areas. As in vision, therefore, the responses in early auditory cortex can be influenced strongly by attentional, task-dependent properties.

A different form of attentional modulation has been studied in speech perception, by looking at the neural correlates of varying the attentional demands of speech perception. Specifically, the extent to which the pattern of neural activation changes when speech is presented in different levels of a masking sound, and in different kinds of masking stimulus—energetic versus informational—was investigated (Scott et al., 2004). In this study, subjects were to listen to a female speaker throughout all the trials. In all conditions, there was also a masking stimulus to be ignored by the subjects: this was either continuous speech-weighted noise (for energetic masking) or a male speaker (for informational masking). These maskers were presented at four different SNR levels, equated for intelligibility across the two conditions as far as possible (as informational masking produces less masking than energetic). This study revealed that an area in left ventral prefrontal cortex varied in activity with the level of the energetic masker—as the masker was louder, this area was more activated. As predicted from behavioral studies, there were no areas specifically sensitive to the level of the informational masker (Brungart, 2001). There were, however, extensive areas in bilateral superior temporal lobe regions that were activated by the masking speaker, regardless of the level at which it was presented. This we took to represent processing of the unattended masking male speaker—processing which we suggest underlies phenomena like the cocktail party effect, where unattended auditory stimuli are processed perceptually to some degree (Cherry, 1953). A recent study by Zatorre, Bouffard, and Belin (2004) showed a similar effect in right STG by varying the number of auditory sources of sound. This suggests that more than one coherent stream of speech can be represented and processed in the left and right dorsolateral temporal lobes, and that attentional selection (or "streaming") may operate in these regions. In contrast, there were level-independent responses to the energetic masker in prefrontal and parietal areas that have been commonly seen in nonauditory and nonlinguistic attentional tasks. We interpret this to mean that when speech is hard to perceive due to competition at the auditory periphery, domain general attentional resources are recruited to help comprehension.

Conclusions

In the human brain, both hierarchical and parallel processing of sound can be seen. Neural responses to structure in sound are seen in regions lateral to primary auditory cortex, in an apparently heterogeneous fashion—the responses lateral to PAC can be driven by different kinds of modulation in the sound, and may also be influenced by task instructions. Regions lateral and anterior to PAC, in the STG and STS are broadly associated with prelexical and phonological processing of speech, and regions posterior to PAC are associated with sensorimotor links, repetition, and aspects of verbal working memory. Attentional modulation can be identified in early auditory cortex, and there is some evidence that multiple streams of auditory objects, including speech from different speakers, are represented in the STG. Contextual influences on speech perception are mediated by areas beyond the dorsolateral temporal lobes, in the left inferior and medial frontal lobe and parietal lobe, consistent with aspects of semantic and syntactic processing. In this discussion we wish to highlight some issues arising from this review that may be of particular relevance to approaches to CAPD.

Speech-Specific Processing?

When speech is contrasted with an acoustically matched baseline, responses are seen in the left STS (Narain et al., 2004; Scott et al., 2000). A parametric approach also has identified that in the STG, responses are seen not only to intelligible speech, but also to acoustic structure, whereas beyond STG, in the STS, and frontal cortex, responses are purely sensitive to the intelligibility of the speech, and not to the acoustic detail (Davis & Johnsrude, 2003, Scott et al., 2006). Does this mean that we can link speech-specific processing to STS? It may be harder to distinguish acoustic from speech related processing than this might suggest. In Scott et al. (2006), the number of channels in noise-vocoded speech were manipulated parametrically. This revealed (along with STS and temporal pole activation) a region in lateral STG, lying lateral and anterior to PAC, which responded to increasing channels of noise-vocoded speech. Importantly, this peak lies within the area of lateral STG that also responds to AM and FM changes, perhaps consistent with the role of amplitude modulation in noise vocoding. This response was also reduced for increasing channels of rotated noise-vocoded speech, suggesting that the response is being driven by lexical as well as acoustic factors. This peak is also very close to the STG peak identified by Jacquemot et al. (2003) as sensitive to language specific phonological information. Thus, this lateral STG area may represent a specific tuning of modulation or structure processing for the structure of speech. It may also represent an "entry point" for top-down modulation of the incoming speech signal, once the system has identified that linguistic information is present. This can be disambiguated by further work, but for the present it is worth noting that speech-related processing may occur early in the auditory cortex (though not in PAC) and that it may well overlap with more basic auditory processing. The difference may be one of degree rather than kind, as responses to lexical information tend to be greater than responses to purely acoustic stimulation. It is also worth noting that whereas STS shows a response that is specific to intelligible speech (from consonant vowel combinations, to words and sentences,) it is also sensitive to nonverbal cues such as gesture, eye gaze, and facial movements. Perhaps techniques with finer spatial resolutions will be able to distinguish these apparently grossly heterogeneous responses.

Auditory Cortex

Functional imaging studies have successfully established that, unlike the predictions of some earlier theorists, speech is not processed "differently" from its earliest encoded entry into the cortex. Instead, speech-specific processing seems to increase with distance from primary auditory cortex. Indeed, it has not been simple to establish the exact role of auditory cortex; for example, ablating auditory cortex does not result in cortical deafness, but is does affect how properties of that sound can be heard. In electrophysiologic work, its has been shown that the response in primary auditory cortex is very plastic and context dependent (Ulanovsky, Las, & Nelken, 2003), suggesting that rather than extracting veridical properties of a sound, PAC represents an auditory object whose invariant characteristics are processed in lateral STG. Such a representation would be dependent on both information from the ascending auditory pathways as well as from top-down modulations. As noted earlier, the responses to cells that do extract more invariant properties of a sound tend to show a heterogeneous response. Developing our understanding of the responses and properties of these areas will help us to understand the potential consequences of, for example, poorly coordinated or incoherent signals entering auditory cortex from the ascending auditory pathway.

"Top-Down" Modulation and Integration

At several points in this review we have seen examples of how nonperceptual systems interact with the processing of speech and sound, in terms of attention, in terms of difficulty, and in the integration with linguistic information. These tend to be associated with activation of brain areas outwith the temporal lobe, either in typically linguistic areas in the angular gyrus, inferior frontal gyrus, areas associated with semantic processing in the medial frontal cortex, or areas associated with nonlinguistic, "executive," attentional processing in the dorsal frontal lobe, frontal pole, and right parietal cortex. This likely reflects the recruitment of "top-down" knowledge for interaction with the incoming perceptual system, either in a relatively "automatic" way (e.g., the influence of predictability on speech intelligibility; Obleser, Wise, Dresner, & Scott, 2007) or deliberate, controlled fashion (e.g., paying attention to speech embedded in noise, although it is hard to hear).

Final Remarks

The rapid progress of in vivo brain imaging techniques in the last 10 years has opened many new possibilities for the investigation of structure–function relationships in the auditory system. Even though the methodology is constantly being developed further, it has now become possible to look for consistent patterns of results in meta-analyses across different imaging studies (Indefrey & Cutler, 2004; Scott & Johnsrude, 2003). It is hoped that the functional neuroimaging approach will move on from simple structure–function mapping and ultimately inform our thinking about the cognitive architecture of auditory and speech perception. We suggest that there are promising first results in this area, and especially so in the interaction of the auditory system with other cognitive domains. These still are early days for our understanding of the "normal" cortical processing of speech, and even though it may be too early to generate very specific hypotheses in the investigation of CAPD, such investigations nonetheless can now be put into the context of a neuroanatomic, functional hierarchy in the speech perception system.

References

Binder, J. R., Frost, J. A., Hammeke, T. A., Bellgowan, P. S. F., Springer, J. A., Kaufman, J. N., et al. (2000). Human temporal lobe activation by speech and nonspeech sounds. *Cerebral Cortex, 10,* 512–528.

Binder, J. R., Frost, J. A., Hammeke, T. A., Cox, R. W., Rao, S. M., & Prieto, T. (1997). Human brain language areas identified by functional magnetic resonance imaging. *Journal of Neuroscience, 17,* 353–362.

Brechmann, A. & Scheich, H. (2005). Hemispheric shifts of sound representation in auditory cortex with conceptual listening. *Cerebral Cortex, 15,* 578–587.

Brungart, D. S. (2001). Informational and energetic masking effect in the perception of two simultaneous talkers. *Journal of the Acoustical Society of America, 109,* 1101–1109.

Buchsbaum, B. R., Hickok, G., & Humphries, C. (2001). Role of left temporal gyrus in phonological processing for speech perception and production. *Cognitive Science, 25,* 663–678.

Cacace, A. T., & McFarland, D. J. (2005). The importance of modality specificity in diagnosing central auditory processing disorder. *American Journal of Audiology, 14,* 112–123.

Callan, D. E., Tajima, K., Callan, A. M., Kubo, S., R Masaki, & Akahane-Yamada, R. (2003). Learning-induced neural plasticity associated with improved identification performance after training of a difficult second-language phonetic contrast. *NeuroImage, 19,* 113–124.

Cherry, E. C. (1953). Some experiments on the recognition of speech, with one or two ears. *Journal of the Acoustical Society of America, 25,* 975–979.

Davis, M. H., & Johnsrude, I. S. (2003). Hierarchical processing in spoken language comprehension. *Journal of Neuroscience, 23*(8), 3423–3431.

Dehaene-Lambertz, G., Dehaene, S., & Hertz-Pannier, L. (2002). Functional neuroimaging of speech perception in infants. *Science, 298,* 2013–2015.

Dehaene-Lambertz, G., Hertz-Pannier, L., Dubois, J., M«eriaux, S., Roche, A., Sigman, M., et al. (2006). Functional organization of perisylvian activation during presentation of sentences in preverbal infants. *Proceedings of the National Academy of Sciences of the United States of America, 103*(38), 14240–14245.

Dehaene-Lambertz, G., Pallier, C., Serniclaes, W., Sprenger-Charolles, L., Jobert, A., & Dehaene, S. (2005). Neural correlates of switching from auditory to speech perception. *NeuroImage, 24*(1), 21–33.

Dupoux, E., Kakehi, K., Hirose, Y., Pallier, C., & Mehler, J. (1999). Epenthetic vowels in Japanese: A perceptual illusion? *Journal of Experimental Psychology: Human Perception and Performance, 25*(6), 1568–1578.

Eggermont J. J. (1998). Representation of spectral and temporal sound features in three cortical fields of the cat. Similarities outweigh differences. *Journal of Neurophysiology, 80,* 2743–2764.

Eggermont, J. J. (2001). Between sound and perception: Reviewing the search for a neural code. *Hearing Research, 157,* 1–42.

Engelien, A., Yang, Y., Engelien, W., Zonana, J., Stern, J., & Silbersweig, D. A. (2002). Physiological mapping of human auditory cortices with a silent event-related fMRI technique. *NeuroImage, 16,* 944–953.

Formisano, E., Kim, D. S., Di Salle, F., van de Moortele, P. F., Ugurbil, K., & Goebel, R. (2003). Mirror-symmetric tonotopic maps in human primary auditory cortex. *Neuron, 40,* 859–869.

Gaskell, M. G., & Marslen-Wilson, W. D. (1997). Integrating form and meaning: A distributed model of speech perception. *Language and Cognitive Processes, 12,* 613–656.

Giraud, A. L., Lorenzi, C., Ashburner, J., Wable, J., Johnsrude, I., Frackowiak, R., et al. (2000). Representation of the temporal envelope of sounds in the human brain. *Journal of Neurophysiology, 84,* 1588–1598.

Golestani, N., & Zatorre, R. J. (2004). Learning new sounds of speech: Reallocation of neural substrates. *NeuroImage, 21,* 494–506.

Hagoort, P., Hald, L., Bastiaansen, M., & Petersson, K. M. (2004). Integration of word meaning and world knowledge in language comprehension. *Science, 304*(5669), 438–441.

Hall, D. A., Johnsrude, I. S., Haggard, M. P., Palmer, A. R., Akeroyd, M. A., & Summerfield, A. Q. (2002). Spectral and temporal processing in human auditory cortex. *Cerebral Cortex, 12,* 140-149.

Harms, M. P., Guinan, J. J., Sigalovsky, I. S., & Melcher, J. R. (2005). Human auditory cortex as shown by fmri determine multisecond time patterns of activity in short-term sound temporal envelope characteristics. *Journal of Neurophysiology, 93,* 210-222.

Harms, M. P., & Melcher, J. R. (2002). Sound repetition rate in the human auditory pathway: Representations in the waveshape and amplitude of fmri activation. *Journal of Neurophysiology, 88,* 1433-1450.

Hart, H. C., Palmer, A. R., & Hall, D. A. (2003). Amplitude and frequency-modulated stimuli activate common regions of human auditory cortex. *Cerebral Cortex, 13,* 773-781.

Hickok, G., Buchsbaum, B., Humphries, C., & Muftuler, T. (2003). Auditory-motor interaction revealed by fMRI: Speech, music, and working memory in area spt. *Journal of Cognitive Neuroscience, 15,* 673-682.

Hickok, G., Erhard, P., Kassubek, J., Helms-Tillery, A. K., Naeve-Velguth, S., Strupp, J. P., Strick, P. L., & Ugurbil, K. (2000). An fMRI study of the role of left posterior superior temporal gyrus in speech production: Implications for the explanation of conduction aphasia. *Neuroscience Letters, 287,* 156-160.

Hickok, G., & Poeppel, D. (2000). Towards a functional neuroanatomy of speech perception. *Trends in Cognitive Sciences, 4,* 131-138.

Indefrey, P., & Cutler, A. (2004). Prelexical and lexical processing in listening. In M. S. Gazzaniga (Ed.), *The cognitive neurosciences* (3rd ed., pp. 759- 774). Cambridge, MA: MIT Press.

Jacquemot, C., Pallier, C., LeBihan, D., Dehaene, S., & Dupoux, E. (2003). Phonological grammar shapes the auditory cortex: A functional magnetic resonance imaging study. *Journal of Neuroscience, 23,* 9541-9546.

Jacquemot, C., & Scott, S. K. (2006). What is the relationship between phonological short-term memory and speech processing? *Trends in Cognitive Sciences, 10*(11), 480-485.

Jäncke, L., Wüstenberg, T., Scheich, H., & Heinze, H. J. (2002). Phonetic perception and the temporal cortex. *NeuroImage, 15,* 733-746.

Kaas, J. H., & Hackett, T. A. (1999). "What" and "where" processing in auditory cortex. *Nature Neuroscience, 2*(12), 1045-1047.

Kaas, J. H., & Hackett, T. A. (2000). Subdivisions of auditory cortex and processing streams in primates. *Proceedings of the National Academy of Sciences of the United States of America, 97*(22), 11793-11799.

Kaas, J. H., Hackett, T. A., & Tramo, M. J. (1999). Auditory processing in primate cerebral cortex. *Current Opinion in Neurobiology, 9,* 164-170.

Liebenthal, E., Binder, J. R., Piorkowski, R. L., & Remez, R. E. (2003). Short-term reorganization of auditory analysis induced by phonetic experience. *Journal of Cognitive Neuroscience, 15*(4), 549-558.

McClelland, J. L., & Elman, J. L. (1986). The TRACE model of speech perception. *Cognitive Psychology, 18,* 1-86.

McQueen, J. M. (2005). Speech perception. In K. Lamberts & R. Goldstone (Eds.), *The handbook of cognition* (pp. 255-275). London: Sage.

Moore, D. R. (2006). Auditory processing disorder (APD): Definition, diagnosis, neural basis, and intervention. *Audiological Medicine, 4,* 4-11.

Narain, C., Scott, S. K., Wise, R. J. S., Rosen, S., Leff, A., Iversen, S. D., et al. (2003). Defining a left-lateralized response specific to intelligible speech using fMRI. *Cerebral Cortex, 13,* 1362-1368.

Nelken, I. (2004). Processing of complex stimuli and natural scenes in the auditory cortex. *Current Opinion in Neurobiology, 14,* 474-480.

Norris, D. (1994). Shortlist: A connectionist model of continuous speech recognition. *Cognition, 52,* 189-234.

Norris, D., & Wise, R. (2000). The study of prelexical and lexical processes in comprehension: Psycholinguistics and functional neuroimaging. In M. S. Gazzaniga (Ed.), *The new cognitive neurosciences.* Cambridge, MA: MIT Press.

Obleser, J., Elbert, T., Lahiri, A., & Eulitz, C. (2003). Cortical representation of vowels reflects acoustic dissimilarity determined by formant frequencies. *Cognitive Brain Research, 15*, 207-213.

Obleser, J., Lahiri, A., & Eulitz, C. (2004). Magnetic brain response mirrors extraction of phonological features from spoken words. *Journal of Cognitive Neuroscience, 16*, 31-39.

Obleser, J., Wise, R. J. S., Dresner, M. A., & Scott, S. K. (2007). Functional integration across brain regions improves speech perception under adverse listening conditions. *Journal of Neuroscience, 27*(9), 2283-2289.

Peña, M., Maki, A., Kovaãiç, D., Dehaene-Lambertz, G., Koizumi, H., Bouquet, F., et al. (2003). Sounds and silence: An optical topography study of language recognition at birth. *Proceedings of the National Academy of Sciences of the United States of America, 100*(20), 11702-11705.

Price, C. J., & Friston, K. (1997). Cognitive conjunction: A new approach to brain activation experiments. *NeuroImage, 5*, 261-270.

Rauschecker, J. P. (1998). Cortical processing of complex sounds. *Current Opinion in Neurobiology, 8*, 516-521.

Rauschecker, J. P., & Tian, B. (2000). Mechanisms and streams for processing of "what" and "where" in auditory cortex. *Proceedings of the National Academy of Sciences of the United States of America, 97*(22), 11800-11806.

Remez, R. E., Fellowes, J. M., & Rubin, P. E. (1997). Talker identification based on phonetic information. *Journal of Experimental Psychology: Human Perception and Performance, 23*, 651-666.

Rodd, J. M., Davis, M. H., & Johnsrude, I. S. (2005). The neural mechanisms of speech comprehension: fMRI studies of semantic ambiguity. *Cerebral Cortex, 15*, 1261-1269.

Rosen, S. (2005). "A riddle wrapped in a mystery inside an enigma": Defining central auditory processing disorder. *American Journal of Audiology, 14*, 139-142.

Scott, S. K., Blank, C. C., Rosen, S., & Wise, R. J. S. (2000). Identification of a pathway for intelligible speech in the left temporal lobe. *Brain, 123*, 2400-2406.

Scott, S. K., & Johnsrude, I. S. (2003). The neuroanatomical and functional organization of speech perception. *Trends in Neurosciences, 26*, 100-107.

Scott, S. K., Rosen, S., Lang, H., & Wise, R. J. S. (2006). Neural correlates of intelligibility in speech investigated with noise-vocoded speech—a positron emission tomography study. *Journal of the Acoustical Society of America, 120*, 1075-1083.

Scott, S. K., Rosen, S., Wickham, L. & Wise, R. J. S. (2004) A positron emission tomography study of the neural basis of informational and energetic masking effects in speech perception. *Journal of the Acoustical Society of America, 115*, 813-821.

Scott, S. K., & Wise, R. J. S. (2004). The functional neuroanatomy of prelexical processing in speech perception. *Cognition, 92*, 13-45.

Shannon, R. V., Zeng, F. G., Kamath, V., Wygonski, J., & Ekelid, M. (1995). Speech perception with primarily temporal cues. *Science, 270*, 303-304.

Sharp, D. J., Scott, S. K., & Wise, R. J. S. (2003). Monitoring and the controlled processing of meaning: Distinct prefrontal systems. *Cerebral Cortex, 14*, 1-10.

Stevens, K. N. (2002). Toward a model for lexical access based on acoustic landmarks and distinctive features. *Journal of the Acoustical Society of America, 111*, 1872-1891.

Thivard, L., Belin, P., Zilbovicius, M., Poline, J., & Samson, Y. (2000). A cortical region sensitive to spectral motion. *NeuroReport, 11*(13), 2969-2972.

Ulanovsky N., Las L., & Nelken I. (2003) Processing of low-probability sounds by cortical neurons. *Nature Neuroscience, 6*, 391-398.

Warren, J. E., Wise, R. J. S., & Warren, J. D. (2005) Sounds do-able: Auditory-motor transformations and the posterior temporal plane. *Trends in Neurosciences, 28*, 636-643.

Wessinger, C. M., VanMeter, J., Tian, B., Van Lare, J., Pekar, J., & Rauschecker, J. P. (2001). Hierarchical organization of the human auditory cortex revealed by functional magnetic resonance imaging. *Journal of Cognitive Neuroscience, 13*, 1-7.

Wise, R. J. S., Chollet, F., Hadar, U., Friston, K., Hoffner, E., & Frackowiak, R. J. S. (1991). Distribution of cortical neural networks involved in word comprehension and word retrieval. *Brain*, *114* (4), 1803–1817.

Wise, R. J. S., Scott, S. K., Blank, S. C., Mummery, C. J., Murphy, K., & Warburton, E. A. (2001). Separate neural subsystems within "Wernicke's area." *Brain*, *124*, 83–95.

Yang, Y., Engelien, A., Engelien, W., Xu, S., Stern, E., & Silbersweig, D. A. (2000). A silent event-related functional MRI technique for brain activation studies without interference of scanner acoustic noise. *Magnetic Resonance in Medicine*, *43*, 185–190.

Zatorre, R. J. (1997). Cerebral correlates of human auditory processing. In J. Syka (Ed.), *Acoustical signal processing in the central auditory system*. New York: Plenum Press.

Zatorre, R. J., Bouffard, M., & Belin, P. (2004). Sensitivity to auditory object features in human temporal neocortex. *Journal of Neuroscience*, *24*, 3637–3642.

CHAPTER 4

Cortical Processing Streams and Central Auditory Plasticity

JOSEF P. RAUSCHECKER

Introduction

It has recently been demonstrated by micro-electrode studies in nonhuman primates and neuroimaging studies in humans that central auditory processing follows two major pathways, both originating in primary auditory cortex: (1) an anteroventral route into anterior superior temporal (ST) cortex for the identification of auditory objects, including speech, and (2) a posterodorsal stream into posterior ST and parietal cortex for the analysis of spatial aspects of sound, including motion in space. As reviewed in this chapter, both cortical processing streams display marked adaptive plasticity to environmental stimulation and a cross-modal ability for reorganization after early sensory deprivation or injury. The remarkable success story of cochlear implants in the deaf is just one example of that plasticity. Improvement of auditory processing after early blindness

is another example. Tinnitus may be considered an example of maladaptive central auditory plasticity following peripheral injury. On closer inspection, however, tinnitus is a combination of lesion-induced reorganization and central gating of auditory processing by nonauditory brain regions.

Auditory Processing Streams

Evidence from Nonhuman Primate Studies

Work on auditory cortex in nonhuman primates in recent years has made it abundantly clear that primary auditory cortex (A1) is surrounded by multiple specialized fields processing different aspects of our sound environment. An anterior stream is devoted to pattern aspects of hearing, that is, for the identification of particular complex sounds; a posterior stream, projecting to parietal cortex and beyond, is involved in processing spatial aspects of sound, including motion in space (Figure 4–1; see also Rauschecker & Tian, 2000; Tian, Reser, Durham, Kustov, & Rauschecker, 2001).

The anterior "what"-stream originates in primary auditory cortex (including area R, the rostral core area) and, via the anterolateral area (AL) of the lateral belt cortex, projects to the ventrolateral prefrontal cortex (Romanski, Tian, Fritz, Mishkin, Goldman-Rakic, & Rauschecker, 1999), which previ-

ously has been identified as the neural basis for object working memory (Goldman-Rakic, 1996). The "what"-stream also includes the rostral parabelt and other rostral ST areas all the way to the rostral pole of ST cortex (Kaas & Hackett, 2000). It seems to parallel an anteroventral processing stream in vision, which originates in primary visual cortex (V1) and projects into inferotemporal (IT) cortex (Ungerleider & Mishkin, 1982). The latter includes mechanisms and neurons selective for the processing of complex visual objects, such as faces, hands, houses, or visual scenes in general (Haxby, Maisog, & Courtney, 1999; Kanwisher,

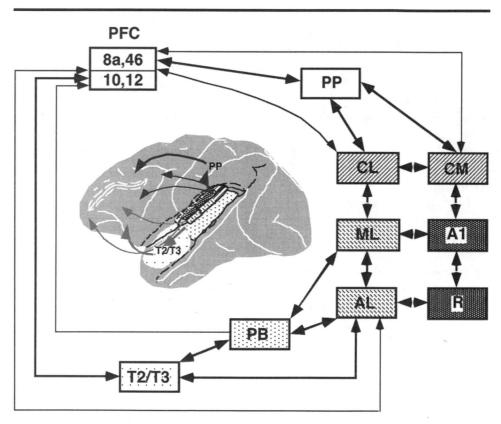

Figure 4–1. Dual pathways for "what" (*gray arrows*) and "where" (*black arrows*) in cortical auditory processing (from Rauschecker & Tian, 2000; modified and extended from Rauschecker, 1998b). Abbreviations, see text.

McDermott, & Chun, 1997; Martin, Wiggs, Ungerleider, & Haxby, 1996). Similarly, the auditory "what"-stream is thought to underlie the processing of behaviorally relevant complex sounds ("auditory objects"), including speech sounds, which are tied to semantic meaning. Auditory and visual "what"-streams interact throughout the border zone of the superior temporal sulcus (STS), whereby the dorsal bank of the STS is largely auditory and the ventral bank is visual (Bruce, Desimone, & Gross, 1981). Nonhuman primate studies have demonstrated selective integration of face and voice processing along anterior regions of the STS (Ghazanfar & Logothetis, 2003).

The posterior "where"-stream originates in primary auditory cortex as well, but projects posteriorly and dorsally, first into areas of the caudal belt (caudomedial area, CM, and caudolateral area, CL) (Kaas & Hackett, 2000). Both of these areas contain neurons that are sharply tuned to the spatial location of a sound presented in the free field (Recanzone, 2000; Tian et al., 2001). The caudal belt and parabelt project to the ventral intraparietal (VIP) area in the inferior parietal cortex (Lewis & Van Essen, 2000), which has been shown previously to contain neurons related to auditory saccades (Andersen, 1997; Bremmer, Schleck, Shah, Zatiris, Kubischik, Hoffman, et al., 2001; Stricanne, Andersen, & Mazzoni, 1996). The caudal belt cortex also projects directly to the dorsolateral prefrontal cortex (DLPFC) (Romanski et al., 1999), which is known to play a role in spatial working memory (Goldman-Rakic, 1996).

Despite these specializations within nonprimary auditory cortex, however, A1 is the basis for many fundamental aspects of hearing as well as hearing disorders. It has been shown recently, for instance, that habituation of neuronal responses in A1 may be the basis for "stream segregation," a psychophysical phenomenon that has often been considered as crucial for auditory figure-ground discrimination (Micheyl, Tian, Carlyon, & Rauschecker, 2005). It can be assumed that deficits in A1 can influence higher functions of hearing fundamentally in many ways. Lesion studies in animals have shown, for instance, that A1 plays a role in sound localization as well as frequency discrimination (Beitel & Kaas, 1993), which would be expected, as A1 is in such a pivotal position from which specialized processing streams originate. Lesions of nonprimary auditory cortex in both cats and monkeys, on the other hand, reveal more selective loss of function corresponding to the physiologic and anatomic dual-pathway model of auditory processing outlined above (Malhotra, Hall, & Lomber, 2004). Lesions of rostral ST cortex, for instance, impair frequency discrimination in rhesus monkeys, whereas lesions of caudal ST cortex impair sound localization (Harrington, Heffner, & Heffner, 2001). Similarly, lesions of the anterior versus posterior auditory fields in cats result in a double-dissociation of auditory pattern discrimination and sound localization, respectively (Lomber, Malhotra, & Hall, 2007).

Evidence from Human Studies

Lesions

Neuropsychological studies in humans have confirmed a similar dichotomy. Infarcts in anterior ST cortex cause auditory agnosias, in which people fail to identify familiar sounds (Vignolo, 1982). In contrast, lesions in posterior ST and posterior parietal (PP) cortex cause auditory spatial deficits (Clarke,

Bellmann, Meuli, Assal, & Steck, 2000) as well as deficits in the perception of auditory motion (Griffiths, Rees, Rees, Green, Witton, Rowe, et al., 1998). Many of these results challenge the traditional view of auditory cortex posterior to Heschl's gyrus (including the planum temporale) being selectively involved in the processing of spoken speech (the "Wernicke-Geschwind" model). It has become clear that posterior ST cortex is involved in the processing of many different types of complex sounds with spectro-temporal variation besides speech, including music and motion in space (Warren, Zielinski, Green, Rauschecker, & Griffiths, 2002). Furthermore, functions of phonological decoding, which have traditionally been assigned to posterior ST cortex, are represented even more selectively in anterior portions of ST cortex (Dronkers, Wilkins, Van Valin, Redfern, & Jaeger, 2004). Phonemic discrimination between real words and nonsense syllables in relation to auditory comprehension was little affected in "Wernicke aphasics" with lesions of posterior ST cortex, whereas this ability was severely impaired in "anterior aphasics" with lesions of anterior ST cortex (Blumstein, Baker, & Goodglass, 1977). This fits well with the idea that anterior temporal lobe lesions lead to "semantic dementia" (Mummery, Patterson, Price, Ashburner, Frackowiak, & Hodges, 2000).

Neuroimaging

Although lesion studies may not provide the necessary resolution to distinguish between fine functional differences, modern neuroimaging techniques, such as positron emission tomography (PET) and functional magnetic resonance imaging (fMRI), have provided conclusive evidence for the functional parcellation of auditory-responsive brain regions. Anterolateral areas of the ST cortex are activated by intelligible speech or speechlike sounds (Alain, Arnott, Hevenor, Graham, & Grady, 2001; Binder, Frost, Hammeke, Bellgowan, Springer, Kaufman, et al., 2000; Binder, Liebenthal, Possing, Medler, & Ward, 2004; Maeder, Meuli, Andriani, Bellman, Fornari, Thiran, et al., 2001; Obleser, Boecker, Drzezga, Haslinger, Hennenlotter, Roettinger, et al., 2006; Scott, Blank, Rosen, & Wise, 2000) or other auditory objects (Zatorre, Bouffard, & Belin, 2004). Thus, it has become more and more obvious also for human auditory cortex that behaviorally relevant auditory patterns, including speech sounds, are identified and discriminated selectively within an anterior auditory "what'-stream" and not in the "planum temporale," which is located posterior to Heschl's gyrus. Auditory areas in the planum temporale constitute an early processing stage and are involved in a variety of auditory functions (Obleser et al., 2006).

Further posterior in the superior temporal gyrus (STG) and STS of humans are regions of the caudal belt and parabelt (projecting dorsally into the inferior posterior parietal cortex) that are specifically active during auditory spatial or auditory motion discriminations tasks (Ahveninen, Jääskeläinen, Raij, Bonmassar, Devore, Hämäläinen, et al., 2006; Arnott, Binns, Grady, & Alain, 2004; Brunetti, Belardinelli, Caulo, Del Gratta, Della Penna, Ferretti, et al., 2005; Degerman, Rinne, Salmi, Salonen, & Alho, 2006; Deouell, Heller, Malach, D'Esposito, & Knight, 2007; Jääskeläinen, Ahveninen, Bonmasser, Dale, Ilmonierni, Lin, et al., 2004; Krumbholz, Schönwiesner, Rubsamen, Zilles, Fink, & von Cramon, 2005; Krumbholz, Schönwiesner, von Cramon, Rubsamen, Shah, Zilles, et al., 2005; Maeder, Meuli, Adriani, Bellman, Fornari, Thiran, et al., 2001; Tata & Ward, 2005a, 2005b; Warren et al., 2002; Zatorre, Bouffard, Ahad, & Belin, 2002; Zimmer & Macaluso, 2005).

Based on meta-analysis, Arnott et al. (2004) reviewed evidence from auditory fMRI and PET studies to determine the reliability of the auditory dual-pathway model in humans. Activation coordinates from 11 "spatial" studies (i.e., where listeners made localization judgments on sounds that could occur at two or more perceptually different positions) and 27 "nonspatial" studies (i.e., where listeners completed nonspatial tasks involving sounds presented from the same location) were entered into the analysis. Almost all temporal lobe activity observed during spatial tasks was confined to posterior areas. In addition, all but one of the spatial studies reported activation within the inferior parietal lobule, as opposed to only 41% of the nonspatial studies. Finally, inferior frontal activity (Brodmann's areas 45 and 47) was reported in only 9% of the spatial studies, but in 56% of the nonspatial studies. These results support an auditory dual-pathway model in humans in which nonspatial sound information (e.g., sound identity) is processed primarily along an anteroventral stream whereas sound location is processed along a posterodorsal stream, that is, within areas posterior to primary auditory cortex.

In conclusion, it appears that, as in the visual system, studies of nonhuman primates can serve as excellent models for human studies. Conversely, human imaging studies can provide useful guidance for microelectrode studies in nonhuman primates, which permit analyses at much higher spatial and temporal resolution than would be possible in most human studies, with some exceptions (Howard, Volkov, Abbas, Damasio, Ollendieck, & Granner, 1996; Howard, Volkov, Mirsky, Garell, Noh, Granner, et al., 2000). Imaging-guided microelectrode studies in monkeys (Tsao, Freiwald, Tootell, & Livingstone, 2006) can further complement these approaches.

Central Auditory Plasticity

Adaptive Plasticity

Many important functions of the auditory system can only be fully appreciated with cortical plasticity in mind. For instance, even with an innate capacity for language, normal speech can hardly be acquired without auditory feedback and a capacity for learning. Likewise, a system capable of localizing sound at extraordinary precision, using various sets of cues, cannot accomplish this without resorting to tuning mechanisms that recalibrate the system continually, especially during the growth phase of the head and outer ears.

Speech Perception: Influence of Early Phonetic Environment

Communication sound processing in animals sometimes appears to be hard-wired. In particular, emotionally driven calls in nonhuman primates do not seem to be modulated much by the animal's auditory experience (Hauser, 1996; Seyfarth, Cheney, & Marler, 1980; Zoloth, Petersen, Beecher, Green, Marler, Moody, et al., 1979). However, other vocalization classes that have more sophisticated social functions are more modifiable (Hauser, 1992). Similar differences seem to hold in songbirds, where some species display hard-wired patterns, whereas others produce lengthy sequences of learned songs, often taught to young birds by a parent (Doupe & Kuhl, 1999). In these cases, experience clearly modifies the tuning properties of neurons during recognition learning, giving rise to plastic representations of behaviorally meaningful auditory objects (Gentner & Margoliash, 2003). Humans, though endowed with an innate capacity for language, acquire language in a process that takes the better part of their childhood (~12 years) (Lenneberg, 1967). Human speech and language has almost exclusive social importance and is, therefore, almost entirely plastic in most of its components.

The most obvious demonstration of experiential factors in language acquisition is the fact that infants raised in different cultures or by different parents can acquire the language of their surrounding phonetic environment without impairment (Jusczyk & Hohne, 1997; Werker & Logan, 1985). The inability to distinguish (and, therefore, to produce) the characteristic sounds for "r" and "l" by speakers of some Asian languages is thus due to the absence of the distinguishing features in their early auditory environment (Lively, Logan, & Pisoni, 1993). Once acquired through early exposure, such a predisposition can only be reversed through intensive training (Logan, Lively, & Pisoni, 1991), which provides further evidence for the existence of a sensitive period of language acquisition.

Compelling studies to prove the influence of early auditory experience on speech development and phonetic perception have been designed by Kuhl and coworkers (Kuhl, 2000). Infants in different countries (Sweden, Russia, and the United States) initially do not show a preference for phonemes unique to their own language. By about 6 months of age, however, they suddenly develop this preference (Kuhl, Williams, Lacerda, Stevens, & Lindblom, 1992). Work by Jusczyk and colleagues shows that language-specific preferences for prosodic cues, which are necessary for the segmentation of the speech stream into perceptual units, also develop between 6 and 9 months of age (Jusczyk & Hohne, 1997).

As discussed above, functional imaging studies point to an involvement of cortical areas in the anterior STG with the processing of speech as well as other auditory object information (Binder, Frost, Hammeke, Bellgowan, Springer, Kaufman, et al., 2000; Binder et al., 2004; Rauschecker & Tian, 2000; Scott et al., 2000; Zatorre et al., 2004). Neurophysiologically, one has to imagine that neurons specific for certain speech sounds are created by combining input from lower order neurons in earlier regions, which contain feature detectors for elements of speech (Kanwal & Rauschecker, 2007; Rauschecker, 1999b). How the invariance of speech perception against changes of pitch or naturally imposed distortions is guaranteed by neural mechanisms is one of the great challenges of auditory neuroscience. Some investigators postulate that invariance is not possible without learning to generalize from the multitude of experienced samples, in other words, neuronal plasticity in the best sense. Auditory cortical plasticity enables the formation of such combinations under the influence of an early phonetic environment. Such self-organization processes ultimately lead to the establishment of phonological representations in higher order computational maps (Kohonen & Hari, 1999).

The study of bilingual subjects is particularly instructive with regard to self-organization of language representations in the brain. Preneurosurgical mapping in a group of epileptic patients has demonstrated that two languages occupy largely overlapping brain space in individuals with low proficiency in the second language (Ojemann & Whitaker, 1978). As the same patients were remapped several years later (before a second surgery had to be undertaken), after their proficiency in the second language had increased, the amount of separation of the two language representations had increased accordingly. This result is in perfect agreement with a functional imaging study on bilingual subjects, which demonstrates that the two languages show little overlap, as long as the subjects were fluent in the second language (Kim, Relkin, Lee, & Hirsch, 1997).

Effects of Musical Training

The conclusions that can be drawn from language acquisition studies apply also to the acquisition of musical abilities. Although there is undoubtedly an inherited component in "musicality," the capacity to appreciate and make music, is universal for the human species; early experience and training makes a significant difference in how much of the brain is engaged in music processing. Early musical training in children seems to be closely related to the development of absolute pitch and a concomitant expansion of auditory cortex (Gaab & Schlaug, 2003; Gaser & Schlaug, 2003; Schlaug, Jancke, Huang, & Steinmetz, 1995). Although a structural expansion could perhaps be ascribed to genetic factors as well as to experiential ones, specific and rapid functional changes are less readily explained by genetics (Pantev, Oostenveld, Engelien, Ross, Roberts, & Hoke, 1998; Pantev, Ross, Fujioka, Trainor, Schulte, & Schulz, 2003; Shahin, Bosnyak, Trainor, & Roberts, 2003; Trainor, Shahin, & Roberts, 2003). Experience-dependent plasticity for the perception of harmonic sounds is greatest before the age of eight or nine (Pantev et al., 1998). The timing of this "sensitive period" corresponds strikingly to that of phonological development mentioned earlier (Johnson & Newport, 1989).

In search for a possible neurophysiologic substrate, one is again confronted with the view that preferences of higher order neurons for specific types of complex sounds are brought about by combining features of lower order neurons. The binding of the lower order features is dependent on coincident timing and, thus, coactivation of neurons, as postulated originally by Hebb (1949) (for review see Rauschecker, 1991). Activity-dependent mechanisms are also suggested by monkey studies that train the animals with particular combinations of tones and find an overrepresentation of these frequencies in the auditory cortex (Recanzone, Schreiner, & Merzenich, 1993). Subsequent studies in monkeys have demonstrated that the map expansions can be facilitated by concomitant electrical stimulation of the basal forebrain, which leads to excretion of acetylcholine, a neurotransmitter that has been implicated in plasticity and learning in a number of systems (Kilgard & Merzenich, 1998; Weinberger, 2003).

The Success Story of Cochlear Implants

Profoundly deaf individuals that still have an intact auditory nerve have profited from the dramatic advances made over the past 30 years in the field of cochlear implants (CIs) (Loeb, 1985; Rauschecker, 1999b, 2002a, 2002b). The CI is a microelectrode array implanted in the cochlea that directly stimulates the auditory nerve. With more than 40,000 patients worldwide, the success of these devices is nothing short of miraculous; most adults are able to converse on the telephone, and most children are able to be educated in mainstream classrooms. Despite the relatively crude CI signal, delivered by a discrete and limited number of stimulating electrodes, most implant listeners are capable of excellent language understanding. Processing by the auditory cortex fills in much of the missing information, just as the visual cortex fills in the blanks left by our blind spot or by illusory contours. In other words, auditory cortex, by means of its adaptive plasticity, learns to interpret the impoverished signal.

Obviously, a difference exists between patients that become deaf before or after acquiring speech (pre- and postlingual deafness, respectively). Whereas the postlingually deaf "re-connect" almost immediately after receiving their CI, success in prelingually deaf individuals depends on age of implantation. As with corrections of early visual defects, such as cataract or strabismus, the maxim is "the earlier the better" (Svirsky, Robbins, Kirk, Pisoni, & Miyamoto, 2000). Thus, another fundamental and encouraging lesson can be learned from CI research about the plasticity of neural representations of auditory information in the brains of young children—that is, in response to sound, the stimulated auditory cortex can recruit neurons from adjacent regions of the brain and can form new neuronal connections. In contrast, if the implant is performed too late, visual input will have already occupied auditory territories that could otherwise get involved in the above reorganization process, providing an example of how cross-modal plasticity can potentially have a negative influence on cochlear implant performance.

Studies in congenitally deaf cats confirm the malleability of the auditory cortex, which is molded by auditory experience from an early age (Klinke, Kral, Heid, Tillein, & Hartmann, 1999). If environmental sounds transmitted via a microphone and CI are used to stimulate the central auditory pathways of young deaf cats, the animals soon begin to respond with appropriate behaviors to these sounds and their auditory cortex begins to develop normal activation patterns. Much less plasticity is observed in congenitally deaf animals that are exposed to sound at an older age (Klinke et al., 1999). These results are very much in tune with

the visual deprivation literature (Rauschecker & Singer, 1981; Wiesel, 1982) and indicate the existence of a sensitive period during early postnatal development of the central auditory system, especially the auditory cortex (Kral, Hartmann, Tillein, Heid, & Klinke, 2001; Rauschecker, 1999a).

Cortical Reorganization in Congenital Deafness

Processes analogous to the auditory compensation in the blind can be demonstrated in congenitally deaf subjects. Results from event-related potential (ERP) as well as neuroimaging techniques have shown that the brain of deaf subjects is reorganized profoundly. Visual motion areas in the right parietal cortex thought to be involved in the initial decoding of visual motion cues in American Sign Language (Obleser et al., 2006) are expanded (Neville & Lawson, 1987). At the same time, "auditory" cortex in the ST cortex is also activated by visual sign language (Nishimura, Haskikawa, Doi, Iwaki, Watanabe, Kusuoka, et al., 1999; Petitto, Zatorre, Gauna, Nikelski, Dostie, & Evans, 2000) and other visual stimuli (Finney, Clementz, Hickok, & Dobkins, 2003; Finney, Fine, & Dobkins, 2001) but is not activated by the presentation of English words, as it normally is in hearing subjects (Neville, Bavelier, Corina, Rauschecker, Karni, Lalwani, et al., 1998).

In addition to visual inputs, vibrotactile activation via the somatosensory system has also been found in the auditory cortex of congenitally deaf humans (Levänen & Hamdorf, 2001; Levänen, Jousmaki, & Hari, 1998). In these studies, the stimuli were applied to palm and fingers and were registered with magnetoencephalography (MEG).

In neurobiological terms, the mechanisms responsible for cross-modal reorganization during visual or auditory deprivation are bound to be quite similar. As has been argued previously, the neural mechanisms are even likely the same for reorganization within and across modalities.

Auditory Cortical Plasticity During the Life Span

Otitis media is an infection of the middle ear, frequently occurring in infants and small children (repeatedly in nearly one-third of all infants before the age of three (Gravel, Wallace, & Ruben, 1996), whose long-term effect on hearing should not be underestimated. Infections typically lead to an attenuation of auditory input by 20 dB or more. This results in significant distortions of speech, especially at higher frequencies (Dobie & Berlin, 1979). As a result, it has been found that masking thresholds are severely altered in children with a history of otitis media (Moore, Hutchings, & Meyer, 1991). The question arises, therefore, whether this very common disease, is a major cause of perceptual and, ultimately, language deficits. This is plausible in view of the effects of visual deprivation on visual cortical development (Wiesel, 1982). Similarly, auditory deprivation resulting from peripheral causes, such as otitis media, could exert lasting effects on the development of auditory cortex, rendering cortical neurons unresponsive to sound, and should therefore be observed more carefully (Moore, Hartley, & Hogan, 2003). Unfortunately, comparatively little animal experimentation has been done to establish sensitive periods in auditory cortex, as they have been known to exist in visual cortex for some time (Blakemore, 1991; Hubel & Wiesel, 1970). Although some of the effects of early hearing impairment may be reversible, if hearing is restored (Gravel, Roberts, Roush, Grose, Besing,

Berchinal, et al., 2006; Moore, Hine, Jiang, Matsuda, Parsons, & King, 1999), we do not know enough about possible permanent damage to discount these risks (Xu, Kotak, & Sanes, 2007).

Impairments of speech discrimination in noisy environments, especially in the presence of multiple speakers, are becoming increasingly apparent in the elderly population (Sommers, 1997). The solution of this "cocktail-party" situation probably involves top-down processing from the auditory cortex (similar to the classic "figure-ground discrimination" in the visual domain (Rauschecker, 1998a). The mechanisms for top-down modulation in the auditory corticothalamic system have been studied extensively in recent years (Suga & Ma, 2003).

Backward masking is another function altered with increasing age (Gehr & Sommers, 1999). One can easily imagine that an auditory cortex deprived of the proper input would lead to impairment in just these functions. Clearly, much more research needs to be devoted to central auditory plasticity during the life span.

Auditory Processing in the Blind: Evidence for Cross-Modal Plasticity

One of the auditory functions that are improved as a result of early blindness in both humans and animals is localization of sounds. Cats that are binocularly lid-sutured from birth for several months certainly do not show any signs of overt behavioral impairments in spatial behavior, as one would predict if vision was needed for its development. Quantitative measurements of sound localization behavior confirm this impression. Sound localization error was measured in a task that required the cats to walk toward a sound source that varied randomly in azimuth location in order to get a food reward. The error was consistently smaller in visually deprived cats as compared to sighted controls (Rauschecker & Kniepert, 1994). The improvement was largest for lateral and rear positions of space, but even in straight-ahead positions, where the localization error is already small in normal controls, no deterioration by any means was found. Identical results have been found in visually deprived ferrets (King & Parsons, 1999; King & Semple, 1996), thus confirming the earlier cat studies. Similar findings have also been reported for blind humans (Lessard, Pare, Lepore, & Lassonde, 1998; Muchnik, Efrati, Nemeth, Malin, & Hildesheimer, 1991; Röder, Teder-Salejarvi, Sterr, Rösler, Hillyard, & Neville, 1999). The study by Röder et al. (1999) confirmed the animal studies even in quite specific detail in that it found the improvements to be most significant in lateral azimuth positions and no deterioration whatsoever in straight-ahead positions. These studies also fit extremely well with the classical findings by Rice and colleagues, who analyzed the echolocation abilities of blind humans and found them to be improved particularly in lateral positions of space (Rice, Feinstein, & Schusterman, 1965; Rice, 1970).

The neurophysiologic correlate of these behavioral changes in the auditory system of blind cats may be found in the anterior ectosylvian sulcus (AES). In the AES region, visual responses in the fundus of the AES virtually disappeared. Neurons in this region, however, did not become unresponsive, but were replaced by neurons with brisk responses to auditory and tactile stimuli. Apparently, auditory and somatosensory areas within the AES had expanded at the expense of formerly visual territory (Rauschecker & Korte, 1993). Auditory spatial tuning (i.e., the tuning for the location of a sound source in free field) was significantly

sharper in the whole AES region when compared to sighted controls. Visually deprived cats had close to 90% spatially tuned cells (with a spatial tuning ratio of better than 2:1 between best and worst location). In addition, neurons with spatial tuning ratios of 10:1 or better were more abundant in blind cats (Korte & Rauschecker, 1993). The increased number of auditory cortical neurons, together with their sharpened spatial filtering characteristics, is likely to improve the sampling density of auditory space and provide the neural basis for the improved spatial abilities of early blind cats and ferrets (Rauschecker, 1995, 2002a, 2002b).

In a study by Weeks, Horwitz, Aziz-Sultan, Tian, Wessinger, Cohen, et al. (2000), congenitally blind and sighted human subjects were tested in a virtual auditory space environment (simulating quasifree-field sound with standardized head-related transfer functions and headphones), and their regional cerebral blood flow (rCBF) was measured in a whole-head PET scanner. The task was (a) to decide whether two subsequent sounds were coming from the same or a different azimuth position in space, or (b) to move a joy-stick into the presumed direction. Both tasks yielded similar results.

In all subjects (sighted or blind) posterior inferior parietal cortex was activated, which provides clear evidence for an involvement of this region in auditory spatial processing. It was confirmed by independent studies that this parietal region (presumably the human analogue of monkey area VIP), in fact, contains a unimodal auditory area (Bushara, Weeks, Ishii, Catalan, Tian, Rauschecker, et al., 1999; Weeks, Aziz-Sultan, Bushara, Tian, Wessinger, Dang, et al., 1999). It is part of a dorsal auditory processing stream (Rauschecker & Tian, 2000) and receives its input from auditory belt and parabelt cortex in the posterior superior temporal gyrus (Lewis & Van Essen,

2000). Both sighted and blind subjects also activated frontal areas, owing to the delayed matching task involving working memory, which are also part of the auditory "where" stream (Romanski et al., 1999).

In blind subjects, occipital cortex was activated in addition to the above areas. Activation zones originated in posterior parietal cortex and extended all the way into Brodmann areas 18 and 19, as determined on the basis of Talairach coordinates (Talairach & Tournoux, 1988). The expansion was most extensive in the right hemisphere, which testifies to its special involvement in spatial processes (Mesulam, 1999). Similar results of auditory activation in the occipital cortex of blind subjects were obtained using event-related potential techniques (Kujala, Alho, Kekoni, Hämäläinen, Reinikainen, Salonen, et al., 1995; Kujala, Alho, Paavilainen, Summala, & Näätänen, 1992).

The surprising activation of occipital, formerly visual cortical areas in blind subjects raises two fundamental questions: Why was such activation not found in visually deprived cats? And is the auditory activation of occipital areas in the blind due to feed-forward, bottom-up activation from auditory areas, or is it due to feedback input from higher order, parietal cortical regions, homologous to the AES in cats? The answer to the first question is simple: occipital areas in visually deprived cats were *never* tested with auditory stimuli. It is, therefore, quite possible that auditory activity would also be found in visually deprived cats. Some earlier studies in fact reported auditory activation of visual cortex even in normal cats (Fishman & Michael, 1973; Spinelli, Starr, & Barrett, 1968) but these reports were never taken very seriously, because the activation was sparse and was generally attributed to unspecific effects of anesthesia or arousal. Auditory projections to visual cortex had also been demonstrated in very young kittens (Innocenti & Clarke, 1984), but a stabilization of these transitory connections by visual deprivation has not been shown. Recent anatomical data with more sensitive tracers have demonstrated, however, that a direct projection from auditory to visual cortex does exist in adult rhesus monkeys (Falchier, Clavagnier, Barone, & Kennedy, 2002; Rockland & Ojima, 2003). These results may be interpreted in favor of a more metamodal organization of the brain (Pascual-Leone & Hamilton, 2001), which could be utilized for compensatory plasticity.

Interregional analysis of the PET imaging data by Weeks et al. (2000) suggests that feedback connections from the inferior parietal lobule (IPL) could also provide a stronger auditory signal in blind than in sighted individuals and perhaps be responsible for the auditory activation in the occipital lobe. Whereas visual cortex provides the strongest source of input to the right IPL in sighted subjects, auditory cortex in the ST region provides most of the input to the IPL in blind subjects. Thus, the IPL region is dominated by auditory input in the blind, which must be reflected in the signal carried by the back-projection from IPL to occipital cortex.

Tinnitus-Related Changes in the Brain

Lesion-Induced Reorganization of Auditory Cortex

Tinnitus, the hearing of a disturbing tone or noise in the absence of a real sound source, is in many ways comparable to the experience of phantom pain, which can still be felt in an amputated limb. Tinnitus can be thought of as an auditory phantom phenomenon, in which the firing of central auditory neurons still conveys specific perceptual experiences, even though the corresponding sensory receptor cells that used to encode them have long been destroyed (Rauschecker, 1999a).

One of the most promising theories on the origin of tinnitus is that of a plastic reorganization in the auditory cortex following peripheral trauma (Jastreboff, 1990; Jastreboff, Brennan, Coleman, & Sasaki, 1988; Rauschecker, 1999a). According to this hypothesis, the process leading to tinnitus begins with a sensorineural hearing loss. This could be a cochlear lesion from loud noise exposure or age-related hair cell loss within a certain frequency range (usually high frequencies). Although the loss of hair cells causes elevated thresholds in that frequency range, neighboring frequency portions may actually be amplified because their central representation expands into the vacated frequency range.

Indeed, preliminary evidence exists from MEG and PET studies for an expansion of the frequency representation in auditory cortex around the tinnitus frequency (Lockwood, Salvi, & Burkard, 2002; Lockwood, Salvi, Burkard, Galantowicz, Coad, & Wack, 1999; Mühlnickel, Elbert, Taub, & Flor, 1998). These results however, await confirmation with high-resolution fMRI (Leaver, Renier, Purcell, Constanzo, Fieger, Morgan, et al., 2006).

The assumption that the ultimate origin of tinnitus must be central is underscored by the fact that tinnitus persists after transection of the auditory nerve, such as after acoustic neurinoma removal (Matthies & Samii, 1997; Seidman & Jacobson, 1996). Other recent findings compatible with a central origin of tinnitus include a change in the firing pattern of auditory cortical neurons but not of more peripheral stations

(Norena & Eggermont, 2003). Furthermore, studies using 2-deoxyglucose and c-fos autoradiography in gerbils treated with salicylate, which is known to generate tinnitus, demonstrate reduced activity in the inferior colliculus but increased activation in portions of auditory cortex (Wallhäusser-Franke, Braun, & Langner, 1996; Wallhäusser-Franke, Mahlke, Oliva, Braun, Wenz, & Langer, 2003).

The origin of tinnitus according to the above hypotheses is based on the same mechanisms as cortical reorganization after lesions of the cochlea (Irvine, Rajan, & Brown, 2001; Rajan, Irvine, Wise, & Heil, 1993). As has been shown in animal studies, the resulting loss of hair cells in a specific part of the cochlea leads to a characteristic cortical reorganization of auditory cortex. Frequency regions neighboring to the lesioned part expand into the vacated space and become "overrepresented" compared to other frequency regions. In addition, these regions lose intracortical inhibitory input from the deafferented cortical region. Cortical neurons with input from frequency ranges next to the cutoff frequency thus display permanently elevated spontaneous activity levels. Similar effects are observed after loud noise exposure or aging (the latter especially in the high-frequency region). It is assumed that the same synaptic mechanisms are responsible for reorganization after lesions and in tinnitus that lead to reorganization from experiential effects of auditory training (Calford, Rajan, & Irvine, 1993; Edeline & Weinberger, 1993).

Similarly, plastic reorganization of A1 has often been considered the basis for tinnitus (Jastreboff, 1990; Rauschecker, 1999b). The idea here is that a lesion in the peripheral representation of certain sound frequencies (as a result of damage to the inner hair cells) leads to filling-in by neighboring frequencies at the central level (Rajan & Irvine,

1998). Different perceptions of the tinnitus signal could result from reorganization in cortical areas with different specializations: Tonal tinnitus may result from reorganization in A1, band-pass noise tinnitus from reorganization in lateral belt areas (see earlier discussion in this chapter).

Increased Gray-Matter Density in Auditory Thalamus

More recently, the possibility has arisen that the reorganization of auditory cortex is accompanied (or even preceded) by changes at the thalamic level. This conjecture has resulted from high-resolution structural MRI studies with voxel-based morphometry (VBM) which have demonstrated a significant increase in gray-matter density in the posterior thalamus, including the medial geniculate nucleus (MGN), but no other part of the auditory system (Mühlau et al., 2006). This matches findings in the somatosensory system by Pons, Garraghty, Ommaya, Kaas, Taub, and Mishkin (1991), who had found massive changes in somatosensory cortex of macaque monkeys after peripheral deafferentation (amputation of an arm). The reorganization at the cortical level was later found to be paralleled by changes in the ventromedial nucleus and mediated by NMDA receptors (Ergenzinger, Glasier, Hahm, & Pons, 1998). By analogy, the reorganization in the central auditory pathways as a result of noise-induced hearing loss would trigger changes at the thalamic level as well as a reorganization of the auditory cortex (Leaver et al., 2006). Whether the thalamic changes precede the changes at the cortical level or vice versa currently cannot be said with certainty. Pons and colleagues (1991) have argued convincingly, however, that the

magnification factor at the thalamic level is much greater than in the cortex, which could help to explain the massive changes seen at the behavioral level.

Limbic System Involvement

Central reorganization of auditory cortex and thalamus in response to peripheral deafferentation may be necessary for the tinnitus sensation to arise; it is almost certainly not sufficient, however, to explain it. If peripheral hearing loss results in central reorganization and this reorganization is the substrate of the tinnitus sensation, how is it possible that only one-third of patients with noise-induced hearing loss develop tinnitus? It seems as if, in addition to the changes in the auditory pathways, a switch exists that can turn the tinnitus sensation on or off.

It has long been assumed that structures in the limbic system associated with the processing of emotions (e.g., the amygdala) have to be involved in tinnitus as well, in particular, for developing the negative emotions and the suffering associated with this condition. The latter have been interpreted as a learned reaction to the tinnitus signal through Pavlovian conditioning (Jastreboff, 1990; Jastreboff, Brennan, Coleman, & Sasaki, 1988). And indeed several imaging studies have pointed to abnormal activation of limbic-related structures in tinnitus patients (Lockwood, Salvi, Coad, Towsley, Wack, & Murphy, 1998).

Most recently, a potential breakthrough in our understanding of tinnitus came to pass when, in a VBM study, Mühlau, Rauschecker, Oestreicher, Gaser, Röttinger, Wohlschläger, et al. (2006) found a highly significant volume loss in the subcallosal area of tinnitus sufferers. (This was the same group of patients, mentioned above, in whom changes in the auditory thalamus were detected.) The subcallosal area overlaps with the limbic-related ventral striatum, and it contains as one of its most interesting components, the nucleus accumbens (NAc). A volume loss in this region would point to a deterioration of function related to it (rather than a learning effect).

Cross-Modal Plasticity and Tinnitus

Available data suggest that tinnitus-related cross-modal interactions are more common than previously anticipated (Cacace, 2003). Tinnitus evoked by gaze changes or orofacial movements has been described numerous times, but is still considered the exception (Lockwood et al., 1998). By contrast, cutaneous-evoked tinnitus (Cacace, Cousins, Parnes, McFarland et al., 1999a; Cacace, Cousins, Parnes, Semenoff et al., 1999b) and craniocervical modulation of tinnitus (Levine, 2000) are much more frequent than previously thought and point to interactions of auditory and somatosensory modalities possibly at an early level, such as the dorsal cochlear nucleus (Levine, 1999).

General Conclusions

Although in many cases neural plasticity presents as adaptive, that is, suitable to improve survival, plasticity sometimes is found to have seemingly negative consequences. For instance, cross-modal plasticity potentially can have a negative influence on cochlear implant performance, particularly in young children, as mentioned above, because competition between synaptic inputs during early development is fierce. Connections established early tend to remain stable and cannot, therefore, be displaced easily at a later stage. Plasticity may exist for beneficial reasons, such as the reorganization of central nervous structures after peripheral lesions, which tends to mend small lesions in the sensory periphery by filling-in at more central levels. As a side effect unintended by nature, such lesion-induced plasticity, however, can also lead to phantom pain and tinnitus, as explained in this chapter. Additional mechanisms may exist to nullify these secondary consequences, but they add another layer of complexity to these sensory systems, which puts the individual at further risk for maladaptation, if the correcting machinery fails. Thus, neural plasticity can display as a "double-edged sword," although epigenetic mechanisms overall are not only beneficial but highly necessary to complement the accomplishments of genetic factors.

Acknowledgments. This review chapter draws substantially from prior reviews by the same author (Rauschecker, 1999a, 2006, 2007) with permission from the respective publishers. Grant support was provided by the National Institutes of Health (grants R01 DC03489, R01 NS052494), the National Science Foundation (grants BCS-0519127 and OISE-0730255), the Tinnitus Research Consortium (TRC), and the Tinnitus Research Initiative (TRI). I would like to thank Jennifer Sasaki for her help with editing this chapter.

References

Ahveninen, J., Jääskeläinen, I. P., Raij, T., Bonmassar, G., Devore, S., Hämäläinen, M., et al. (2006). Task-modulated "what" and "where" pathways in human auditory cortex. *Proceedings of the National Academy of Sciences*, *103*, 14608–14613.

Alain, C., Arnott, S. R., Hevenor, S., Graham, S., & Grady, C. L. (2001). "What" and "where" in the human auditory system. *Proceedings of the National Academy of Sciences, 98*, 12301–12306.

Andersen, R. A. (1997). Multimodal integration for the representation of space in the posterior parietal cortex. *Philosophical Transactions of the Royal Society of London B, Biological Sciences, 352*, 1421–1428.

Arnott, S. R., Binns, M. A., Grady, C. L., & Alain, C. (2004). Assessing the auditory dual-pathway model in humans. *NeuroImage, 22*, 401–408.

Beitel, R. E., & Kaas, J. H. (1993). Effects of bilateral and unilateral ablation of auditory cortex in cats on the unconditioned head orienting response to acoustic stimuli. *Journal of Neurophysiology, 70*, 351–369.

Binder, J. R., Frost, J. A., Hammeke, T. A., Bellgowan, P. S., Springer, J. A., Kaufman, J. N., et al. (2000). Human temporal lobe activation by speech and nonspeech sounds. *Cerebral Cortex, 10*, 512–528.

Binder, J. R., Liebenthal, E., Possing, E. T., Medler, D. A., & Ward, B. D. (2004). Neural correlates of sensory and decision processes in auditory object identification. *Nature Neuroscience, 7*, 295–301.

Blakemore, C. (1991). Sensitive and vulnerable periods in the development of the visual system. *Ciba Foundation Symposiums, 156*, 129–147.

Blumstein, S. E., Baker, E., & Goodglass, H. (1977). Phonological factors in auditory comprehension in aphasia. *Neuropsychologia, 15*, 19–30.

Bremmer, F., Schlack, A., Shah, N. J., Zafiris, O., Kubischik, M., Hoffmann, K., et al. (2001). Polymodal motion processing in posterior parietal and premotor cortex: A human fMRI study strongly implies equivalencies between humans and monkeys. *Neuron, 29*, 287–296.

Bruce, C., Desimone, R., & Gross, C. G. (1981). Visual properties of neurons in a polysensory area in superior temporal sulcus of the macaque. *Journal of Neurophysiology, 46*, 369–384.

Brunetti, M., Belardinelli, P., Caulo, M., Del Gratta, C., Della Penna, S., Ferretti, A., et al. (2005). Human brain activation during passive listening to sounds from different locations: An fMRI and MEG study. *Human Brain Mapping, 26*, 251–261.

Bushara, K. O., Weeks, R. A., Ishii, K., Catalan, M.-J., Tian, B., Rauschecker, J. P., et al. (1999). Modality-specific frontal and parietal areas for auditory and visual spatial localization in humans. *Nature Neuroscience, 2*, 759–766.

Cacace, A. T. (2003). Expanding the biological basis of tinnitus: crossmodal origins and the role of neuroplasticity. *Hearing Research, 175*, 112–132.

Cacace, A. T., Cousins, J. P., Parnes, S. M., McFarland, D. J., Semenoff, D., Holmes, T., et al. (1999a). Cutaneous-evoked tinnitus. II. Review of neuroanatomical, physiological and functional imaging studies. *Audiology and Neuro-otology, 4*, 258–268.

Cacace, A. T., Cousins, J. P., Parnes, S. M., Semenoff, D., Holmes, T., McFarland, D. J., et al. (1999b). Cutaneous-evoked tinnitus. I. Phenomenology, psychophysics and functional imaging. *Audiology and Neuro-otology, 4*, 247–257.

Calford, M. B., Rajan, R., & Irvine, D. R. (1993). Rapid changes in the frequency tuning of neurons in cat auditory cortex resulting from pure-tone-induced temporary threshold shift. *Neuroscience, 55*, 953–964.

Clarke, S., Bellmann, A., Meuli, R. A., Assal, G., & Steck, A. J. (2000). Auditory agnosia and auditory spatial deficits following left hemispheric lesions: evidence for distinct processing pathways. *Neuropsychologia, 38*, 797–807.

Degerman, A., Rinne, T., Salmi, J., Salonen, O., & Alho, K. (2006). Selective attention to sound location or pitch studied with fMRI. *Brain Research, 1077*, 123–134.

Deouell, L. Y., Heller, A. S., Malach, R., D'Esposito, M., & Knight, R. T. (2007). Cerebral responses to change in spatial location of unattended sounds. *Neuron, 55*, 985–996.

Dobie, R. A., & Berlin, C. I. (1979). Influence of otitis media on hearing and development. *Annals of Otology, Rhinology, and Laryngology, 88*(5 Pt. 2 Suppl. 60), 48–53.

Doupe, A. J., & Kuhl, P. K. (1999). Birdsong and human speech: common themes and mechanisms. *Annual Review of Neuroscience, 22,* 567–631.

Dronkers, N. F., Wilkins, D. P., Van Valin, R. D., Jr., Redfern, B. B., & Jaeger, J. J. (2004). Lesion analysis of the brain areas involved in language comprehension. *Cognition, 92,* 145–177.

Edeline, J. M., & Weinberger, N. M. (1993). Receptive field plasticity in the auditory cortex during frequency discrimination training: selective retuning independent of task difficulty. *Behavioral Neuroscience, 107,* 82–103.

Ergenzinger, E. R., Glasier, M. M., Hahm, J. O., & Pons, T. P. (1998). Cortically induced thalamic plasticity in the primate somatosensory system. *Nature Neuroscience, 1,* 226–229.

Falchier, A., Clavagnier, S., Barone, P., & Kennedy, H. (2002). Anatomical evidence of multimodal integration in primate striate cortex. *Journal of Neuroscience, 22,* 5749–5759.

Finney, E. M., Clementz, B. A., Hickok, G., & Dobkins, K. R. (2003). Visual stimuli activate auditory cortex in deaf subjects: Evidence from MEG. *NeuroReport, 14,* 1425–1427.

Finney, E. M., Fine, I., & Dobkins, K. R. (2001). Visual stimuli activate auditory cortex in the deaf. *Nature Neuroscience, 4,* 1171–1173.

Fishman, M. C., & Michael, P. (1973). Integration of auditory information in the cat's visual cortex. *Vision Research, 13,* 1415–1419.

Gaab, N., & Schlaug, G. (2003). Musicians differ from nonmusicians in brain activation despite performance matching. *Annals of the New York Academy of Sciences, 999,* 385–388.

Gaser, C., & Schlaug, G. (2003). Brain structures differ between musicians and non-musicians. *Journal of Neuroscience, 23,* 9240–9245.

Gehr, S. E., & Sommers, M. S. (1999). Age differences in backward masking. *Journal of the Acoustical Society of America, 106,* 2793–2799.

Gentner, T. Q., & Margoliash, D. (2003). Neuronal populations and single cells representing learned auditory objects. *Nature, 424,* 669–674.

Ghazanfar, A. A., & Logothetis, N. K. (2003). Neuroperception: facial expressions linked to monkey calls. *Nature, 423,* 937–938.

Goldman-Rakic, P. S. (1996). The prefrontal landscape: implications of functional architecture for understanding human mentation and the central executive. *Philosophical Transactions of the Royal Society of London B, 351,* 1445–1453.

Gravel, J. S., Roberts, J. E., Roush, J., Grose, J., Besing, J., Burchinal, M., et al. (2006). Early otitis media with effusion, hearing loss, and auditory processes at school age. *Ear and Hearing, 27,* 353–368.

Gravel, J. S., Wallace, I. F., & Ruben, R. J. (1996). Auditory consequences of early mild hearing loss associated with otitis media. *Acta Otolaryngologica, 116,* 219–221.

Griffiths, T. D., Rees, G., Rees, A., Green, G. G., Witton, C., Rowe, D., et al. (1998). Right parietal cortex is involved in the perception of sound movement in humans. *Nature Neuroscience, 1,* 74–79.

Harrington, I. A., Heffner, R. S., & Heffner, H. E. (2001). An investigation of sensory deficits underlying the aphasia-like behavior of macaques with auditory cortex lesions. *NeuroReport, 12,* 1217–1221.

Hauser, M. D. (1992). Articulatory and social factors influence the acoustic structure of rhesus monkey vocalizations: A learned mode of production? *Journal of the Acoustical Society of America, 91,* 2175–2179.

Hauser, M. D. (1996). *The evolution of communication.* Cambridge, MA.: MIT Press.

Haxby, J. V., Maisog, L. M., & Courtney, S. M. (1999). Multiple regression analysis of effects of interest in fMRI time series. In J. Lancaster, P. Fox, & K. Friston (Eds.), *Mapping and modeling the human brain.* New York: Wiley.

Hebb, D. O. (1949). *The organization of behavior: A neurophysiological theory.* New York: Wiley.

Howard, M. A., Volkov, I. O., Abbas, P. J., Damasio, H., Ollendieck, M. C., & Granner, M. (1996). A chronic microelectrode investigation of the tonotopic organization of human auditory cortex. *Brain Research, 724,* 260–264.

Howard, M. A., Volkov, I. O., Mirsky, R., Garell, P. C., Noh, M. D., Granner, M., et al. (2000). Auditory cortex on the human posterior superior temporal gyrus. *Journal of Comparative Neurology, 416,* 79-92.

Hubel, D. H., & Wiesel, T. N. (1970). The period of susceptibility to the physiological effects of unilateral eye closure in kittens. *Journal of Physiology, 206,* 419-436.

Innocenti, G. M., & Clarke, S. (1984). Bilateral transitory projection from auditory cortex in kittens. *Developmental Brain Research, 14,* 143-148.

Irvine, D. R., Rajan, R., & Brown, M. (2001). Injury- and use-related plasticity in adult auditory cortex. *Audiology and Neuro-otology, 6,* 192-195.

Jääskeläinen, I. P., Ahveninen, J., Bonmassar, G., Dale, A. M., Ilmoniemi, R. J. L., S., Lin, F. H., et al. (2004). Human posterior auditory cortex gates novel sounds to consciousness. *Proceedings of the National Academy of Sciences, 101,* 6809-6814.

Jastreboff, P. J. (1990). Phantom auditory perception (tinnitus): mechanisms of generation and perception. *Neuroscience Research, 8,* 221-254.

Jastreboff, P. J., Brennan, J. F., Coleman, J. K., & Sasaki, C. T. (1988). Phantom auditory sensation in rats: an animal model for tinnitus. *Behavioral Neuroscience, 102,* 811-822.

Johnson, J. S., & Newport, E. L. (1989). Critical period effects in second language learning: The influence of maturational state on the acquisition of English as a second language. *Cognitive Psychology, 21,* 60-99.

Jusczyk, P. W., & Hohne, E. A. (1997). Infants' memory for spoken words. *Science, 277,* 1984-1986.

Kaas, J. H., & Hackett, T. A. (2000). Subdivisions of auditory cortex and processing streams in primates. *Proceedings of the National Academy of Sciences, 97,* 11793-11799.

Kanwal, J. S., & Rauschecker, J. P. (2007). Auditory cortex of bats and primates: managing species-specific calls for social communication. *Frontiers in Bioscience, 12,* 4621-4640.

Kanwisher, N., McDermott, J., & Chun, M. M. (1997). The fusiform face area: a module in human extrastriate cortex specialized for face perception. *Journal of Neuroscience, 17,* 4302-4311.

Kilgard, M. P., & Merzenich, M. M. (1998). Cortical map reorganization enabled by nucleus basalis activity. *Science, 279,* 1714-1718.

Kim, K. H., Relkin, N. R., Lee, K. M., & Hirsch, J. (1997). Distinct cortical areas associated with native and second languages. *Nature, 388,* 171-174.

King, A. J., & Parsons, C. (1999). Improved auditory spatial acuity in visually deprived ferrets. *European Journal of Neuroscience, 11,* 3945-3956.

King, A. J., & Semple, D. J. (1996). Improvement in auditory spatial acuity following early visual deprivation in ferrets. *Society for Neuroscience Abstracts.*

Klinke, R., Kral, A., Heid, S., Tillein, J., & Hartmann, R. (1999). Recruitment of the auditory cortex in congenitally deaf cats by long-term cochlear electrostimulation. *Science, 285,* 1729-1733.

Kohonen, T., & Hari, R. (1999). Where the abstract feature maps of the brain might come from. *Trends in Neuroscience, 22,* 135-139.

Korte, M., & Rauschecker, J. P. (1993). Auditory spatial tuning of cortical neurons is sharpened in cats with early blindness. *Journal of Neurophysiology, 70,* 1717-1721.

Kral, A., Hartmann, R., Tillein, J., Heid, S., & Klinke, R. (2001). Delayed maturation and sensitive periods in the auditory cortex. *Audiology and Neuro-Otology, 6,* 346-362.

Krumbholz, K., Schönwiesner, M., Rübsamen, R., Zilles, K., Fink, G. R., & von Cramon, D. Y. (2005). Hierarchical processing of sound location and motion in the human brainstem and planum temporale. *European Journal of Neuroscience, 21,* 230-238.

Krumbholz, K., Schönwiesner, M., von Cramon, D. Y., Rübsamen, R., Shah, N. J., Zilles, K., et al. (2005). Representation of interaural temporal information from left and right auditory space in the human planum temporale and inferior parietal lobe. *Cerebral Cortex, 15,* 317-324.

Kuhl, P. K. (2000). A new view of language acquisition. *Proceedings of the National Academy of Sciences, 97,* 11850-11857.

Kuhl, P. K., Williams, K. A., Lacerda, F., Stevens, K. N., & Lindblom, B. (1992). Linguistic experience alters phonetic perception in infants by 6 months of age. *Science, 255,* 606–608.

Kujala, T., Alho, K., Kekoni, J., Hämäläinen, H., Reinikainen, K., Salonen, O., et al. (1995). Auditory and somatosensory event-related brain potentials in early blind humans. *Experimental Brain Research, 104,* 519–526.

Kujala, T., Alho, K., Paavilainen, P., Summala, H., & Näätänen, R. (1992). Neural plasticity in processing sound location by the early blind: an event-related potential study. *Electroencephalography and Clinical Neurophysiology, 84,* 469–472.

Leaver, A. M., Renier, L., Purcell, J., Costanzo, M., Fieger, A., Morgan, S., et al. (2006). Auditory cortical map plasticity in tinnitus. *Society for Neuroscience Abstracts, 32.*

Lenneberg, E. H. (1967). *Biological foundations of language.* New York: John Wiley & Sons.

Lessard, N., Pare, M., Lepore, F., & Lassonde, M. (1998). Early-blind human subjects localize sound sources better than sighted subjects. *Nature, 395,* 278–280.

Levänen, S., & Hamdorf, D. (2001). Feeling vibrations: enhanced tactile sensitivity in congenitally deaf humans. *Neuroscience Letters, 301,* 75–77.

Levänen, S., Jousmaki, V., & Hari, R. (1998). Vibration-induced auditory-cortex activation in a congenitally deaf adult. *Current Biology, 8,* 869–872.

Levine, R. A. (1999). Somatic (craniocervical) tinnitus and the dorsal cochlear nucleus hypothesis. *American Journal of Otolaryngology, 20,* 351–362.

Levine, R. A. (2000). Somatic modulation of tinnitus: prevalence and properties. *Association for Research in Otolaryngology, 23,* 272A.

Lewis, J. W., & Van Essen, D. C. (2000). Corticocortical connections of visual, sensorimotor, and multimodal processing areas in the parietal lobe of the macaque monkey. *Journal of Comparative Neurology, 428,* 112–137.

Lively, S. E., Logan, J. S., & Pisoni, D. B. (1993). Training Japanese listeners to identify English /r/ and /l/. II: The role of phonetic environment and talker variability in learning new perceptual categories. *Journal of the Acoustical Society of America, 94,* 1242–1255.

Lockwood, A. H., Salvi, R. J., & Burkard, R. F. (2002). Tinnitus. *New England Journal of Medicine, 347,* 904–910.

Lockwood, A. H., Salvi, R. J., Burkard, R. F., Galantowicz, P. J., Coad, M. L., & Wack, D. S. (1999). Neuroanatomy of tinnitus. *Scandinavian Audiology Supplement, 51,* 47–52.

Lockwood, A. H., Salvi, R. J., Coad, M. L., Towsley, M. L., Wack, D. S., & Murphy, B. W. (1998). The functional neuroanatomy of tinnitus: evidence for limbic system links and neural plasticity. *Neurology, 50,* 114–120.

Loeb, G. E. (1985). The functional replacement of the ear. *Scientific American, 252,* 104–111.

Logan, J. S., Lively, S. E., & Pisoni, D. B. (1991). Training Japanese listeners to identify English /r/ and /l/: A first report. *Journal of the Acoustical Society of America, 89,* 874–886.

Lomber, S. G., Malhotra, S., & Hall, A. J. (2007). Functional specialization in non-primary auditory cortex of the cat: Areal and laminar contributions to sound localization. *Hearing Research, 229,* 31–45.

Maeder, P. P., Meuli, R. A., Adriani, M., Bellmann, A., Fornari, E., Thiran, J. P., et al. (2001). Distinct pathways involved in sound recognition and localization: a human fMRI study. *NeuroImage, 14,* 802–816.

Malhotra, S., Hall, A. J., & Lomber, S. G. (2004). Cortical control of sound localization in the cat: Unilateral cooling deactivation of 19 cerebral areas. *Journal of Neurophysiology, 92,* 1625–1643.

Martin, A., Wiggs, C. L., Ungerleider, L. G., & Haxby, J. V. (1996). Neural correlates of category-specific knowledge. *Nature, 379,* 649–652.

Matthies, C., & Samii, M. (1997). Management of 1000 vestibular schwannomas (acoustic neuromas): Clinical presentation. *Neurosurgery, 40,* 1–9; discussion 9–10.

Mesulam, M. M. (1999). Spatial attention and neglect: parietal, frontal and cingulate contributions to the mental representation and attentional targeting of salient extrapersonal events. *Philosophical Transactions of the Royal Society of London B Biological Sciences, 354,* 1325–1346.

Micheyl, C., Tian, B., Carlyon, R. P., & Rauschecker, J. P. (2005). Perceptual organization of tone sequences in the auditory cortex of awake macaques. *Neuron, 48,* 139–148.

Moore, D. R., Hartley, D. E., & Hogan, S. C. (2003). Effects of otitis media with effusion (OME) on central auditory function. *International Journal of Pediatric Otorhinolaryngology, 67*(Suppl. 1), S63–S67.

Moore, D. R., Hine, J. E., Jiang, Z. D., Matsuda, H., Parsons, C. H., & King, A. J. (1999). Conductive hearing loss produces a reversible binaural hearing impairment. *Journal of Neuroscience, 19,* 8704–8711.

Moore, D. R., Hutchings, M. E., & Meyer, S. E. (1991). Binaural masking level differences in children with a history of otitis media. *Audiology, 30,* 91–101.

Muchnik, C., Efrati, M., Nemeth, E., Malin, M., & Hildesheimer, M. (1991). Central auditory skills in blind and sighted subjects. *Scandinavian Audiology, 20,* 19–23.

Mühlau, M., Rauschecker, J. P., Oestreicher, E., Gaser, C., Röttinger, M., Wohlschläger, A. M., et al. (2006). Structural brain changes in tinnitus. *Cerebral Cortex, 16,* 1283–1288.

Mühlnickel, W., Elbert, T., Taub, E., & Flor, H. (1998). Reorganization of auditory cortex in tinnitus. *Proceedings of the National Academy of Sciences, 95,* 10340–10343.

Mummery, C. J., Patterson, K., Price, C. J., Ashburner, J., Frackowiak, R. S., & Hodges, J. R. (2000). A voxel-based morphometry study of semantic dementia: Relationship between temporal lobe atrophy and semantic memory. *Annals of Neurology, 47,* 36–45.

Neville, H. J., Bavelier, D., Corina, D., Rauschecker, J. P., Karni, A., Lalwani, A., et al. (1998). Cerebral organization for language in deaf and hearing subjects: biological constraints and effects of experience. *Proceedings of the National Academy of Sciences, 95,* 922–929.

Neville, H. J., & Lawson, D. (1987). Attention to central and peripheral visual space in a movement detection task: An event-related potential and behavioral study. II. Congenitally deaf adults. *Brain Research, 405,* 268–283.

Nishimura, H., Haskikawa, K., Doi, K., Iwaki, T., Watanabe, Y., Kusuoka, H., et al. (1999). Sign language "heard" in the auditory cortex. *Nature, 397,* 116.

Norena, A. J., & Eggermont, J. J. (2003). Changes in spontaneous neural activity immediately after an acoustic trauma: implications for neural correlates of tinnitus. *Hearing Research, 183,* 137–153.

Obleser, J., Boecker, H., Drzezga, A., Haslinger, B., Hennenlotter, A., Roettinger, M., et al. (2006). Vowel sound extraction in anterior superior temporal cortex. *Human Brain Mapping, 27,* 562–571.

Ojemann, G. A., & Whitaker, H. A. (1978). The bilingual brain. *Archives of Neurology, 35,* 409–412.

Pantev, C., Oostenveld, R., Engelien, A., Ross, B., Roberts, L. E., & Hoke, M. (1998). Increased auditory cortical representation in musicians. *Nature, 392,* 811–814.

Pantev, C., Ross, B., Fujioka, T., Trainor, L. J., Schulte, M., & Schulz, M. (2003). Music and learning-induced cortical plasticity. *Annals of the New York Academy of Sciences, 999,* 438–450.

Pascual-Leone, A., & Hamilton, R. (2001). The metamodal organization of the brain. *Progress in Brain Research, 134,* 427–445.

Petitto, L. A., Zatorre, R. J., Gauna, K., Nikelski, E. J., Dostie, D., & Evans, A. C. (2000). Speech-like cerebral activity in profoundly deaf people processing signed languages: implications for the neural basis of human language. *Proceedings of the National Academy of Sciences, 97,* 13961–13966.

Pons, T. P., Garraghty, P. E., Ommaya, A. K., Kaas, J. H., Taub, E., & Mishkin, M. (1991). Massive cortical reorganization after sensory deafferentation in adult macaques. *Science, 252,* 1857–1860.

Rajan, R., Irvine, D. R., Wise, L. Z., & Heil, P. (1993). Effect of unilateral partial cochlear lesions in adult cats on the representation of lesioned and unlesioned cochleas in primary auditory cortex. *Journal of Comparative Neurology, 338,* 17–49.

Rajan, R., & Irvine, D. R. F. (1998). Neuronal responses across cortical field A1 in Plasticity induced by peripheral auditory organ damage. *Audiology and Neuro-Otology, 3,* 123–144.

Rauschecker, J. P. (1991). Mechanisms of visual plasticity: Hebb synapses, NMDA receptors, and beyond. *Physiological Reviews, 71,* 587–615.

Rauschecker, J. P. (1995). Compensatory plasticity and sensory substitution in the cerebral cortex. *Trends in Neuroscience, 18,* 36–43.

Rauschecker, J. P. (1998a). Cortical control of the thalamus: Top-down processing and plasticity. *Nature Neuroscience, 1,* 179–180.

Rauschecker, J. P. (1998b). Cortical processing of complex sounds. *Current Opinions in Neurobiology, 8,* 516–521.

Rauschecker, J. P. (1999a). Auditory cortical plasticity: A comparison with other sensory systems. *Trends in Neuroscience, 22,* 74–80.

Rauschecker, J. P. (1999b). Making brain circuits listen. *Science, 285,* 1686–1687.

Rauschecker, J. P. (2002a). Auditory reassignment. In F. Boller & J. Grafman (Eds.), *Handbook of neuropsychology. Vol. 9: Plasticity and rehabilitation* (2nd ed, pp. 167–176). Amsterdam: Elsevier.

Rauschecker, J. P. (2002b). Crossmodal consequences of visual deprivation. In G. Calvert, C. Spence, & B. E. Stein (Eds.), *Handbook of multisensory processes* (pp. 695–702). Cambridge, MA: MIT Press.

Rauschecker, J. P. (2006). Plasticity in auditory functions. In M. Selzer, S. Clarke, L. Cohen, P. Duncan, & F. Gage (Eds.), *Textbook of neural repair and rehabilitation, Vol. 1. Neural repair and plasticity* (pp. 162–179). Cambridge: Cambridge University Press.

Rauschecker, J. P. (2007). Cortical processing of auditory space: pathways and plasticity. In F. Mast & L. Jäncke (Eds.), *Spatial processing in navigation, imagery, and perception* (pp. 189–410). New York: Springer-Verlag.

Rauschecker, J. P., & Kniepert, U. (1994). Enhanced precision of auditory localization behavior in visually deprived cats. *European Journal of Neuroscience, 6,* 149–160.

Rauschecker, J. P., & Korte, M. (1993). Auditory compensation for early blindness in cat cerebral cortex. *Journal of Neuroscience, 13,* 4538–4548.

Rauschecker, J. P., & Singer, W. (1981). The effects of early visual experience on the cat's visual cortex and their possible explanation by Hebb synapses. *Journal of Physiology, 310,* 215–239.

Rauschecker, J. P., & Tian, B. (2000). Mechanisms and streams for processing of "what" and "where" in auditory cortex. *Proceedings of the National Academy of Sciences, 97,* 11800–11806.

Recanzone, G. H. (2000). Spatial processing in the auditory cortex of the macaque monkey. *Proceedings of the National Academy of Sciences, 97,* 11829–11835.

Recanzone, G. H., Schreiner, C. E., & Merzenich, M. M. (1993). Plasticity in the frequency representation of primary auditory cortex following discrimination training in adult owl monkeys. *Journal of Neuroscience, 13,* 87–103.

Rice, C. E. (1970). Early blindness, early experience, and perceptual enhancement. *Research Bulletin of the American Foundation for the Blind, 22,* 1–22.

Rice, C. E., Feinstein, S. H., & Schusterman, R. J. (1965). Echo-detection ability of the blind: size and distance factor. *Journal of Experimental Psychology, 70,* 246–251.

Rockland, K. S., & Ojima, H. (2003). Multisensory convergence in calcarine visual areas in macaque monkey. *International Journal of Psychophysiology, 50,* 19–26.

Röder, B., Teder-Salejarvi, W., Sterr, A., Rösler, F., Hillyard, S. A., & Neville, H. J. (1999). Improved auditory spatial tuning in blind humans. *Nature, 400,* 162–166.

Romanski, L. M., Tian, B., Fritz, J., Mishkin, M., Goldman-Rakic, P. S., & Rauschecker, J. P. (1999). Dual streams of auditory afferents target multiple domains in the primate prefrontal cortex. *Nature Neuroscience, 2,* 1131–1136.

Schlaug, G., Jancke, L., Huang, Y., & Steinmetz, H. (1995). In vivo evidence of structural brain asymmetry in musicians. *Science, 267,* 699–701.

Scott, S. K., Blank, C. C., Rosen, S., & Wise, R. J. (2000). Identification of a pathway for intelligible speech in the left temporal lobe. *Brain, 123*(Pt. 12), 2400–2406.

Seidman, M. D., & Jacobson, G. P. (1996). Update on tinnitus. *Otolaryngology Clinics of North America, 29,* 455–465.

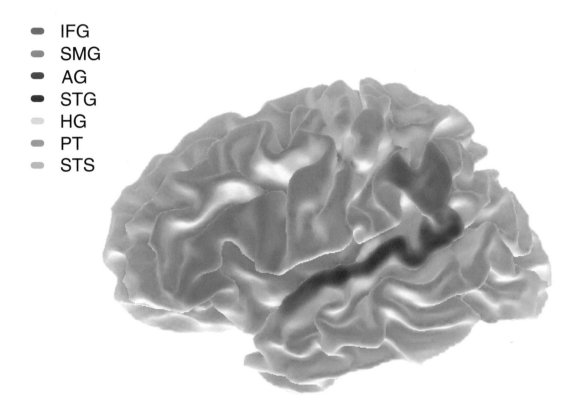

Plate 3–1. Surface view of the left hemisphere. Approximate macroanatomic locations of cortical regions that are engaged in auditory and speech processing are highlighted in color. IFG, inferior frontal gyrus; SMG, supramarginal gyrus; AG, angular gyrus; STG, superior temporal gyrus; HG, transverse temporal gyrus (Heschl's gyrus); PT, planum temporale; STS, superior temporal sulcus.

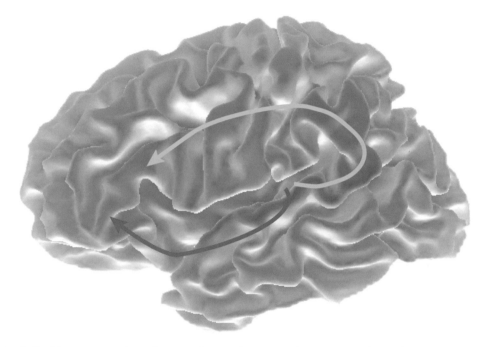

Plate 3–2. Two processing streams from primary auditory cortex have been proposed on the basis of electrophysiologic work in nonhuman primates, and functional neuroimaging in humans. The ventral pathway (*red*) runs along STG, anterior STS, and ventrolateral IFG. The dorsal pathway (*green*) comprises PT, posterior STG, AG, SMG, and posterior IFG. The respective roles of the ventral and dorsal pathways have not yet become clearly established, although the former has been associated with extracting linguistic meaning from acoustic-phonetic structure, whereas the latter has been suggested to form a link of perception with production and aspects of verbal working memory.

Gray Matter R1
on the Superior Temporal Lobe

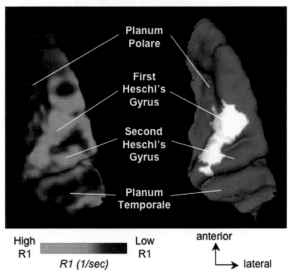

Plate 5–1. High R1 overlapping Heschl's gyrus may coincide with primary auditory cortex. *Left:* A spatial map of R1 over the right superior temporal lobe of one subject. R1 is indicated in color on a dark blue (low R1) to light blue (high R1) scale. The distribution of R1 suggests that gray matter myelin content is generally least anteriorly (in planum polare), intermediate posteriorly (on planum temporale), and greatest on the posteromedial aspect of Heschl's gyrus. *Right:* R1 map after thresholding to show only the region of highest R1 (*white*). The location of this region (the posteromedial part of Heschl's gyrus) is typical of the location of primary auditory cortex (koniocortex).

Mapping Gray Matter Thickness

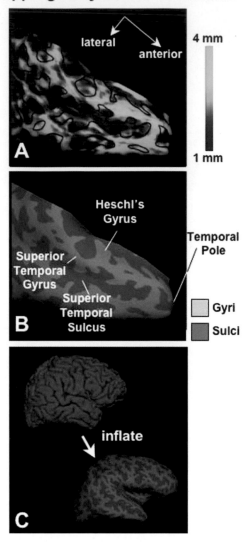

Plate 5–2. A. Spatial map of gray matter thickness displayed on a computationally inflated view of the temporal lobe. Thickness is indicated in gradations of blue. Black lines indicate the borders between sulci and gyri in the underlying anatomy. The anatomy can be seen in (**B**) where cortex of sulci and gyri is displayed in light and dark gray, respectively. **C.** Side view of a cortical surface resconstruction before (*top, left*) and after (*bottom, right*) inflation. The thickness map was obtained from T1-weighted images of the whole brain (MPRAGE, 1.5 Tesla scanner, voxel size: 1 mm × 1 mm × 1 mm) using FreeSurfer (Dale et al., 1999; Fischl et al., 1999). Thickness values were determined using the original, uninflated cortex. One subject.

Seyfarth, R. M., Cheney, D. L., & Marler, P. (1980). Monkey responses to three different alarm calls: Evidence of predator classification and semantic communication. *Science, 210,* 801–803.

Shahin, A., Bosnyak, D. J., Trainor, L. J., & Roberts, L. E. (2003). Enhancement of neuroplastic P2 and N1c auditory evoked potentials in musicians. *Journal of Neuroscience, 23,* 5545–5552.

Sommers, M. S. (1997). Speech perception in older adults: the importance of speech-specific cognitive abilities. *Journal of the American Geriatric Society, 45,* 633–637.

Spinelli, D. N., Starr, A., & Barrett, T. W. (1968). Auditory specificity in unit recordings from cat's visual cortex. *Experimental Neurology, 22,* 75–84.

Stricanne, B., Andersen, R. A., & Mazzoni, P. (1996). Eye-centered, head-centered, and intermediate coding of remembered sound locations in area LIP. *Journal of Neurophysiology 76,* 2071–2076.

Suga, N., & Ma, X. (2003). Multiparametric corticofugal modulation and plasticity in the auditory system. *Nature Reviews Neuroscience, 4,* 783–794.

Svirsky, M. A., Robbins, A. M., Kirk, K. I., Pisoni, D. B., & Miyamoto, R. T. (2000). Language development in profoundly deaf children with cochlear implants. *Psychological Science, 11,* 153–158.

Talairach, J., & Tournoux, P. (1988). *A coplanar sterotaxic atlas of the human brain.* Stuttgart, Germany: Thieme-Verlag.

Tata, M. S., & Ward, L. M. (2005a). Early phase of spatial mismatch negativity is localized to a posterior "where" auditory pathway. *Experimental Brain Research, 167,* 481–486.

Tata, M. S., & Ward, L. M. (2005b). Spatial attention modulates activity in a posterior "where" auditory pathway. *Neuropsychologia, 43,* 509–516.

Tian, B., Reser, D., Durham, A., Kustov, A., & Rauschecker, J. P. (2001). Functional specialization in rhesus monkey auditory cortex. *Science, 292,* 290–293.

Trainor, L. J., Shahin, A., & Roberts, L. E. (2003). Effects of musical training on the auditory cortex in children. *Annals of the New York Academy of Sciences, 999,* 506–513.

Tsao, D. Y., Freiwald, W. A., Tootell, R. B., & Livingstone, M. S. (2006). A cortical region consisting entirely of face-selective cells. *Science, 311,* 670–674.

Ungerleider, L. G., & Mishkin, M. (1982). Two cortical visual systems. In D. J. Ingle, M. A. Goodale, & R. J. W. Mansfield (Eds.), *Analysis of visual behavior* (pp. 549–586). Cambridge, MA: MIT Press.

Vignolo, L. A. (1982). Auditory agnosia. *Philosophical Transactions of the Royal Society of London B Biological Sciences, 298,* 49–57.

Wallhäusser-Franke, E., Braun, S., & Langner, G. (1996). Salicylate alters 2-DG uptake in the auditory system: A model for tinnitus? *NeuroReport, 7,* 1585–1588.

Wallhäusser-Franke, E., Mahlke, C., Oliva, R., Braun, S., Wenz, G., & Langner, G. (2003). Expression of c-fos in auditory and non-auditory brain regions of the gerbil after manipulations that induce tinnitus. *Experimental Brain Research, 153,* 649–654.

Warren, J. D., Zielinski, B. A., Green, G. G. R., Rauschecker, J. P., & Griffiths, T. D. (2002). Analysis of sound source motion by the human brain. *Neuron, 34,* 1–20.

Weeks, R., Horwitz, B., Aziz-Sultan, A., Tian, B., Wessinger, C. M., Cohen, L., et al. (2000). A positron emission tomographic study of auditory localisation in the congenitally blind. *Journal of Neuroscience, 20,* 2664–2672.

Weeks, R. A., Aziz-Sultan, A., Bushara, K. O., Tian, B., Wessinger, C. M., Dang, N., et al. (1999). A PET study of human auditory spatial processing. *Neuroscience Letters, 262,* 155–158.

Weinberger, N. M. (2003). The nucleus basalis and memory codes: auditory cortical plasticity and the induction of specific, associative behavioral memory. *Neurobiology, Learning, and Memory, 80,* 268–284.

Werker, J. F., & Logan, J. S. (1985). Cross-language evidence for three factors in speech perception. *Perception and Psychophysics, 37,* 35–44.

Wiesel, T. N. (1982). Postnatal development of the visual cortex and the influence of environment. *Nature, 299,* 583–591.

Xu, H., Kotak, V. C., & Sanes, D. H. (2007). Conductive hearing loss disrupts synaptic and spike adaptation in developing auditory cortex. *Journal of Neuroscience, 27,* 9417–9426.

Zatorre, R. J., Bouffard, M., Ahad, P., & Belin, P. (2002). Where is 'where' in the human auditory cortex? *Nature Neuroscience, 5,* 905–909.

Zatorre, R. J., Bouffard, M., & Belin, P. (2004). Sensitivity to auditory object features in human temporal neocortex. *Journal of Neuroscience, 24,* 3637–3642.

Zimmer, U., & Macaluso, E. (2005). High binaural coherence determines successful sound localization and increased activity in posterior auditory areas. *Neuron, 47,* 893–905.

Zoloth, S. R., Petersen, M. R., Beecher, M. D., Green, S., Marler, P., Moody, D. B., et al. (1979). Species-specific perceptual processing of vocal sounds by monkeys. *Science, 204,* 870–873.

CHAPTER 5

Imaging Gray Matter Structure in Living Humans: Implications for Understanding Auditory Processing

JENNIFER R. MELCHER

This chapter describes our group's recent structural MRI studies of the auditory cortex in humans. These studies took a preliminary look at how several relatively new approaches can be used to discern, in living humans, the internal architecture of auditory cortical gray matter. Our studies were motivated by functional MRI work—our own and that of many others—and a desire to relate fMRI activation patterns directly to the architecturally distinct areas known to reside within the gray matter of the superior temporal lobe and comprise auditory cortex (von Economo, 1929; Galaburda & Sanides, 1980). The primary objective of the work described here was to establish whether structural MRI of the gray matter could be used to delineate auditory

cortical areas directly in individual, living subjects.

However, the work we describe also has implications for understanding the structural bases of auditory behavior. One of the oldest neuroscientific approaches for understanding the brain's role in any form of behavior (including auditory) involves correlating brain abnormalities with behavioral impairments (Efron, 1963; Zatorre, 1988). The insights to be gained from this approach expanded dramatically with the development of noninvasive brain imaging techniques, including MRI. They have further expanded as MRI technology and image analysis tools have matured. At this point in time, MR images showing striking distinctions between tissues (e.g., gray and white matter) are more or less expected, and the resolution of structure within the approximately 3 millimeter thickness of the gray matter has been clearly demonstrated (Duyn et al., 2007). These and other capabilities make it possible to detect even subtle and highly localized brain abnormalities and compare them with behavioral measures. Here, we illustrate some of the capabilities of MRI and also suggest new questions that could be addressed regarding the relationship between cortical gray matter structure and auditory behavior.

In the following sections, three types of structural MRI results are summarized. The first were obtained by mapping an intrinsic MR property of tissue that is sensitive to myelin. We reasoned this approach might allow the delineation of at least one division of auditory cortex, koniocortex (i.e., primary auditory cortex), as the gray matter of koniocortex contains a high concentration of myelinated fibers, higher than any other part of the gray matter of the superior temporal lobe. This approach did indeed provide a promising marker for koniocortex and, in addition, revealed intriguing hemispheric differences in gray matter myelination of the temporal lobe. A second set of results involves mapping gray matter thickness, an aspect of the gray matter known to change during learning and covary with behavior (Anderson, Eckburg, & Relucio, 2002; Milad et al., 2005). Our studies did not examine thickness in relation to behavioral performance, but nevertheless provide some basic information that may be of use to others wishing to do so. The third set of results illustrate the detail with which the internal (i.e., laminar) structure of gray matter can be discerned using high spatial resolution (~100 μm) MRI, and a way that auditory areas other than koniocortex might be delineated. However, to begin, we first present some background.

Background

In both humans and nonhuman primates, the auditory cortical areas of the superior temporal lobe form several major distinctions: a core area with histologic features of primary sensory cortex (i.e., koniocortex or Brodmann area 41), belt areas flanking the core medially and laterally, and lateral parabelt areas (e.g., Kaas, Hackett, & Tramo, 1999; Hackett, Chapter 2 of this volume). These areas (and subareas thereof) have been distinguished based on a variety of anatomic criteria: cytoarchitectonic, myeloarchitectonic, immunohistochemical, and connectional (Brodmann, 1909; Galaburda & Sanides, 1980; Hackett, Preuss, & Kaas, 2001; Hopf, 1968; Rivier & Clarke, 1997; von Economo, 1929). The myelin-stained histologic material in Figure 5–1 illustrates some of the differences between areas. The gray matter of the auditory core, containing primary auditory cortex, is characterized by high myelin content reflecting a high density of thalamocortical fibers running perpendicular to the deeper gray matter layers. The medial, and especially, the lateral belt flanking the core are characterized by a concentration of staining within the gray matter input layer (IV). The histologic sections displayed in Figure 5–1 were chosen because they are stained for myelin, to which MRI is highly sensitive. Thus, they illustrate structural attributes of tissue that can potentially be discerned using MRI. Our structural MRI studies sought to resolve two particular attributes, the overall difference in gray matter myelin content between core and belt, and the concentration of myelination defining layer IV.

Histologic studies of human auditory cortex have established general positional relationships between the different architectural divisions of auditory cortex and the gross morphology of the superior temporal

Human Auditory Cortex: Histology

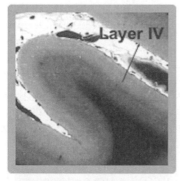

lateral belt

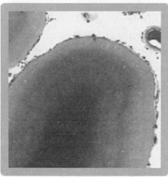

core

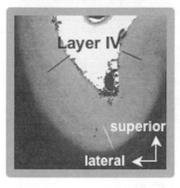

medial belt

Figure 5–1. Myelin-stained histologic sections through the lateral belt (*top*), core (*middle*), and medial belt (*bottom*) of human auditory cortex. The sections (coronal) are from a brain processed according to the method of Yakovlev (1970) and described in detail by Fullerton and Pandya (2007; brain 1). Irina Sigalovsky and Barbara Fullerton (Eaton-Peabody Laboratory, Massachusetts Eye and Ear Infirmary, Boston, MA) provided these photomicrographs.

lobe. The organizational center of auditory cortex, the core region, generally overlaps posteromedial Heschl's gyrus, in particular, the more anterior gyrus when there are two (e.g., Rademacher, Caviness, Steinmetz, & Galaburda, 1993). The lateral belt and parabelt areas extend laterally onto the planum temporale and superior temporal gyrus, whereas the medial belt extends into the circular sulcus.

However, histologic studies have also demonstrated considerable intersubject variability in the disposition and extent of the core (and therefore presumably the surrounding belt areas) relative to Heschl's gyrus (Rademacher et al., 1993, 2001; Sweet, Anton, Petersen, & Lewis, 2005). This variability, and a strong interest in relating the functions of auditory cortex to its structure, has led to methods for coregistering auditory cortical functions to the various anatomically defined divisions (i.e., mapping functionally imaged brains into normalized coordinates, into surface-based coordinates or onto atlases indicating the probability that a given brain region coincides with a cytoarchitectonically defined area) (Fischl, Sereno, & Dale, 1999; Rademacher et al., 2001; Talairach & Tournoux, 1988). These methods, being approximate, may obscure relationships between structure and function that would be seen if gray matter architecture and function could be related to one another directly on an individual basis. The results presented here are a step toward making direct architectural/functional comparisons.

Spatially Mapping an Intrinsic MR Property Sensitive to Myelin

Our interest in mapping intrinsic MR properties of the gray matter (e.g., longitudinal and transverse relaxation rate) stems from the sensitivity of these properties to various aspects of gray matter composition (e.g., myelin and iron content) including aspects that change during development, with disease, or between cortical areas (Besson, Greentree, Foster, & Rimmington, 1989; Steen, Reddick, & Ogg, 2000; Vymazal et al., 1999; Yoshiura et al., 2000). Our experiments (Sigalovsky, Fischl, & Melcher, 2006) mapped a particular intrinsic MR tissue property, R1 (i.e., the reciprocal of T1). R1, the longitudinal relaxation rate for protons excited in the imaging process, can depend on various microscopic tissue properties (e.g., see Gore & Kennan, 1999). However, a predominant factor influencing R1 is tissue myelin content, a point illustrated by the contrast between gray and white matter in R1-weighted images. Our approach involved first estimating R1 for each voxel in the brain (by systematically varying the flip angle of the radiofrequency excitation and using the resulting variations in image signal to estimate R1; Fischl et al., 2004). R1 was then averaged across the depth of the gray matter at finely spaced points covering the cortical surface, and spatially mapped over the surface of the superior temporal lobe (Color Plate 3, left). Note that the resulting maps do not show how R1 varies across the depth of the gray matter, but rather show the spatial distribution of overall R1 over a 2-D "sheet" covering the superior temporal lobe.

A Putative Marker for Primary Auditory Cortex

Mappings of R1 over the superior temporal lobe of normal human subjects showed several trends, including low R1 on planum polare, intermediate levels of R1 on planum temporale, and high R1 on Heschl's gyrus, particularly posteromedially as illustrated in Color Plate 5–1 (left). The high R1 overlapping Heschl's gyrus is especially intrigu-

ing because it forms a distinct region defined by a sharp decline in R1 medially and laterally (Figure 6 in Sigalovsky et al., 2006). The R1 value approximately midway in this decline was used as a the cutoff for the thresholded R1 map in Color Plate 5–1 (right) showing only the highest R1 on the superior temporal lobe. A distinct region of high R1 overlapping Heschl's gyrus (the first when there were two) was a consistent finding across subjects and hemispheres.

The high R1 overlapping Heschl's gyrus resembles koniocortex in several ways. (1) The high R1 has the same general location as koniocortex, and also differs in location from subject-to-subject in a manner expected based on histologic localizations of koniocortex (e.g., compare Figure 5 in Sigalovsky et al., 2006 with Figure 2 in Rademacher et al., 2001). (2) Koniocortex is an area of especially heavy myelination (e.g., Figure 5–1, middle panel), and so, presumably are regions of high R1. (3) And finally, the heavy myelination of koniocortex rapidly gives way to lower myelination medially and laterally (Hackett et al., 2001; Hopf, 1968) as does R1 at the edges of the high R1 overlapping Heschl's gyrus. We concluded that high R1 may provide a marker for koniocortex in individual, living subjects.

Hemispheric Differences

In addition to varying across the superior temporal lobe, R1 also differed between hemispheres. Planum temporale, superior temporal gyrus, superior temporal sulcus, and to some extent posteromedial Heschl's gyrus, showed greater R1 on the left. (Anterolateral Heschl's gyrus and a region corresponding roughly to the medial belt showed no difference between hemispheres.) The finding of greater R1 on the left in some areas is interesting in light of functional data suggesting that the left hemisphere is preferentially involved in the processing of rapid temporal changes in acoustic signals (Efron, 1963; Liégeois-Chauvel, de Graaf, Laguitton, & Chauvel, 1999; Zatorre & Belin, 2001). In particular, the hemispheric differences in gray matter R1 suggest a left-right difference in gray matter myelination. Because myelin plays a crucial role in maintaining the timing of neural activity, greater myelination on the left could increase the precision of neural timing, thus providing the left hemisphere with an enhanced ability (over the right) to discriminate and follow rapid acoustic changes. More generally, greater gray matter myelination on the left could be a substrate for the left hemisphere's specialized processing of speech and language, as well as rapid acoustic changes.

Spatially Mapping Gray Matter Thickness

In addition to mapping R1, we also mapped gray matter thickness, a basic morphologic parameter, and an interesting one because of its dependence on the neural composition of the gray matter, for example, cell number, size, and packing density. We set out to determine whether thickness could be used to delineate auditory cortical areas and, in the process, established some basic facts about gray matter thickness on the superior temporal lobe.

Quantification of gray matter thickness was performed using automated methods and began with images optimized for showing contrast between gray and white matter (Fischl & Dale, 2000; MacDonald, Kabani, Avis, & Evans, 2000). Thickness was estimated from these high-contrast images by first segmenting the gray matter from adjacent white matter and cerebrospinal fluid (CSF), then determining the shortest distance between the gray matter/CSF and gray matter/white matter surfaces at finely spaced points covering the cortical surface. Importantly, these calculations were based on a 3-D representation of the cortex, so the resulting thickness values were free of the overestimation inherent in measuring thickness from 2-D slices (histologic or MR). (In 2-D slices, much of the gray matter will be intersected obliquely, resulting in a systematic overestimation of thickness.) Sample thickness data for the temporal lobe of one subject are shown in Color Plate 5–2A. Thickness (coded in color) has been spatially mapped over the computationally inflated cortical surface (Color Plates 5–2B and 5–2C). The inflation allows the thickness of gray matter in sulci and on gyri, to be appreciated in a single view. The map illustrates the well-documented fact that the gray matter of gyri is generally thicker than that of sulci (Blinkov & Glezer, 1968; von Economo, 1929). This qualitative observation can also be expressed quantitatively as a correlation between the thickness of cortical gray matter and its surface curvature (r~0.6; Sigalovsky et al., 2006).

When we examined whether thickness maps might be used to isolate cortical areas in the same manner as R1 maps were used, the results were not promising. For instance, circumscribed regions of either high or low thickness as might correspond to a cortical area were not seen, even after adjusting the maps to compensate for the correlation between thickness and cortical curvature. Despite this negative result, the findings for thickness nevertheless provided confirmation of the validity of the methods in that gray matter thickness was generally greater on the temporal lobe than in the rest of the cerebrum and tended to increase from posterior to anterior as described previously in histologic material (von Economo, 1929). The absolute values for gray matter thickness were also in approximate agreement with thickness values based on histology

(~3 mm; von Economo, 1929), but tended to run slightly less, perhaps because of the overestimation inherent in measuring thickness from 2-D tissue slices (as von Economo did).

Although mapping gray matter thickness may not be useful for delineating auditory cortical areas, it may still prove highly informative in studies of auditory cortical processing. Thickness mapping has provided insights into numerous central nervous system processes including learning, extinction of conditioning, cognitive aspects of aging, and the progression of neurologic or psychiatric disease (Draganski et al., 2004; Milad et al., 2005; Narr et al., 2005; Rosas et al., 2002; Sailer et al., 2003; Salat et al., 2004; Sowell et al., 2003; Thompson et al., 2004). Among the large number of studies examining gray matter thickness in human subjects, almost none have examined thickness in direct relation to either auditory or speech processing (Kang, Yund, & Woods, 2003; Sigalovsky et al., 2006). Interesting, but unaddressed questions include whether thickness changes occur during auditory training, during language acquisition or following damage to the auditory periphery, to name only a few examples.

Imaging the Internal Structure of Gray Matter

Although R1 mapping may provide a marker for koniocortex in human subjects, it still leaves us without a means for distinguishing other cortical areas. High-resolution imaging of the laminar structure of the gray matter may ultimately help fill this gap. Using submillimeter spatial resolution, it is possible to obtain images of gray matter laminar structure showing detail approaching that of low-magnification microscopic images of myelin stained tissue. Figures 5–2 and 5–3

Laminar Structure of Gray Matter (postmortem tissue)

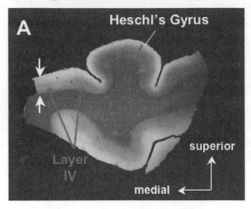

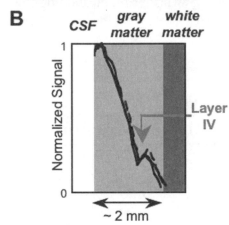

Figure 5–2. A. MR image of postmortem human material showing the laminar structure of the gray matter on and adjacent to Heschl's gyrus. The imaging plane is approximately coronal. The image resolution (100 × 100 × 100 μm) allows details of the gray matter (e.g., layer IV) to be discerned. **B.** Image signal versus depth within the gray matter (*between white arrows in [A]*). Image obtained in collaboration with Graham Wiggins at the Athinoula A. Martinos Center for Biomedical Imaging, Massachusetts General Hospital, Charlestown.

illustrate this with images of postmortem tissue and living brains, respectively (Barbier et al., 2002; Duyn et al., 2007; Eickhoff

Laminar Structure
of Human Cortical Gray Matter (in vivo)

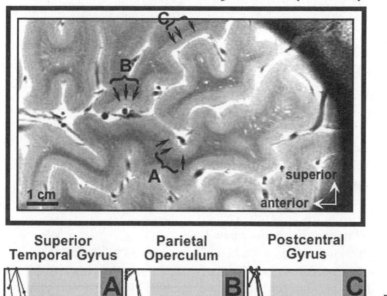

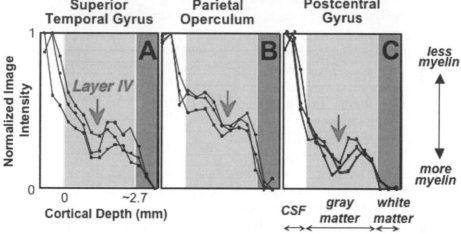

Figure 5–3. Layer IV of the gray matter in a living subject. Imaging time approximately 7 minutes. *Top:* Arrows point to bands of low signal intensity within the gray matter of auditory and nonauditory regions in a sagittal, T2-weighted image. The bands likely reflect concentrated myelin within layer IV. *Bottom:* Image signal intensity plotted vs. cortical depth in (**A**) superior temporal gyrus, (**B**) parietal operculum, (**C**) postcentral gyrus. The dips in signal within the gray matter correspond to the bands of low signal intensity (i.e., layer IV). In-plane resolution: 350 × 270 μm. Slice thickness: 1.5 mm. Image sequence: turbo spin echo. Scanner field strength: 3 tesla. Phased array surface coil. Image obtained in collaboration with Lawrence Wald at the Athinoula A. Martinos Center for Biomedical Imaging, Massachusetts General Hospital, Charlestown.

et al., 2005; Walters et al., 2003). In both examples, there is visible structure within the gray matter, including bands of low signal intensity corresponding to layer IV. It remains to be seen whether high-resolution MRI can robustly and routinely capture subtle differences in laminar profile between non-primary areas of living cortex. However, the emerging data are promising.

Future Directions

Being able to delimit auditory koniocortex and perhaps, eventually, other architectonic areas directly in individual, living humans should enable new advances in our understanding of the relationship between cortical structure and function. However, structural imaging of cortical gray matter also opens other possibilities. For instance, changes in gray matter myelination that occur in auditory cortex early in life could be tracked in ways not possible from limited amounts of histologic material. Given the important role that myelin plays in maintaining the timing of neural activity, it may prove interesting to examine MR indicators of myelin (e.g., R1) in people with auditory temporal processing deficits. More generally, insights into the structural substrates behind human hearing and speech perception might be obtained by assessing gray matter structural variables in patients with auditory psychophysical deficits or communication disorders. In sum, structural MRI approaches like those illustrated here present an opportunity to better understand the relationship between cortical gray matter structure and many diverse aspects of auditory behavior.

Acknowledgments. The author thanks Irina Sigalovsky, Lawrence Wald, Graham Wiggins, Haobing Wang, and Barbara Fullerton for their help in obtaining (and in the case of I.S. and H.W., analyzing) the images in the figures. She also thanks Barbara Norris for her assistance in preparing the figures. This work was supported in part by NIH/NIDCD R21 DC006071 and P30 DC005209.

References

Anderson, B. J., Eckburg, P. B., & Relucio, K. I. (2002). Alterations in the thickness of motor cortical subregions after motor-skill learning and exercise. *Learning and Memory*, *9*, 1–9.

Barbier, E. L., Marrett, S., Danek, A., Vortmeyer, A., van Gelderen, P., Duyn, J., et al. (2002). Imaging cortical anatomy by high-resolution MR at 3.0T: Detection of the stripe of Gennari in visual area 17. *Magnetic Resonance in Medicine*, *48*, 735–738.

Besson, J. A. O., Greentree, S. G., Foster, M. A., & Rimmington, J. E. (1989). Regional variation in rat brain proton relaxation times and water content. *Magnetic Resonance Imaging*, *7*, 141–143.

Blinkov, S., & Glezer, I. (1968). *The human brain in figures and tables: A quantitative handbook*. New York: Basic Books.

Brodmann, K., (1909). *Brodmann's "localisation in the cerebral cortex."* London: Smith-Gordon.

Dale, A. M., Fischl, B., & Sereno, M. I. (1999). Cortical surface-based analysis. I. Segmentation and surface reconstruction. *NeuroImage*, *9*, 179–194.

Draganski, B., Gaser, C., Busch, V., Schuierer, G., Bogdahn, U., & May, A. (2004). Neuroplasticity: changes in grey matter induced by training. *Nature*, *427*, 311–312.

Duyn, J. H., van Gelderen, P., Li, T.-Q., de Zwart, J. A., Koretsky, A. P., & Fukunaga, M. (2007). High-field MRI of brain cortical substructure based on signal phase. *Proceedings of the National Academy of Sciences*, *104*, 11796–11801.

Efron, R. (1963). Temporal perception, aphasia and Déjá Vu. *Brain*, *86*, 403–424.

Eickhoff, S., Walters, N. B., Schleicher, A., Kril, J., Egan, G. F., Zilles, K., et al. (2005). High-resolution MRI reflects myeloarchitecture and cytoarchitecture of human cerebral cortex. *Human Brain Mapping*, *24*, 206–215.

Fischl, B., & Dale, A. M. (2000). Measuring the thickness of the human cerebral cortex from magnetic resonance images. *Proceedings of the National Academy of Sciences*, *97*, 11050–11055.

Fischl, B., Salat, D. H., van der Kouwe, A. J. W., Makris, N., Ségonne, F., Quinn, B. T., et al. (2004). Sequence-independent segmentation of magnetic resonance images. *NeuroImage*, *23*, S69–S84.

Fischl, B., Sereno, M. I., & Dale, A. M. (1999). Cortical surface-based analysis. II: Inflation, flattening, and a surface-based coordinate system. *NeuroImage*, *9*, 195–207.

Fullerton, B. C., & Pandya, D. N. (2007). Architectonic analysis of the auditory-related areas of the superior temporal region in human brain. *Journal of Comparative Neurology*, *504*, 470–498.

Galaburda, A., & Sanides, F. (1980). Cytoarchitectonic organization of the human auditory cortex. *Journal of Comparative Neurology*, *190*, 597–610.

Gore, J. C., & Kennan, R. P. (1999). Physical and physiological basis of magnetic relaxation. In D. D. Stark & W. G. Bradley, Jr. (Eds.), *Magnetic resonance imaging* (Vol. 1, pp. 33–42). St. Louis, MO: Mosby.

Hackett, T. A., Preuss, T. M., & Kaas, J. H. (2001). Architectonic identification of the core region in auditory cortex of macaques, chimpanzees, and humans. *Journal of Comparative Neurology*, *441*, 197–222.

Hopf, A. (1968). Photometric studies on the myeloarchitecture of the human temporal lobe [in German]. *J Hirnforsch.* 10, 285–297.

Kaas, J. H., Hackett, T. A., & Tramo, M. J. (1999). Auditory processing in primate cerebral cortex. *Current Opinion in Neurobiology*, *9*, 164–170.

Kang, X., Yund, B., & Woods, D. (2003). Cortical thickness measurements of human auditory cortex. *Abstracts for the International Society for Magnetic Resonance in Medicine.*

Liégeois-Chauvel, C., de Graaf, J.B., Laguitton, V., & Chauvel, P. (1999). Specialization of left auditory cortex for speech perception in man depends on temporal coding. *Cerebral Cortex*, *9*, 484–496.

MacDonald, D., Kabani, N., Avis, D., & Evans, A. C. (2000). Automated 3-D extraction of inner and outer surfaces of cerebral cortex from MRI. *NeuroImage*, *12*, 340–356.

Milad, M. R., Quinn, B. T., Pitman, R. K., Orr, S. P., Fischl, B., & Rauch, S. L. (2005). Thickness of ventromedial prefrontal cortex in humans is correlated with extinction memory. *Proceedings of the National Academy of Sciences*, *102*, 10706–10711.

Narr, K. L., Toga, A. W., Szeszko, P., Thompson, P. M., Woods, R. P., Robinson, D., et al. (2005). Cortical thinning in cingulated and occipital cortices in first episode schizophrenia. *Biological Psychiatry*, *58*, 32–40.

Rademacher, J., Caviness, V. S., Jr., Steinmetz, H., & Galaburda, A. M. (1993). Topographical variation of the human primary cortices: implications for neuroimaging, brain mapping, and neurobiology. *Cerebral Cortex*, *3*, 313–329.

Rademacher, J., Morosan, P., Schormann, T., Schleicher, A., Werner, C., Freund, H.-J., et al. (2001). Probabilistic mapping and volume measurement of human primary auditory cortex. *NeuroImage*, *13*, 669–683.

Rivier, F., & Clarke, S. (1997). Cytochrome oxidase, acetylcholinesterase, and NADPH-diaphorase staining in human supratemporal and insular cortex: evidence for multiple auditory areas. *NeuroImage*, *6*, 288–304.

Rosas, H. D., Liu, A. K., Hersch, S., Glessner, M., Ferrante, R. J., Salat, D. H., et al. (2002). Regional and progressive thinning of the cortical ribbon in Huntington's disease. *Neurology*, *58*, 695–701.

Sailer, M., Fischl, B., Salat, D., Tempelmann, C., Schonfeld, M. A., Busa, E., et al. (2003). Focal thinning of the cerebral cortex in multiple sclerosis. *Brain*, *126*, 1734–1744.

Salat, D. H., Buckner, R. L., Snyder, A. Z., Greve, D. N., Desikan, R. S., Busa, E., et al. (2004). Thinning of the cerebral cortex in aging. *Cerebral Cortex 14*, 721–730.

Sigalovsky, I. S., Fischl, B., & Melcher, J. R. (2006). Mapping an intrinsic MR property of gray matter in auditory cortex of living humans: A possible marker for primary cortex and hemispheric differences. *NeuroImage*, *32*, 1524–1537.

Sowell, E. R., Peterson, B. S., Thompson, P. M., Welcome, S. E., Henkenius, A. L., & Toga, A. W. (2003). Mapping cortical change across the human life span. *Nature Neuroscience, 6,* 309–315.

Steen, R. G., Reddick, W. E., & Ogg, R. J. (2000). More than meets the eye: Significant regional heterogeneity in human cortical T1. *Magnetic Resonance Imaging, 18,* 361–368.

Sweet, R. A., Anton, K., Petersen, D., & Lewis, D. A. (2005). Mapping auditory core, lateral belt, and parabelt cortices in the human superior temporal gyrus. *Journal of Comparative Neurology, 491,* 270–289.

Talairach, J., & Tournoux, P. (1988). *Co-planar stereotaxic atlas of the human brain.* New York: Thieme Medical.

Thompson, P. M., Hayashi, K. M., Sowell, E. R., Gogtay, N., Giedd, J. N., Papoport, J. L., et al. (2004). Mapping cortical change in Alzheimer's disease, brain development, and schizophrenia. *NeuroImage, 23*(Suppl. 1), S2–S18.

von Economo, C. (1929). *The cytoarchitectonics of the human cerebral cortex.* London: Oxford University Press.

Vymazal, J., Righini, A., Brooks, R. A., Canesi, M., Mariani, C., Leonardi, M., & Pezzoli, G. (1999). T1 and T2 in the brain of healthy subjects, patients with Parkinson disease, and patients with multiple system atrophy: Relation to iron content. *Radiology, 211,* 489–496.

Walters, N. B., Egan, G. F., Kril, J. J., Kean, M., Waley, P., Jenkinson, M., et al. (2003). *In vivo* identification of human cortical areas using high-resolution MRI: An approach to cerebral structure-function correlation. *Proceedings of the National Academy of Sciences, 100,* 2981–2986.

Yakovlev, P. I. (1970). Whole brain serial histological sections. In G. C. Tedeschi (Ed.), *Neuropathology: Methods and diagnosis* (pp. 371–378). Boston: Little Brown.

Yoshiura, T., Higano, S., Rubio, A., Shrier, D. A., Kwok, W. E., Iwanaga, S., et al. (2000). Heschl and superior temporal gyri: Low signal intensity of the cortex on T2-weighted MR images of the normal brain. *Radiology, 214,* 217–221.

Zatorre, R. J. (1988). Pitch perception of complex tones and human temporal-lobe function. *Journal of the Acoustical Society of America, 84,* 566–572.

Zatorre, R. J., & Belin, P. (2001). Spectral and temporal processing in human auditory cortex. *Cerebral Cortex, 11,* 946–953.

CHAPTER 6

Models of Central Auditory Processing Abilities and Disorders

DENNIS J. MCFARLAND AND ANTHONY T. CACACE

Introduction

Development and evaluation of tests of central auditory processing must be based on explicit theories of sensory information processing. Only with explicit theories can we develop specific hypotheses about relationships among tests that can be evaluated, analyzed, and interpreted in an unambiguous manner. Theoretically based predictions provide the opportunity for practical solutions to be realized and for science to advance. If done properly, the consolidation of the experimental data can be formalized into a comprehensive theory and ultimately produce evidence-based diagnosis and treatment.

These types of initiatives are not new but can be traced to the process of scientific inquiry, in which idea inception follows a path from hypothesis generation, to experimentation, consensus, and finally to knowledge that can be shared with the scientific community. In this context, and based on our interpretation of available literature, we have concluded that the area of CAPD/APD is stalled somewhere between the experimentation and consensus stages of development (Cacace & McFarland, 2005). In fact, over the course of many decades, it is fair to say that progress in this area has been slow to materialize and this field of inquiry continues to be controversial. Why is this the case and how can we improve the status quo?

To understand the current state of affairs, we outline positions and discuss/critique models from different professional points of view that have been used over the years to define the area of CAPD/APD. Regardless of the different professional work domains and academic training of individuals in these areas, we maintain that a key conceptual element for distinguishing CAPD/APD from other conditions is based on the premise that CAPD/APD is an auditory perceptual dysfunction. If we accept this proposition, then it is also reasonable to assume that perceptual dysfunctions are modality specific (McFarland & Cacace, 1995). Based on this argument, it follows that the primary dysfunction in this disorder should be linked directly to the processing of acoustic information; deficits should not be apparent or at least should be manifest to a lesser degree when matched tasks are presented to other sensory modalities. In this way, CAPD/APD can be distinguished from cognitive, language-based, and supramodal attentional problems which are not characterized by modality specific perceptual dysfunctions. In order for this approach to be effective, multimodal testing is advocated. We maintain that evaluating matched tasks in multiple sensory modalities is necessary to make the appropriate diagnosis. The logic expressed in this statement is simple but powerful. This is an important concept to keep in mind because there is no "gold standard" in CAPD/APD assessment and therefore, we must be particularly vigilant when making a diagnosis. From a diagnostic point of view, in order to assure "adequacy of truth," we must demonstrate that the performance in question is indeed specific to the auditory modality. This factor alone would help clear up much of the uncertainty that plagues the literature on this topic. As noted in Chapter 12, and as we reiterate again here, it is a distinct possibility that deficits in information processing might be more generalized in nature and include effects in multiple sensory modalities. If this is the case, then the information processing disorder in question would require more appropriate descriptions, like "amodal processing disorder," "supramodal processing disorder," "polysensory processing disorder," or "pansensory processing disorder." Therefore, as we

view CAPD/APD through the eyes of different professional domains, we encourage readers to question whether models that limit testing to a single sensory modality can actually reach a valid conclusion regarding the specificity of the deficit? This is a reasonable request for responsible clinicians to consider and this question should be pursued rigorously on a case-by-case basis. If, regrettably, all that can be expected from a *unimodal* battery of tests is an "indeterminate" diagnosis, then there is ample justification to abandon this approach and replace it with a better and more valid framework.

Auditory processing and its disorders have been discussed in several distinct but related literatures, which include the fields of audiology, speech-language pathology, education, psychology (mostly in the areas of individual differences and neuropsychology), occupational therapy, and others. As a caveat, Bellis (2004) states

> *Although one may find many speech and language, psychological, and educational tests that include the term "auditory processing" in their titles, these are not to be considered diagnostic tests for APD. Instead, only those tests that exercise sufficient acoustic control and have been shown to be sensitive to disorders of the central auditory nervous system—while, at the same time, minimizing higher-order confounds such as language, memory, cognition, and related factors—should be used for APD diagnosis.* (p. 22)

Although ensuring sensitivity and minimizing confounds is indeed good advice, to our knowledge, it has not been shown empirically that the tests typically used by audiologists do this any better than tests used by other professions. In addition, the scope of practice for speech-language pathologists includes "assessment and diagnosis" of "sensory awareness related to communication" (ASHA, 2001).

Clearly, any discussion of testing and theory in these specific fields is somewhat arbitrary because each is complex and each encompasses many issues. In addition, there is some degree of overlap as the concepts and methods are not entirely distinct. For example, psychologists and speech-language pathologists might both use scales from the Goldman-Fristoe-Woodcock battery. Likewise, many individuals in the past have been educated and dually certified as audiologists and speech-language pathologists. However, as audiology transitions to doctoral level status (Au.D. or Ph.D.), it is probable that joint certification will be less likely in the future. Nonetheless, it is important to consider similarities and differences in the approaches taken to auditory processing in these different areas. The review that follows is representative, but not exhaustive; the intent is to illustrate the kinds of tests and concepts each of these fields uses in the study of auditory processing and its disorders.

Auditory Processing in the CAPD/APD Literature

Early tests of central auditory processing used stimuli such as filtered speech (Bocca, 1958) and dichotic digits (Kimura, 1961), as well as nonspeech tests such as sound localization and temporal-order discrimination (see Jerger, Weikers, Sharbrough, & Jerger, 1969; also see Jerger, Chapter 1, this volume, for a historical overview). In large part, these initial studies examined effects in individual subjects with documented damage to the central auditory nervous system. Also noteworthy is the fact that in early reports, circa 1960s, imaging studies were not as refined as they are in current day practice, lesions (typically tumors) reported in these studies were not well circumscribed; they extended beyond classical auditory areas, and therefore purported results may not be limited to specific auditory areas and should be viewed cautiously. Subsequent writings in the field of CAPD/APD have discussed differential patterns of performance deficits for lesions located in different parts of the auditory nervous system. Proponents of this site-of-lesion approach suggested different syndromes associated with lesions to general regions such as the cochlea, brainstem, and cortex (e.g., Musiek & Baran, 1986; Musiek & Pinherio, 1987; Tobin, 1985). As this literature evolved, similarity of test scores between subjects with structural lesions and those with functional deficits was used as a means of validating the use of CAPD/APD tests in individuals without demonstrable lesions (e.g., Jerger, Johnson, & Loiselle, 1988). However, this approach became problematic given the uncertainty about the exact nature of deficient test performance. In addition, there is a bewildering array of patterns to the test profiles of the individual case reports that make up much of the CAPD/ APD literature (e.g., Musiek, Geurkink, & Kietel, 1982). Finally, alternative structure-function formulations began to appear (e.g., Katz, 1992).

Subsequent classifications of CAPD/ APD types have been based on the characteristics of the tests, rather than on site(s)-of-lesion. This could be construed as the approach embraced by the ASHA model, which has resulted from a number of consensus conferences. The resultant model listed several auditory related tests and processes: sound localization, auditory discrimination, auditory pattern recognition, temporal aspects of audition, auditory performance decrements with competing acoustic signals, and auditory performance decrements with degraded acoustic signals (ASHA, 1996). Exploratory and confirmatory factor analyses have been used in an attempt to support the ASHA point of view. Based on a four-factor model, Domitz and Schow (2000) and Schow, Seikel, Chermak, and Berent (2000) have reported results that purport to recover basic auditory abilities from this methodology. Although potentially useful, this work is problematic for several reasons. Most notably, the authors failed to consider alternative models in their analysis. For example, McFarland and Cacace (2002) reanalyzed the data of Schow et al. (2000) and found that a single-factor model could just as easily account for the pattern of intercorrelations among tests as the four-factor model suggested by Schrow et al. (2000). Although Schow et al. (2000) suggest that these scales measure a number of distinct abilities; they do not provide any data to support this assertion. Thus, Schow et al. (2000) have the task of validating four measures in order to justify this claim. This involves showing that the tests in question correlate with what they are theoretically expected to correlate with (e.g., other measures of the purported auditory ability). In addition, this validation process involves demonstrating that test results are modality-specific (Cacace & McFarland, 1998; McFarland & Cacace, 1995) and do not correlate with matched tests in other sensory modalities. To date, the four-factor model has not been validated and the results remain tenuous. In addition to validating what these tests measure, it is also important to determine what they predict in terms of useful outcomes (e.g., success in school such as math and reading skill, activities of daily living, etc.). Although it is possible to categorize auditory abilities and tests in many ways, it is necessary and just as important to establish the utility of any

proposed system. These types of issues have been discussed by Watson and Kidd (Chapter 13, this volume).

Problems inherent in "test validation by consensus conferences" are highlighted by the succession of task force reports that have appeared in recent years. The first of these occurred in 1996 (ASHA, 1996) and suggested the categories discussed above. This was followed by the Brouton Conference, held at the University of Texas at Dallas (Jerger & Musiek, 2000). The Brouton Conference embraced explicitly the concept of modality specificity as a defining characteristic of CAPDs/APDs. Subsequently, another ASHA committee rejected modality specificity as a defining characteristic of auditory processing disorders (ASHA, 2005). However, there have been several commentaries questioning the veracity contained in various aspects of these proposals (e.g., Cacace & McFarland, 2005; Katz et al, 2002; Moore, 2006).

Other models have also been proposed over the years. One of which is the categorical model of Katz, also known as "the Buffalo model" and another is the Bellis/Ferre model. In a recent discussion of these models, Butras, Loubert, Dupris, Marcoux, Dumont, and Baril (2007), point out that neither of these models are based on data published in peer-reviewed articles, both share common categories, both refer to neuroanatomic substrate that could be dysfunctional, but neither provide any direct evidence to support these proposed neuroanatomic substrates of APDs. The model proposed by Katz (i.e., the Staggered Spondiac Word test, SSW), which has been in use for over four decades, is based solely on speech stimuli (Katz, 1962). According to the author, the SSW test can be applied in locating abnormalities within the brain and in evaluating APDs associated with learning and other disabilities (e.g., Katz & Smith, 1991).

As far as its characteristics are concerned, it can be construed as a combined monotic and dichotic test paradigm that uses two spondaic words as stimuli that partially overlap in time. To illustrate the task, if we use the words like *hotdog* and *baseball* as stimuli; the initial syllable (*hot*) is heard monotically in the left ear, the second syllable of the first word and the first syllable of the second word (*dog* and *base*) are heard simultaneously in both ears (dichotic presentation) and *ball* is heard monotically in the right ear. Response requirements are based on the sequential reproduction of verbal material in the order in which they were perceived. Forty pairs of words are presented and percent correct performance is quantified for each syllable in the monotic and dichotic conditions. Based on patterns of SSW data with learning-impaired children, four diagnostic categories have been proposed in which presumed auditory-based disorders segregate, these include: auditory decoding, auditory tolerance fading memory, auditory integration, and organization. As we have noted in a previous interchange, one of the primary problems with this model is that Katz has never published any specific details on how these categories were established or how they were validated (Cacace & McFarland, 2005b). Based on this fact alone, the validity of this model is suspect. Moreover, on theoretical grounds it is difficult to reconcile how decoding, memory, integration, and organization would reflect abilities that would be specific to the auditory modality. Additional concerns about what these categories actually mean and how a single 10-minute test would allow for differential placement into one of these categories remain unanswered. Of particular interest is the category of "tolerance fading memory." Tolerance fading memory is an idiosyncratic term used only by proponents of the Buffalo model despite the fact that there is a huge literature on memory. This category is most difficult to conceptualize, since no details are provided in terms of how it was established, how it was linked to brain dysfunction in individuals, and how it related to, or is correlated with, other tests of memory function or memory decay. This last concern relates to the fact that none of these areas have been cross-validated with any other tests. Therefore, this model cannot to be taken seriously unless basic relationships with other relevant tests are established. It should be rejected at this point in time due to lack of empirical evidence. Moreover, there are data from a variety of sources to suggest that dichotic tests are highly sensitive to other factors like attention and memory, and therefore these measures are not well suited and, for that matter, are less than optimal for studying disorders of auditory perception. In sum, the "Buffalo model" is an example whereby a theoretical position is posited but the model is not well suited to reach a logical conclusion regarding CAPDs/APDs. The descriptions are ill conceived and there is no direct empirical evidence to support the different categories at this time.

The SSW test arose to prominence at a time when diagnostic assessment of brain function was not well developed in comparison to today's standards (e.g., imaging methodology). Within this same time frame, Kimura (1967) introduced a "structural" pathway model of dichotic listening to explain the effects of temporal lobectomy. At that time, Kimura also observed asymmetries in dichotic tests performance in normal individuals. According to the structural pathway model, contralateral pathways were stronger than ipsilateral pathways. During simultaneous presentation to both ears, the contralateral pathways inhibit the ipsilateral pathways. A right-ear advantage, typically seen in normal right-handed individuals, is in accorded with the left hemisphere being dominant for speech. From this logic, it follows that information from the left ear presumably had a more arduous course, having first been processed by the right hemisphere and then having to cross the corpus callosum in order to reach the language-dominant left hemisphere.

An alternative to the pathway model is the suggestion that asymmetries observed with dichotic presentation of verbal materials reflects the perceived position of events or objects in space, rather than characteristics of afferent pathways (Bradshaw, Burden, & Nettleton, 1986; Phillips & Gates, 1982). According to this view, performance deficits resulting from lateralized cerebral damage can be caused by *hemispatial neglect*. Bisaich, Perani, Valler, and Berti (1986) reported results from a sample of individuals on a binaural auditory lateralization task that involved making interaural intensity judgments. They noted that right-handed and left-handed subjects with brain damage but without visual field deficits showed lateralization deficits in the hemispace both contralateral and ipsilateral to the lesion. The authors argue that the co-occurrence of visual neglect and auditory lateralization deficits is consistent with an interpretation in terms of a distortion of the inner representation of egocentric space (i.e., a defect in spatial attention). Harris (1994) interpreted a high correlation between scores on dichotic speech perception tests and central masking in subjects with brain damage as indicating these tests measure "auditory attention." In the Harris study, an interpretation in terms of language lateralization was ruled out by the nonverbal nature of the central masking task (use of pure tones and white noise). The importance of language was evaluated by manipulating the verbal content of stimuli. Pinek and Brouchon (1992) demonstrated that two types of auditory spatial deficits could be dissoci-

ated following right parietal lobe damage; sound localization deficits, determined by a head turning response, involved both hemifields and thus were consistent with what would be expected from a pathway model. Sound localization deficits, determined by a manual pointing response in the same patients, tended to appear in the left hemifield and were accompanied by visual neglect, consistent with a generalized spatial deficit. Such results suggest that a given individual can have either a sensory specific pathway dysfunction or a more generalized supramodal spatial deficit. An appropriate test protocol, such as one assessing multiple sensory modalities, should provide the means for differentiating between these alternatives. Because of the complexities involved in applying dichotic listening tests in central auditory testing including the issues related to auditory neglect, we must consider the fact that ear and side of stimulus presentation are confounded (Spierer, Meuli, & Clarke, 2007). Distinguishing a spatial deficit from a sensory perceptual pathway dysfunction becomes an important consideration and requires a more complex design. Indeed, to address the specificity issue and to better understand this area, it becomes necessary to perform more than just dichotic tests alone, which would include some type of localization or lateralization task. Additional issues regarding the neglect phenomenon are considered further in the section on Neuropsychology.

Speech and Language Pathology

Speech-language pathologists often administer tests that are designed to assess auditory abilities. There is a wide assortment of these, but examples include the Goldman-Fristoe-Woodcock battery (Baran & Gengel,

1984), the Test for the Auditory Comprehension of Language (Hassan & Jammal, 2005), and the Auditory Comprehension Test for Sentences (Flanagan & Jackson, 1997). These tests generally involve oral presentation of speech stimuli with the intent of evaluating receptive language skills.

As noted earlier, one concern that has been expressed with the use of such tests for identification of CAPD/APDs is the apparent lack of control for acoustic factors (e.g., Bellis, 2004). Although this is a valid concern, it remains to be demonstrated empirically exactly how important this issue is for the psychometric properties (reliability and validity) of assessment instruments. If it turns to be a major problem, then it should be correctable easily with modern technology. For example, in both busy private practices or in school system environments, computerized testing could easily provide better control over stimulus presentation and the use of noise-canceling headphones could provide better control over the acoustic environment in which testing is performed, particularly if the background noise is continuous. As we mentioned previously and reiterate again here, it is questionable whether or not speech materials should be the primary focus of auditory processing assessment (e.g., Moore, 2006).

Individuals within the speech-language community often make a distinction between auditory processing and language processing. This distinction may be conceptualized in terms of low-level acoustic characteristics that are contrasted to speech perception. Rees (1973) has suggested that purported tests of auditory function are often influenced by language abilities. Likewise, Kamhi (2004) suggests that words are the basic units of language, rather than individual speech sounds. This approach calls into question the idea of using auditory tests to assess fundamental abilities on which speech perception might depend.

As we have discussed in detail elsewhere (McFarland & Cacace, 1995), the fundamental question here concerns the extent to which a given disorder can be shown to be modality specific. Certainly language skills, such as knowledge of vocabulary, may be amodal in nature and affect both speech perception and reading. These abilities are not properly referred to as being auditory skills. However, the modality specificity of the skills involved in speech perception is an issue that must be decided by empirical studies rather than by debate and certainly not by consensus conferences.

Although tests of auditory function used by the speech-language pathologist may not control for acoustic factors, they are generally better characterized in terms of their psychometric properties than many of the CAPD/APD tests employed by audiologists. For example, the studies cited earlier by Baran and Gengel (1984), Hassan and Jammal (2005), and Flanagan and Jackson (1997) were concerned with issues of reliability and/or validity. Indeed, tests used by speech-language pathologists are likely to have published norms and statistics. In contrast, and with a few exceptions such as the SCAN test, this is a shortcoming of many tests of CAPD/APD used by audiologists (McFarland & Cacace, 2005). Indeed, this problem applies to the current ASHA recommendations as well (ASHA, 2005).

The Educational Literature

Professionals in special education and educational psychology are routinely involved in assessing the skills of their clients with learning disabilities. This may include assessment of auditory skills. A popular approach within this field is the Dunn and Dunn model (Lovelace, 2005), which holds that students differ in terms of learning styles. There are several hypothesized facets to learning styles, but one dimension consists of perceptual preferences, which include auditory, visual, tactile, and kinesthetic modalities. Lovelace (2005) summarizes data which suggest that matching students' learning styles with appropriate instruction improves academic achievement. However, not all conceptualizations of learning styles emphasize perceptual factors (e.g., Zhang & Sternberg, 2005).

There are many tests of learning styles available, some of which include *perceptual* preferences, which tend to be based on questions about personal preferences. In a review of this literature, Tiedermann (1989) concluded that there is a limited amount of evidence to support using these tests. However, one interesting feature of the learning styles approach is that the use of any particular style does not necessarily imply that there is a disability. As such, this line of thinking can be applied to the design of instruction for all students regardless of their level of achievement.

The Individual Differences Literature

In psychology, research in the field of individual differences has a long tradition, going back over eight decades (e.g., Spearman, 1927). In his seminal work, Spearman postulated a general factor "g" that represents an ability common to all cognitive tasks. Support for this notion comes from the fact that nearly all correlations between cognitive tests are positive, the so-called "positive manifold" and this general factor represents what is commonly referred to as "intelligence." There has also been a long and continuing debate within the field of individual differences concerning whether intelligence is best viewed as a single entity

or as a collection of specific abilities (e.g., Guilford, 1959). One alternative view holds that there are both general and specific abilities, which are organized in a hierarchical manner (Vernon, 1950).

Particularly relevant to the conceptualization of auditory processing, concerns the relationship between *g* and sensory discrimination. Although it was assumed for many years that the two were independent, more recent studies suggest that *g* may have an influence on basic sensory discrimination abilities (see Deary, 2004, for a review). As *g* is a general, supramodal construct, this would imply that tests of basic sensory skills measure more than simply modality-specific processes. However, the view that sensory discrimination makes more than a trivial contribution to *g* is not universally held (Acton & Schroeder, 2001). This debate is in part about the size of the correlations between a general cognitive factor and sensory discrimination performance.

Carroll (1993) reanalyzed data from a large number of studies concerned with human abilities. He has interpreted the results as supporting a hierarchical model, which includes a general factor, G, secondary factors (Gc and Gf), representing crystallized and fluid intelligence, as well as a number of other specific factors. One of these consistently identified factors is related to auditory abilities, which is designated as Ga (auditory processing). The utility of this conceptualization is supported by research that suggests that both Gc and Ga predict the development of reading skills (Vanderwood, McGew, Flanagan, & Keith, 2002).

Many different models for the structure of human abilities have been suggested, and many of these do *not* include auditory factors. However, Tulsky and Price (2003) have recently reanalyzed the data that served as the basis for norming the Weschler Adult Intelligence Scale (WAIS-III) and the Weschler Memory Scale (WMS-III) and found that a

6-factor model that included auditory memory as a construct best fit the scale of intercorrelational data. This study illustrates how notions of modality-specific processes are becoming more popular in the field of human abilities. Currently, there is controversy concerning the relationship between constructs such as intelligence and working memory (e.g., Ackerman, Beiri, & Boyle, 2005) and we can expect to see further theoretical developments in this area as well.

Another issue in the field of individual differences of interest to auditory processing skills concerns the relationship between speeded perceptual-motor tasks and general intelligence. Researchers have reported a relationship between intelligence and "inspection time," defined as the duration of stimulus exposure required for individuals to discriminate between two alternative stimuli (Vickers, Nettelbeck, & Willson, 1972). Although initial studies of this phenomenon used visual stimuli, a number of more recent reports employed auditory stimuli (e.g., McCrory & Cooper, 2005; Parker, Crawford, & Stephen, 1999). Careful examination of these tasks indicates that they are, in fact, related to tasks employed for the evaluation of CAPDs/APDs. For example, the study by McCrory and Cooper (2005) required subjects to determine the order of two tones separated by a brief silent interval. The task used by Parker, Crawford, and Stephen (1999) required subjects to use phase differences between the ears to localize sound in space. These are examples of auditory temporal processing and localization tasks identified, for example, by the ASHA task force as being useful for the identification of CAPDs/APDs (ASHA, 1996, 2005).

The fact that these auditory tasks correlate with general intelligence suggests that they measure more than just modality-specific processes. However, there is alternative evidence indicating that these types of tasks are not only measures of amodal abilities. The work of Hirsh and Sherrick (1961) is widely cited as showing that temporal order judgments require the same amount of separation in both vision and audition. However, in a contemporary extension of this work in which auditory (level and frequency) and visual (size, orientation, and color) tasks were used, McFarland, Cacace, and Setzen (1998) found large differences between temporal order thresholds in the auditory and visual modalities, as well as in submodalities within audition and vision. These results suggest that temporal resolution also involves perceptual mechanisms specific to a given submodality. Fink, Ulbrich, Churan, and Wittmann, (2006) extended these results by showing that the pattern of intercorrelations among several temporal-order tasks cannot be explained solely on the basis of a single underlying ability. These results suggest that temporal-order tasks measure both modality specific abilities and more generalized amodal abilities. Furthermore, the extent to which a given auditory temporal-order task depends on intelligence may vary with the specific stimulus feature used (Olsson, Bjorkman, Haag, & Juslin, 1988).

Researchers in the field of individual differences have at times employed tasks very similar to some of those used by audiologists to measure CAPDs/APDs. Results suggest a relationship between some of these tasks and the penultimate amodal ability, intelligence. In addition, some theorists postulate specific auditory abilities.

Neuropsychology

The Speech-Sounds Perception Test (SSPT) and Seashore Rhythm Tests (SRTs) are part of the Halstead-Reitan Neuropsychological Test Battery (Reitan & Wolfson, 1993). For the SSPT, tape-recorded nonsense syllables are presented to individuals who are instructed to select the presented sound from four written choices. The SRT requires participants to determine whether or not two segmental rhythmic beats are the same or different. Thus, the traditional neuropsychology exam may involve assessment of auditory processing. Whereas these tests were originally designed to detect brain damage, more recent use has been concerned with identifying functional impairments. To this end, Berger (1998) reported that these tests are related to a verbal comprehension factor from the WAIS.

Neuropsychological testing at times also involves the use of dichotic presentation of stimuli, a paradigm that is commonly used in many CAPD/APD testing batteries. However, the scoring and interpretation differs between these fields. Neuropsychologists have typically used this paradigm as an index of language lateralization or as an index of neglect. These tests are not commonly employed clinically, but have generated a large amount of research. The modality specificity of effects is a topic of interest in this field.

Neglect refers to a lack of responding to stimuli on one side of the body. It has most often been described for the visual modality, using an "extinction" test where stimuli are presented simultaneously in both visual fields. Neglect to the contralateral side or hemifield is commonly found following damage to the right parietal lobe, but it may also appear following other brain lesions. Robertson et al. (1997) showed that unilateral (hemispatial) neglect is also associated with auditory sustained attention to nonspatially lateralized stimuli. Pavani, Ladavas, and Driver (2002) showed that patients with visuospatial neglect also have deficits in auditory localization but not in pitch discrimination. These studies demonstrate the concern in this literature with identifying critical components of behavioral tasks that cause deficient performance. Diagnosis is viewed as a form of hypothesis testing and critical features of behavioral tests are manipulated to test alternative hypotheses.

Dodrill (1997) has suggested that neuropsychology has not made the same kind of progress in recent years as other fields in the clinical neurosciences. To support this, he notes that the same tests are in use today as were used 30 years ago. This contrasts markedly with fields such as neuroradiology. Dodrill (1997) attributes this lack of progress in neuropsychology to widely held myths, like the notion that neuropsychologists have a good knowledge of the constructs that their tests measure. When asked where they learned this, he contends that most neuropsychologists would say that they learned this from their mentors. When asked where their mentors learned this "the answer is likely to be that someone dreamed it up" (p. 3). Thus, there is recognition by some neuropsychologists that further work is necessary to define the constructs used in this field.

Occupational Therapy (OT) Literature

Occupational therapists also assess sensory functioning. An example of an instrument used by this profession is the Adult Sensory Profile (Brown, Tollefson, Dunn, Cromwell, & Filion, 2001). This instrument makes use of individuals' subjective ratings of how they react to various situations. Constructs measured by this test include sensory responsiveness, sensation seeking, and sensation avoidance. Brown and colleagues provide validating evidence in the form of the opinions of expert judges.

Sensory defensiveness is seen as the result of sensory modulation dysfunction, which, in turn, is a problem in the capacity to regulate and organize the degree, intensity, and nature of response to sensory input in a graded manner. Auditory defensiveness can be characterized as oversensitivity to certain sounds and may involve irritable or fearful responses to noises like vacuum cleaners, motors, and so forth (Stagnitti, Raison, & Ryan, 1999). Oversensitivity might correspond to what audiologist consider as hyperacusis. Treatment in adults consists of insight and sensory stimulation (Pfeiffer & Kinnealey, 2003).

Summary and Conclusions

As this brief review illustrates, tests and theories of auditory processing have been independently developed in several professional domains including audiology, speech-language pathology, education, psychology, and occupational therapy. Although all of these groups purport to have measures of auditory processing, the details of the tests vary with respect to content, how they are validated, and how auditory processing is conceptualized.

Tests devised by audiologists reflect concern with precise control of the acoustic stimulus. Some other areas use imprecise presentation of materials, whereas others involve spoken language on the part of the examiner. It remains to be determined how crucial precise control of the stimulus is for the assessment of auditory processing. In some cases the need for precise control is obvious, such as with temporal-order tasks, sound-localization/lateralization tasks, modulation detection, establishing just noticeable difference thresholds for duration, frequency, and level, tests of forward and backward masking, and/or other psychoacoustic paradigms too numerous to mention. In other cases this is less apparent, such as with the assessment of auditory verbal memory. Ultimately, empirical studies would best answer these questions. In any case, recent advances in the incorporation of psychometric testing with portable computer hardware/software should provide many opportunities for better instruments to evolve.

The numerous disciplines using tests of auditory abilities differ greatly in the extent to which issues of standardization, reliability, and validity are considered. These issues are thought to be very important in the field of individual differences. In contrast, standardization, reliability, and validity are generally given much less attention by audiologists who develop tests of auditory processing. This is particularly noteworthy, as the recent ASHA position statement (ASHA, 2005) does not even mention these issues. Without information about reliability and validity, there is no way for professionals to evaluate the utility of a given test.

The way auditory processing is conceptualized also differs between these fields. For example, neuropsychologists tend to view test performance as the product of several distinct abilities. Neuropsychologists vary characteristics of the test in order to evaluate alternative hypotheses about a given patients deficit (Franzen, 1989). In contrast, audiologists often take the inclusive approach by which they infer that any test using auditory stimuli is a measure of an "auditory behavior" (Bellis, 2004). Most fields attempt to detect deficits, but the approach in the field of education emphasizes preferences that are not considered either good or bad.

Research comparing the correlation between test scores on various measures of auditory processing will clarify how they are related. Although uncommon, there are some examples in the literature. Riccio, Cohen, Garrison, and Smith (2005) examined the correlations between several measures of CAPD/APD and several measures of attention and memory. They found that CAPD/APD measures significantly correlated with each other and with some measures of attention and memory. They concluded that CAPD/APD measures include elements of attention and memory, but also additional elements not tapped by these measures. Maerlender, Wallis, and, Isquith (2004) correlated scores of a dichotic digits test used for CAPD/APD assessment with the digit-span subtest of the WISC. They found that the two were related and concluded that tests of auditory working memory might be a more sensitive test for evaluation of central auditory disorders. They further state that "the validity of the CAPD diagnosis, and its acceptance across disciplines, will rest on validation through the use of multiple measures to form a nomothetical net that is meaningful across disciplines" (p. 325).

At another level, it is important to have theoretical conceptualizations and definitions of auditory processing and its disorders that can span several disciplines. Probably the best candidate is the conceptualization arising from basic research in neuroscience. Although these are continuingly evolving, there is general consensus about the nature of the auditory nervous system and the kinds of information processing that is done there (e.g., Leonard, Eckert, & Bishop, 2005).

References

Ackerman, P. L., Beiri, M. E., & Boyle, M. O. (2005). Working memory and intelligence: the same or different constructs? *Psychological Bulletin, 131*, 30–60.

Acton, G. S., & Schroeder, D. H. (2001). Sensory discrimination as related to general intelligence. *Intelligence, 29*, 263–271.

American Speech-Language-Hearing Association. (1996). Central auditory processing: Current status of research and implications for clinical practice. *American Journal of Audiology, 5*, 41–54.

American Speech-Language-Hearing Association. (2001). *Scope of practice in speech-language pathology.* Rockville, MD: Author.

American Speech-Language-Hearing Association. (2005). (Central) auditory processing disorders—the role of the audiologist [Position statement]. Available at http://www.asha.org/members/deskref-journals/deskref/default

Baran, J. A., & Gengel, R. (1984). Test-retest reliability of three G-F-W subtests. *Language, Speech, and Hearing Services in the Schools, 15*, 199–204.

Bellis, T. J. (2004). Redefining auditory processing disorder: An audiologist's perspective. *ASHA Leader, 6*, 22–23.

Berger, S. (1998). The WAIS-R factors: Usefulness and construct validity in Neuropsychological assessment. *Applied Neuropsychology, 5*, 37–42.

Bisiach, E., Perani, D., Valler, G., & Berti, A. (1986). Unilateral neglect: Personal and extrapersonal. *Neuropsychologia, 24*, 759–767.

Bocca, E. C. (1958). Clinical aspects of cortical deafness. *Laryngoscope, 68*, 301–309.

Bradshaw, J. L., Burden, V., & Nettleton, N. C. (1986). Dichotic and dichhaptic techniques. *Neuropsychologia, 24*, 79–90.

Brown, C., Tollefson, N., Dunn, W., Cromwell, R., & Filion, D. (2001). The adult sensory profile: measuring patterns of sensory processing. *American Journal of Occupational Therapy, 55*, 75–82.

Cacace, A. T., & McFarland, D. J. (1998) Central auditory processing disorder in school-aged children: A critical review. *Journal of Speech, Language and Hearing Research, 51*, 355–373.

Cacace, A.T., & McFarland, D. J. (2005a). The importance of modality specificity in diagnosing central auditory processing disorder. *American Journal of Audiology, 14*, 112–123.

Cacace, A. T., & McFarland, D. (2005b). Response to Katz and Tillery (2005), Musiek, Chermak, and Bellis (2005), and Rosen (2005). *American Journal of Audiology, 14*, 145–150.

Carroll, J. B. (1993). *Human cognitive abilities: A survey of factor-analytic studies*. Cambridge, UK: Cambridge University Press.

Deary, I. (2004). Sensory discrimination and intelligence: Testing Spearman's other hypothesis. *American Journal of Psychology, 117*, 1–18.

Dodrill, C. B. (1997). Myths of neuropsychology. *Clinical Neuropsychologist, 11*, 1–17.

Domitz, D. M., & Schow, R. L. (2000). A new CAPD battery- multiple auditory processing assessment: Factor analysis and comparison with SCAN. *American Journal of Audiology, 9*, 1–11.

Fink, M., Ulbrich, P., Churan, J., &Wittmann, M. (2006). Stimulus-dependent processing of temporal order. *Behavioral Processes, 71*, 344–352.

Flanagan, J. L., & Jackson, S. T. (1997). Test-retest reliability of three aphasia tests: Performance of non-brain-damaged older adults. *Journal of Communication Disorders, 30*, 33–43.

Franzen, M. D. (1989). *Reliability and validity in neuropsychological assessment*. New York: Springer.

Guildford, J. P. (1959). *Personality*, New York: McGraw-Hill.

Harris, J. (1994). Brain lesions, central masking, and dichotic speech perception. *Brain and Language, 46*, 96–197,

Hassan, K. E., & Jammal, R. (2005). Validation and development of norms for the test for auditory comprehension of language-revised (TACL-R) in Lebanon. *Assessment in Education, 12*, 183–202.

Jerger, J., Weikers, N. J., Sharbrough, F. W., 3rd, & Jerger, S. (1969). Bilateral lesions of the temporal lobe: A case study. *Acta Otolaryngologica, Supplement, 258*, 1–51.

Jerger, J., & Musiek F. (2000). Report of the Consensus Conference on the Diagnosis of Auditory Processing Disorders in Children. *Journal of the American Academy of Audiology, 11*, 467–474.

Jerger, S., Johnson, K., & Loiselle, L. (1988). Pediatric central auditory dysfunction. Comparison of children with confirmed lesions versus suspected processing disorders. *American Journal of Otology, 9*(Suppl.), 63–71.

Jutras, B., Loubert, M., Dupuis, J. L., Marcous, C., Dumont, V., & Baril, M. (2007). Applicability of central auditory processing models. *American Journal of Audiology, 16*, 100–106.

Kamhi, A. G. (2004). A meme's eye view of speech-language pathology. *Language, Speech and Hearing Services in Schools, 35*, 105–111.

Katz, J. (1992). Classification of auditory processing disorders. In J. Katz, N. A. Stecker, & D. Henderson, (Eds.), *Central auditory processing: A transdisciplinary view* (pp. 81–91). St. Louis, MO: Mosby Year Book.

Katz, J., Johnson, C. D., Tillery, K., Bradham, T., Bradner, S., Delagrange, T., et al. (2002). Clinical and research concerns regarding the 2000 APD consensus report and recommendations. *Audiology Today, 14*, 14–17.

Katz, J., & Smith, P. S. (1991). The Staggered Spondaic Word Test. A ten-minute look at the central nervous system through the ears. *Annals of the New York Academy of Sciences, 620*, 233–251.

Kimura, D. (1961). Some effects of temporal-lobe damage on auditory perception. *Canadian Journal of Psychology, 15*, 156–165.

Leonard, C. M., Eckert, M. A., & Bishop, D. V. M. (2005). The neurobiology of developmental disorders. *Cortex, 41*, 277–281.

Lovelace, M. K. (2005). Meta-analysis of experimental research based on the Dunn and Dunn model. *Journal of Educational Research, 98*, 176–183.

Maerlender, A. C., Wallis, D. J., & Isquith, P. K. (2004). Psychometric and behavioral measures of central auditory function: the relationship between dichotic listening and digit span tasks. *Child Neuropsychology, 10*, 318–327.

McCrory, C., & Cooper, C. (2005). The relationship between three auditory inspection time tasks and general intelligence. *Personality and Individual Differences, 38*, 1835–1845.

McFarland, D. J., & Cacace, A. T. (1995) Modality specificity as a criterion for diagnosing central auditory processing disorders. *American Journal of Audiology, 4,* 32–44.

McFarland, D. J., & Cacace, A. T. (2002). Factor analysis in CAPD and the "unimodal" test battery: Do we have a model that will satisfy? *American Journal of Audiology, 11,* 9–12.

McFarland, D. J. & Cacace, A. T. (2005). Current controversies in CAPD: From Procruste's bed to Pandora's box. In T. K. Parthasarathy (Ed.), *An introduction to auditory processing disorders in children* (pp. 247–263). Mahwah, NJ: Lawrence Erlbaum.

McFarland, D. J., Cacace, A. T., & Setzen, G. (1998). Temporal-order discrimination for selected auditory and visual stimulus dimensions. *Journal of Speech, Language, and Hearing Research, 41,* 300–314.

Moore, D. R. (2006). Auditory processing disorder (APD): Definition, diagnosis, neural basis, and intervention. *Audiological Medicine, 4,* 4–11.

Musiek, F. E., & Baran, J. A. (1986). Neuroanatomy, neurophysiology, and central auditory assessment. Part 1: Brain stem. *Ear and Hearing, 7,* 207–219.

Musiek, F. E., Geurkink, N. A., & Kietel, S. A. (1982). Test battery assessment of auditory perceptual dysfunction in children. *Laryngoscope, 92,* 251–257.

Musiek, F. E., & Pinherio, M. L. (1987). Frequency patterns in cochlear, brainstem, and cerebral lesions. *Audiology, 26,* 79–88.

Olsson, H., Bjorkman, C., Haag, K., & Juslin, P. (1988). Auditory inspection time: On the importance of selecting the appropriate sensory continuum. *Personality and Individual Differences, 25,* 627–634.

Parker, D. M., Crawford, J. R., & Stephen, E. (1999). Auditory inspection time and intelligence: A new spatial localization task. *Intelligence, 27,* 131–139.

Pavani, F., Ladavas, E., & Driver, J. (2002). Selective deficit of auditory localization in patients with visuospatial neglect. *Neuropsychologia, 40,* 291–301.

Pfeiffer, B., & Kinealey, M. (2003). Treatment of sensory defensiveness in adults. *Occupational Therapy International, 10,* 175–184.

Phillips, D. P., & Gates, G. R. (1982). Representation of the two ears in the auditory cortex: A re-examination. *International Journal of Neuroscience, 16,* 41–46.

Pinek, B., & Brouchon, M. (1992). Head turning versus manual pointing to auditory targets in normal subjects and subjects with right parietal damage. *Brain and Cognition, 18,* 1–11.

Rees, N. S. (1973). Auditory processing factors in language disorders: The view from Procrustes' bed. *Journal of Speech and Hearing Disorders, 38,* 304–315.

Reitan, R. M., & Wolfson, D. (1993). *The Halstead-Reitan Neuropsychological Test Battery: Theory and clinical interpretation* (2nd ed.). Tuscon, AZ: Neuropsychology Press.

Riccio, C. A., Cohen, M. J., Garrison, T., & Smith, B. (2005). Auditory processing measures: Correlation with neuropsychological measures of attention, memory, and behavior. *Child Neuropsychology, 11,* 363–372.

Robertson, I. H., Manly, T., Beschin, N., Daini, R., Haeske-Dewick, H., Homberg, V., et al. (1997). Auditory sustained attention as a marker of unilateral spatial neglect. *Neuropsychologia, 35,* 1527–1532.

Schow, R. L., & Chermak, G. D. (1999). Implications from factor analysis for central auditory processing disorders. *American Journal of Audiology,* 8, 137–142.

Schow, R. L., Seikel, J. A., Chermak, G. D., & Berent, M. (2000). Central auditory processes and test measures: ASHA 1996 revisited. *American Journal of Audiology, 9,* 63–68.

Spearman, C. E. (1927). *The abilities of man.* New York: Macmillan.

Spierer, L., Meuli, R., & Clarke, S. (2007). Extinction of auditory stimuli in hemineglect: Space versus ear. *Neuropsychologia, 45,* 540–551.

Stagnitti, K., Raison, P., & Ryan, P. (1999). Sensory defensiveness syndrome: a paediatric perspective and case study. *Australian Occupational Therapy Journal, 46,* 175–187.

Tiedermann, J. (1989). Measures of cognitive styles: a critical review. *Educational Psychologist,* 24, 261–275.

Tobin, H. (1985). Binaural interaction tasks. In M. L. Pinherio & F. E. Musiek (Eds.), *Assessment of central auditory dysfunction: Foundations and clinical correlates* (pp. 155–171). Baltimore: Williams & Wilkins.

Tulsky, D. S., & Price, L. R. (2003). The joint WAIS-III and WMS-III factor structure: development and cross-validation of a six-factor model of cognitive functioning. *Psychological Assessment, 15*, 149–162.

Vanderwood, M. L., McGew, K. S., Flanagan, D. P., & Keith, T. Z. (2002). The contribution of general and specific cognitive abilities to read-ing achievement. *Learning and Individual Differences, 13*, 159–188.

Vernon, P. E. (1950). *The structure of human intelligence*. London: Methun.

Vickers, D., Nettelbeck, T., & Willson, R. J. (1972). Perceptual indices of performance: The measurement of "inspection time" and "noise" in the visual system. *Perception, 1*, 263–295.

Zhang, L., & Sternberg, R. J. (2005). A threefold model of intellectual styles. *Educational Psychology Review, 17*, 1–53.

CHAPTER 7

Challenges in CAPD: An Epidemiologic Perspective

KAREN J. CRUICKSHANKS

Introduction

As scientists and clinicians struggle to improve our understanding of complex brain disorders, including central auditory processing disorders (CAPDs), it is useful to reflect on key insights from epidemiology and the current movement toward evidence-based medicine. This chapter provides a brief overview the importance of standardizing definitions and diagnoses and the variety of systems commonly used to objectively weigh evidence regarding causation and prevention to advance the treatment and prevention of CAPD to the next level of efficacy and impact.

Case Definitions

The importance of consistent nomenclature is well recognized throughout the scientific community. However, in practice, consistent

naming usually evolves over time as multiple investigators report their findings and a consensus builds for a common definition of the disorder. In medicine, the challenges of defining diseases and disorders are compounded for rare disorders and for complex disorders. Early definitions usually are based on the most severe cases leading to modifications as the spectrum of disease becomes apparent. When reliable diagnostic tests are not available, clinicians may rely on a standard set of symptoms, a minimum number of which must be present for diagnosis.

Systematic definitions are essential for consistency in treatment, but also for permitting comparisons across studies and reports. For example, historically, diabetes was considered a single disorder diagnosed by glucose in the urine and other symptoms. Early scientific papers sometimes reported conflicting findings because subjects had different forms of the disease (West, 1978). Depending on the study population's age distribution, some studies included subjects with insulin-dependent diabetes (now called Type 1) and subjects with non-insulin-dependent diabetes (now called Type 2). Significant advances in understanding the etiology of diabetes and developing treatments more effective than starvation diets required the recognition that "diabetes" was a heterogeneous disorder representing different fundamental defects—autoimmune-mediated destruction of the β-cells and insufficient endogenous insulin or defects in insulin sensitivity and ineffective endogenous insulin.

Studies of cardiovascular disease in the 1960s revealed high rates of cerebrovascular disease deaths in the southern United States, patterns that remain to this day (Borhani, 1965). An essential step in determining if the "stroke risk belt" was real required determining if the geographic differences could be due to practice patterns —how physicians labeled deaths in older adults; researchers needed to determine if physicians in the South were misclassifying deaths from other causes as cerebrovascular in origin. By carefully comparing records in a masked fashion, researchers determined that practice patterns could not explain the excess mortality, leading to other studies looking at access to emergency services, quality of hospital care, and other factors as determinants of this geographic variation (Kuller et al., 1969).

Epidemiologists stress the need for clear and consistent case definitions not only to improve comparability across studies but also to arrive at precise estimates of the burden of disease and disability. Without agreement in the field, widely discrepant estimates of the number of people with the disease can be generated leading to misuse of research and health care expenditures, excessive worries about nonexistent epidemics and crises, or unrecognized significant health problems.

One example of the impact of definitions on prevalence estimates comes from an early report from the Framingham Eye Study, on the prevalence of glaucoma, a leading cause of vision impairment (Kahn & Milton, 1980). Kahn and Milton (1980) reported on the prevalence of glaucoma in the study participants using 27 different definitions, combining a small number of examination elements (history, intraocular pressure, visual-field defects, and cup-disc ratios). They demonstrated that the "prevalence" of open-angle glaucoma varied from 0.4% to 11.2% depending on the definition used. Furthermore, they demonstrated that using combination definitions (A and B or C) weakened associations with potential risk factors.

Twelve years later Klein et al. (1992) used an updated set of diagnostic criteria to report the prevalence of glaucoma in the population-based Beaver Dam Eye Study. Estimates ranged from 0 to 2.2%, depending on the definition illustrating the slow time line for consensus-building—after 12 years of research, the field had not yet arrived at a standard definition. Glaucoma remains a poorly understood ocular disorder although new technology has improved consistency in classifying eyes in the subsequent years.

Efforts have been made to define CAPD more clearly and to work toward reducing the heterogeneity included in the classification, but these have been met with some resistance (Cacace & McFarland, 2005; Musiek, Bellis, & Chermak, 2005; Rosen, 2005). Continuing the dialogue is an important step toward accelerating the advancement of ways to treat and prevent CAPD. This book, with its focus on controversies, should stimulate progress toward that common goal.

A recent paper from the Blue Mountains Hearing Study in Australia has illustrated the necessity of arriving at a consensus diagnosis for CAPD (Golding, Carter, Mitchell, & Hood, 2004). In this report, results from the Macquarie Synthetic Sentence Identification Test and the Macquarie Dichotic Sentence Identification Test were used along with the Arthur Boothyroyd (AB) Monosyllabic Word Lists to define the presence/absence of CAPD in a community-based study of older adults. The prevalence of CAPD varied from 2% if abnormal outcomes were obtained for all defined test outcomes ($n = 7$) to 76.4% if any one of the outcomes was abnormal (Golding et al., 2004). A more recent paper, using the number of abnormal results as an index of severity showed a male excess only for those with five to seven abnormalities, illustrating the dangers of overlooking important associations when more inclusive, and hence heterogeneous, definitions are used (Golding et al., 2005).

Diagnosing: The Problems of Test Batteries

Clearly, developing a standard definition and method for diagnosing CAPD is necessary. In 1996, a consensus conference attempted to define CAPD and standardize the assessment of this disorder (Task Force on Central Auditory Processing Consensus Development, 1996). They recommended a battery of tests be used, with a patient failing any one considered to have CAPD. More recently, that approach has been re-endorsed (American Speech-Language-Hearing Association, 2005; Jerger & Musiek, 2000). Aside from the complex challenges of specificity—separating manifestations of auditory processing disorders from other central disorders such as cognitive impairment, visual processing, attention deficit disorders, and autism, topics that are discussed thoroughly elsewhere in this volume—there are fundamental problems in establishing the reliability of tests and in advocating using multiple tests in a parallel fashion (any positive).

Each test has an inherent measurement error; some false positives and false negatives will occur. Determining the sensitivity and specificity of tests requires a gold standard and none exists for CAPD so investigators and clinicians often attempt to estimate test accuracy by comparing results with clinical judgment. Although that may be the best available approach, one should be extremely cautious when applying results from one study to other settings (other clinicians, practice groups, populations, or studies) because the test's effectiveness in detecting cases in other groups will be dependent on the similarity between the new and the original group (including the prevalence of "true CAPD") and the consistency of the original clinician. Without a gold standard, measurement error is poorly quantified.

Following recommendations for multiple tests also incorporates the inherent mathematical problem of parallel testing. As discussed in introductory epidemiology text books, considering a positive on any of the set of tests to be a case increases the sensitivity over the individual test performance but decreases the specificity leading to over-diagnosis (Fletcher, Fletcher, & Wagner, 1988). Figure 7–1 and Table 7–1 illustrate the effect of using two tests A and B, both with good sensitivity and specificity. Essentially some of the cases missed by one test will be detected by the second, improving the sensitivity, while only those negative on both tests will be noncases (decreasing specificity). However, the problem with this approach comes from healthy people being diagnosed as having a disorder when they do not (the false positives). Using parallel testing leads to larger numbers of false positives than a single test due to the decreased specificity.

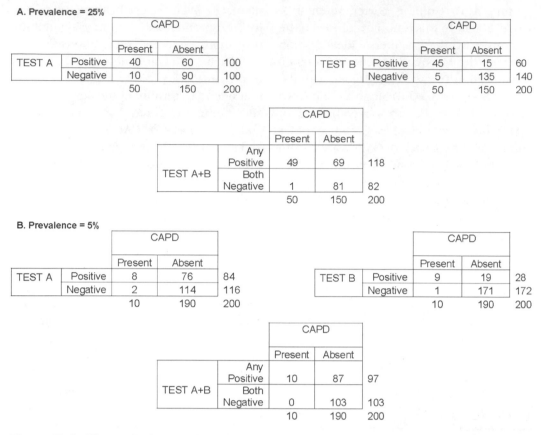

Figure 7–1. Theoretical examples of two tests (A and B). Each test has good sensitivity and correctly identifies most of the cases of CAPD; however, parallel testing (A *or* B are positive *vs.* A *and* B are negative) results in greater misclassification (overdiagnosis) compared to a single test with good specificity (B). When the prevalence of the disorder is lower (5% *vs.* 25% in this example) the positive predictive values are lower and more people are misdiagnosed as having CAPD. Parallel testing leads to inflated prevalence estimates compared to a single test with good specificity (see Table 7–1).

It also is important to remember that the positive predictive value (PPV) is dependent on the prevalence of disorder in the group being tested, as shown in Table 7–1. When the true prevalence of the disease is higher (in this example, 25% vs. 5%), the PPV is higher (42% vs. 10%). Thus, tests that may be acceptable in a high-risk referral population can be useless for measuring disease in a general population. Combining tests in parallel compounds the problem because lower specificity leads to lower PPV. Using parallel testing results in overdiagnosis compared to either single test, which leads to overestimating prevalence. The impact on prevalence estimates is shown in Table 7-1. In this example, although the prevalence is set at 25% or 5%, the test batteries estimate prevalence as 59% or 49%. Closer estimates are obtained when a single test with high sensitivity and specificity is employed; adding tests in parallel increases the error.

TABLE 7–1. Impact of Test Batteries

Test	Sensitivity	Specificity	Positive Predictive Value	Negative Predictive Value	Estimated Prevalence
	%	%	%	%	%
Prev 25%					
A	80	60	40	90	50
B	90	90	75	96	30
A or B	98	54	41.5	99	59
Prev 5%					
A	80	60	9.5	98	42
B	90	90	32	99	14
A or B	100	54	10	~100	48.5

Calculations of test performance characteristics were based on the data presented in Figure 7–1 for two prevalence conditions: A. True Prevalence = 25% and B. True Prevalence = 5%. Performance characteristics are shown for single tests A and B and for parallel testing (either test (A or B) is positive versus both (A and B) are negative).

In this example, when the prevalence of disease is high, combining tests leads to correctly diagnosing 49 subjects, but 69 are treated as having CAPD when they do not. However, when the prevalence is low (5%), all 10 subjects with CAPD are correctly diagnosed, but an additional 87 are misdiagnosed as having CAPD when they do not. Parallel testing in clinical practice can be a serious problem. Using this same strategy in the general population leads to wildly overestimated prevalence rates. The Blue Mountains Hearing Study (Golding et al., 2004) illustrated this problem as they reported a prevalence of 2% when one test is abnormal and 76% when any test outcome is abnormal! With more opportunities to fail, more people fail. Because children are often the focus of testing for CAPD, clinicians should be very concerned about the detrimental effects of over-diagnosing CAPD, which can include the adverse consequences of being inappropriately labeled disordered, costs of treatment that is not needed, and delays in achieving an accurate diagnosis for the presenting symptoms and beginning appropriate treatment. Population-based prevalence and incidence studies, where the goal is an accurate estimate of the burden of disease, should not use parallel testing paradigms to avoid exaggerating the magnitude of the health problem.

Summarizing the Evidence: Guidelines and Systems for Deciding When a Risk Factor Is Causal and When Treatments Work

Scientists throughout the ages have struggled with the problem of determining when we know the cause of the disease and how to treat it. Most often, evidence is gathered slowly over time from a variety of experiments or studies and must be carefully weighed, taking into consideration limitations and flaws in study design, and gaps in the evidence, before reaching conclusions.

Unfortunately, there is no simple solution to this problem. The Henle-Koch postulates were one early attempt to provide a systematic approach to determining if a virus or bacteria was the cause of an infectious disease (Evans, 1978). As reviewed by Evans, these guidelines established the notion, before technologic advances made viewing micro-organisms possible, that the organism should be present in every case, should occur in no other disease, and must be isolated from the body, repeatedly passed, and cause disease in the newly exposed individuals (Evans, 1978). Epidemiologists have built on these original tenets, expanding them to apply to chronic diseases as well.

Although there are many variations of the lists, the criteria for causal associations are often summarized as: Consistency, strength, specificity, temporal relationship, and the coherence of the association (Evans, 1978). These guidelines have been used widely in epidemiology and policy decision-making in combination with weighing the quality of the studies by considering study designs, reliability of measurements, analytic approaches, and possible uncontrolled confounding, to summarize the strength of the scientific evidence and arrive at screening and treatment recommendations.

"Consistency" reflects the need for replication. The same association should have been demonstrated in multiple studies, using strong designs or multiple studies using different designs. Replication suggests that the finding is not due to chance, inherent limitations of one study design or selection factors. Studies with strong designs

and thorough analyses contribute more in weighted systems (see below) than flawed studies or cross-sectional evidence. Although animal models and small experimental studies can contribute to the evidence, usually greater weight is given to prospective study designs in human subjects such as cohort studies and randomized controlled trials.

"Strength" is the size of the association and the precision of the estimate. Larger effects are more likely to be clinically significant and reproducible. Precision is reflected in small confidence intervals. Evidence of a dose-response relationship is an important aspect.

"Specificity" is evident when an exposure is associated with a single disorder (such as asbestos and mesothelioma), and it is more likely to reflect a causal association. However, this guideline is often not met in chronic diseases because of broad systemic effects from environmental and behavioral factors.

"Temporal relationship" is a key line of evidence—that the exposure precedes the development of the disease. Although many important insights can be gained from cross-sectional designs, demonstrating that the exposure came first is important as diseases and disorders can cause alterations in biomarkers which then appear to be associated with the disease in cross-sectional designs.

"Coherence" requires that there be a biologically plausible explanation for the association. Using all the relevant literature and clinical experience, does the association make sense? Unfortunately, scientists are very creative at explaining unexpected findings so it is important to be objective.

These concepts are not rules but guidelines. Often data are lacking for all five elements, even for well-accepted associations, and as we learn more about the multiple health effects of exposures it is likely that specificity is rare. Nonetheless, they are useful to guide the process of summarizing the scientific literature, to judge the state of knowledge and to inform health policy.

Systematic Reviews and Weighting Systems

There are a variety of scales and weighting systems to evaluate when the scientific evidence is sufficient to conclude that screening and/or treatments are appropriate (Guyatt et al., 1995; Higgins & Green, 2006; West et al., 2002). Some establish methods for conducting reviews of clinical trials in a systematic way, others stress factoring in the quality of the study designs when arriving at a conclusion and consider both observational and experimental data, and others address analytic methods such as meta-analysis to calculate an overall effect combining the data from multiple studies. All share their emphasis on human studies and rigorous study designs involving longitudinal data. Although animal models can be extremely useful for understanding potential mechanisms and well-controlled cross-sectional human studies can provide information which supports etiologic hypotheses, it is generally accepted that it is necessary to have prospective human data when weighing evidence for or against screening and treating people and developing clinical practice standards and guidelines.

Three examples of these approaches are the efforts of the United States Preventive Services Task Force (USPSTF), which has been charged with recommending screening and treatment procedures across a wide variety of health issues (USPSTF, 2001; USPSTF, 2004; West et al., 2002); the Evidence-Based Medicine Working Group which outlined strategies for clinicians to use to incorporate the latest scientific evidence into their practices (Guyatt et al., 1995); and an approach used in a recent report from the Institute of Medicine evaluating the impact of noise on hearing and tinnitus in the military (IOM, 2006).

In 2001, the USPSTF evaluated universal newborn hearing screening (USPSTF, 2001). They conducted a systematic search of the literature to identify papers addressing key questions and ranked the studies by the type of design: I, Randomized, controlled trial; II-1, controlled trial without randomization; II-2, Cohort or case-control analytic study; II-3, multiple time series, dramatic uncontrolled experiments; III, Opinions of respected authorities (USPSTF, 2001). The quality or strength of the evidence was then judged to be good, fair, or poor (USPSTF, 2001). Good evidence was defined as "consistent results from well-designed, well-conducted studies in representative populations that directly assess effects on health outcomes." Fair evidence was defined as "sufficient to determine effects on health outcomes, but the strength . . . is limited by the number, quality, or consistency of the individual studies, generalizability to routine practice, or indirect nature . . . " Poor evidence was "insufficient . . . because of limited number or power of studies, important flaws in their design or conduct, gaps in the chain of evidence, or lack of information on important health outcomes" (USPSTF, 1996).

Using this laborious process, the USPSTF concluded that the evidence was not strong enough to recommend for or against routine screening of newborns (USPSTF, 2001). This conclusion was heavily influenced by the lack of evidence that early detection and intervention lead to improved speech and language skills and concerns about whether the benefits outweigh the costs associated with the high false-positive rates for screening methods. The committee emphasized that there had been no prospective, controlled studies of the impact of early intervention. In spite of the widespread acceptance in the hearing science community of the need for newborn hearing screening, an objective evaluation revealed the startling paucity of data supporting this position. Although newborn screening for hearing loss was not supported, the USPSTF has recommended routine screening for rare pediatric vision disorders (USPSTF, 2004) and metabolic disorders where clear evidence of benefits from early treatment exists. It is imperative for hearing researchers to address the critical need for strong scientific evidence and demonstrate the efficacy of early identification and treatments rather than continuing to rely on expert opinion.

More than a decade ago, physicians began to recognize the need to incorporate the rapid growth of scientific information into their clinical decision processes. A working group evolved that published a series of guides to the medical literature designed to assist the busy clinician to evaluate the literature and appropriately apply the information to their own patients (Oxman et al., 1993). An outgrowth of this process has been the proliferation of reports on practice standards to improve the care delivered to patients across practices and the nation. In these standards, randomized controlled trials are essential for the highest recommendation whereas observational studies are considered weaker evidence. These methods have been applied to evaluate numerous treatments for a variety of conditions, including new surgical techniques (Benson et al., 2001). They could be useful to summarize what is known about effective treatments for children with CAPD.

The Institute of Medicine also employs objective criteria for evaluating evidence in their evaluations of important health issues. For example, in the recent review of the hearing effects of noise in the military (IOM, 2006), noting that few longitudinal studies were available, the committee developed a set of criteria to guide their deliberations. They weighed the strength of evidence by considering the number of "strong" studies as well as the design and thoroughness of the analytic approach. The committee repeatedly documented that evidence for widely-held beliefs was insufficient to support conclusions (IOM, 2006). Hearing research has lagged behind other biomedical fields in using strong study designs to address key treatment and screening questions as well as critical etiologic hypotheses. In the field of CAPD, others have identified the need for rigorous methods to identify patients with CAPD and to conduct well-designed randomized controlled trials to demonstrate the efficacy of treatments (Friel-Patti, 1999), but much work remains to be done.

Finally, although these examples all considered evidence from randomized clinical trials as stronger than evidence from population-based observational studies, there is disagreement that trials are inherently better than observational studies (Barrett-Connor, 2004; Benson & Hartz, 2000; Concato, 2004; Concato, Shah, & Horwitz, 2000). Masked randomized controlled trials offer the benefits of reducing potential bias, but they also have limitations. Patients selected for trials are not representative of the broad spectrum of patients with the disease or disorder (leaving questions about the generalizability of the findings), people who choose to enroll in trials are likely to be different from targeted subjects who decline to participate, loss to follow-up and other design flaws limit the utility of the findings.

Properly conducted observational studies, particularly those using population-based designs may provide stronger, more broadly applicable evidence than some trials. Recently, several reports comparing trials and observational studies have demonstrated less heterogeneity in effect estimates than randomized controlled trials (Benson & Hartz, 2000; Concato, 2004; Concato et al., 2000). Perhaps the pendulum is swinging to create a more balanced approach similar to earlier guidelines for causation (Evans, 1978) that considers all of the evidence rather than overemphasizing one line of evidence or study design. Similar findings from studies employing a variety of designs and studying different groups of people provide the consistency required for policy decisions and prevention programs.

the use of multiple tests in parallel, and the challenges of distinguishing other central brain disorders from auditory processing problems) will continue to slow progress in developing a clear understanding of the etiology of CAPD and efficient, effective treatment strategies. It is time for CAPD research to integrate the concepts and approaches that have led to advances treating and preventing other health disorders.

Acknowledgment. The author wishes to thank Lois M. Jollenbeck, Ph.D. and Jane S. Durch, M.S., Senior Program Officers at the Institute of Medicine, National Academy of Sciences for discussions, perspectives, and unique contributions to this chapter.

Summary

Although the CAPD research community has often acknowledged the need for consistent definitions and evidence of treatment effects, there has been little progress in developing consensus on a more objective definition or standardized diagnostic tools that avoid the problems inherent in the use of test batteries. Few randomized controlled trials have been conducted to document the efficacy of interventions and treatments. Adopting standardized systems for objectively evaluating the quality of the evidence supporting widely held principles and beliefs will identify important gaps to be addressed.

It is likely there is considerable heterogeneity in the group of patients currently considered to have CAPD and many patients who are misdiagnosed as having CAPD. Clinicians and researchers must be concerned about the potential for harm from overdiagnosis and misclassification effects. This heterogeneity (from the breadth of manifestations included under the umbrella,

References

American Speech-Language-Hearing Association. (2005). (Central) auditory processing disorders—The role of the audiologist [Position Statement]. Available at http://www.asha.org/members/deskref-journals/deskref/default

Barrett-Connor, E. (2004). Commentary: observation versus intervention—what's different? *International Journal of Epidemiology, 33,* 457–459.

Benson, K., & Hartz, A. J. (2000). A comparison of observational studies and randomized, controlled trials. *New England Journal of Medicine, 342,* 1878–1886.

Benson, W. E., Cruickshanks, K. J., Fong, D. S., Williams, G. A., Bloome, M. A., Frambach, D., et al., (2001). Surgical management of macular holes: A report by the American Academy of Ophthalmology. *American Academy of Ophthalmology, 108,* 1328–1335.

Borhani, N. (1965). Changes and geographic distribution of mortality from cerebrovascular disease. *American Journal of Public Health, 55,* 673–681.

Cacace, A. T., & McFarland, D. J. (2005). The importance of modality specificity in diagnosing central auditory processing disorder. *American Journal of Audiology, 14,* 112–123.

Concato, J. (2004). Observational versus experimental studies: What's the evidence for a hierarchy? *Journal of the American Society for Experimental NeuroTherapeutics, 1,* 341–347.

Concato, J., Shah, N., & Horwitz, R. I. (2000). Randomized, controlled trials, observational studies, and the hierarchy of research designs. *New England Journal of Medicine, 342,* 1887–1892.

Evans, A. S. (1978). Causation and disease: A chronological journey. *American Journal of Epidemiology, 142,* 1126–1135.

Fletcher, R. H., Fletcher, S. W., & Wagner, E. H. (1988). *Clinical epidemiology: The essentials.* Baltimore: Williams & Wilkins.

Friel-Patti, S. (1999). Clinical decision-making in the assessment and intervention of central auditory processing disorders. *Language, Speech, and Hearing Services in Schools, 30,* 345–352.

Golding, M., Carter, N., Mitchell, P., & Hood, L. J. (2004). Prevalence of central auditory processing (CAP) abnormality in an older Australian population: The Blue Mountains Hearing Study. *Journal of the American Academy of Audiology, 15,* 633–642.

Golding, M., Mitchell, P., & Cupples, L. (2005). Risk markers for the graded severity of auditory processing abnormality in an older Australian population: The Blue Mountains Hearing Study. *Journal of the American Academy of Audiology, 16,* 348–356.

Guyatt, G. H., Sackett, D. L., Sinclair J. C., Hayward, R., Cook D. J., & Cook, R. J. (1995). Users' Guides to the Medical Literature: IX. A method for grading health care recommendations. *The Journal of the American Medical Association, 274,* 1800–1804.

Higgins, J. P. T., & Green, S. (2006). Cochrane handbook for systematic reviews of interventions 4.2.6. In J. P. T. Higgins & S. Green, (Eds.), *The Cochrane Library, Issue 4, 2006.* Chichester, UK: John Wiley & Sons.

Institute of Medicine (IOM). (2006). *Noise and military service: Implications for hearing loss and tinnitus.* Humes, L. E., Joellenbeck, L. M., & Durch J. S. (Eds.). Washington, DC: The National Academies Press.

Jerger, J., & Musiek, F. (2000). Report of the Consensus Conference on the Diagnosis of Auditory Processing Disorders in School-Aged Children. *Journal of the American Academy of Audiology, 11,* 467–474.

Kahn, H. A., & Milton, R. C. (1980). Alternative definitions of open-angle glaucoma. *Archives of Ophthalmology, 98,* 2172–2177.

Klein, B. E. K., Klein, R., Sponsel, W. E., Franke, T., Cantor, L. B., Martone, J., & Menage, M. J. (1992). Prevalence of glaucoma: The Beaver Dam eye study. *Ophthalmology, 99,* 1499–1504.

Kuller, L. H., Bolker, A., Saslaw, M. S., Paegel, B. L., Sisk, C., Borhani, N., et al. (1969). Nationwide Cerebrovascular Disease Mortality Study: I. Methods and analysis of death certificates. *American Journal of Epidemiology, 90,* 536–544.

Musiek, F. E, Bellis, T. J., & Chermak, G. D. (2005) Nonmodularity of the central auditory nervous system: Implications for (central) auditory processing disorder. *American Journal of Audiology, 14,* 128–138.

Oxman, A. D., Sackett D. L., & Guyatt G. H. (1993). Users' guides to the medical literature. I. How to get started. *The Journal of the American Medical Association, 270,* 2093–2095.

Rosen, S. (2005). "A riddle wrapped in a mystery inside an enigma": Defining central auditory processing disorder. *American Journal of Audiology, 14,* 139–142.

Task Force on Central Auditory Processing Consensus Development. (1996). Central auditory processing: Current status of research and implications for clinical practice. *American Journal of Audiology, 5,* 41–52.

U.S. Preventive Services Task Force. (2001). Newborn hearing screening: Recommendations and rationale. *American Family Physician, 64,* 1995–1999.

U.S. Preventive Services Task Force. (2004). Screening for visual impairment in children younger than age 5 years: Recommendation statement. *Annals of Family Medicine, 2,* 263–266.

West, K. M. (1978). *Epidemiology of diabetes and its vascular lesions.* New York: Elsevier North-Holland.

West, S., King, V., Carey, T. S., Lohr, K. N., McKoy, N., Sutton, S. F., et al. (2002). *Systems to rate the strength of scientific evidence.* Evidence Report/Technology Assessment No. 47 (Prepared by the Research Triangle Institute-University of North Carolina Evidence-based Practice Center under Contract No. 290-97-0011). AHRQ Publication No. 02-E016. Rockville, MD: Agency for Healthcare Research and Quality.

CHAPTER 8

Issues in the Assessment of Auditory Processing in Older Adults

LARRY E. HUMES

Age-related changes have been documented in the auditory periphery, the auditory portions of the central nervous system, and in many nonauditory portions of the cortex that are believed to mediate various cognitive functions (e.g., CHABA, 1988; Willott, 1991). Each of these age-related changes, in isolation or in combination, may lead to corresponding age-related declines in speech communication (CHABA, 1988; Humes, 1996). Identification of the underlying causes of age-related decline in speech communication is critical to the remediation of these difficulties. For example, if an older person's speech-communication difficulties are primarily due to auditory processing problems occurring in the central nervous system, then fitting this individual with a conventional hearing aid is less likely to prove beneficial.

Establishing the locus of an older adult's speech-communication deficit is probably even more challenging than doing so in

younger adults or in children. This is due, in part, to the fact that many older adults have peripheral sensorineural hearing loss. For example, approximately 25 to 40% of those over the age of 60 years have a hearing loss that is sufficient to cause problems in everyday communication (Cruickshanks et al., 1998; Gates, Cooper, Kannel, & Miller, 1990), whereas the prevalence of even mild amounts of sensorineural hearing loss among school-age children can be as low as <1% (Wake et al., 2006). In addition, the prevalence of Mild Cognitive Impairment among those over the age of 65 years ranges from 3 to 18% (Portet et al., 2006) and increases with age (Lopez et al., 2003). Thus, in the context of somewhat high prevalence of peripheral hearing loss and cognitive impairment in older adults, the challenge of identifying true deficits in the auditory portions of the central nervous system is great.

This task of identifying true deficits in auditory processing is made even more challenging due to the common use of speech stimuli in many behavioral tests of auditory processing administered to the elderly. The speech stimulus is a broadband stimulus that can be impacted critically and negatively by the presence of even mild amounts of high-frequency sensorineural hearing loss; the type of hearing loss most prevalent among older adults. The identification, recognition or comprehension of the speech stimulus, moreover, is a process that involves not only modality-specific auditory processing, but also amodal cognitive processes, such as memory and attention. As a result, cognitive deficits may have an impact on performance measures from older adults that are obtained using speech as the test stimulus. In addition, most speech-based measures of auditory processing make the listening task more difficult by either degrading the speech stimulus directly or by adding background stimuli to it. Doing so, however, can also place additional demands on cognitive resources and increase the likelihood of cognitive contributions to observed age-related decrements in performance. For example, a memory task using auditory stimuli can be made more difficult for young, normal-hearing listeners by simply adding background noise to the stimuli (Pichora-Fuller, Schneider, & Daneman, 1995; Rabbit, 1968; Surprenant, 2007). Thus, degrading the input places greater demands on cognitive function, even in young, normal-hearing adults. Finally, the response task used with the performance measure may also place additional demands on cognitive processing. For example, a performance measure requiring the repetition of entire sentences composed of several words could place extra demands on memory processes compared to one involving the repetition of a single word at the end of the sentence.

In summary, age-related decreases in hearing sensitivity, auditory processing, and cognitive function have all been documented. To ascertain the role played by age-related declines in auditory processing it is important to understand the roles played by the other factors, peripheral sensorineural hearing loss and age-related declines in cognition. As applied to clinical assessment of auditory processing disorders in the elderly, these issues are central to the concept of test validity. That is, is a measure of "(central) auditory processing" actually measuring modality-specific, higher level auditory processing or is performance on a particular task determined primarily by peripheral hearing loss or amodal cognitive function?

The next section of this chapter reviews the impact of peripheral hearing loss in older adults on various measures of speech communication. Again, the focus is placed on measures of speech communication because these stimuli, usually degraded in some manner, are used in the overwhelming majority of tests designed to measure (central) auditory processing in older adults. Following this section, a review of the impact of cognitive function on measures of (central) auditory processing in older adults is provided. Finally, the chapter concludes with a section devoted to other assessment issues of importance to the clinical measurement of auditory processing in older adults, such as test reliability and test battery structure.

The Important Role Played by Peripheral Sensorineural Hearing Loss

Numerous studies from many laboratories around the world have now documented the very prominent role played by the peripheral high-frequency sensorineural hearing loss, so common among older adults, in measures of speech understanding obtained from the elderly (Divenyi & Haupt, 1997a, 1997b, 1997c; Dubno, Ahlstrom, & Horwitz, 2000; Dubno, Lee, Matthews, & Mills, 1997; Helfer, 1992; Gordon-Salant & Fitzgibbons, 1993; Helfer & Wilber, 1990; Humes & Christopherson, 1991; Humes, 2002; Humes et al., 1994; Humes & Roberts, 1990; Jerger & Chmiel, 1997; Jerger, Jerger, & Pirozzolo, 1991; Souza & Turner, 1994; van Rooij & Plomp, 1990; van Rooij & Plomp, 1991; van Rooij, Plomp, & Orlebeke, 1989; Wiley et al., 1998). In general, each of these studies examined age, hearing loss and, often, some other auditory-processing or cognitive-processing measures in the same elderly adults. These studies typically found that the primary or sole predictor of performance was the peripheral hearing loss, most often the average hearing loss for pure tones at frequencies of 1000, 2000, and 4000 Hz. Across this large set of studies, average high-frequency hearing loss typically accounted for 65 to 90% of the systematic (explainable or "non-error") variance.

The findings of Jerger, Jerger, and Pirozzolo (1991) illustrate the strong influence of peripheral sensorineural hearing loss on specific speech-recognition measures common to many auditory-processing test batteries used with older adults. In that study, five measures of speech-recognition performance were obtained from 200 older adults. Measures of speech recognition included scores for the predictability-low (PL) and predictability-high (PH) sentences from the Speech Perception in Noise (SPIN) test (Bilger, Nuetzel, Rabinowitz, & Rzeczkowski, 1984; Kalikow, Stevens, & Elliott, 1977), scores for a custom recording of the Psychoacoustic Laboratory Phonetically Balanced (PAL-PB) words, referred to as P-word scores, the Synthetic Sentence Identification (SSI) test (Speaks & Jerger, 1965), and the dichotic version of this test, the Dichotic Sentence Identification (DSI) test (Fifer, Jerger, Berlin, Tobey, & Campbell, 1983). Except for the PB word score, which was obtained in quiet, all other measures were obtained with either a competing multitalker babble (SPIN test) or competing talker (SSI, DSI). Significant negative correlations were observed by Jerger et al. (1991) between average high-frequency hearing loss and each of these five measures of speech-recognition performance despite the use of a presentation of 50 dB sensation level (re: detection threshold for the SPIN multitalker babble). Specifically, for the PB-word, SPIN-PH, and SPIN-PL scores, Pearson-r correlation coefficients with high-frequency hearing loss were -0.76, -0.73, and -0.78, respectively. Importantly, these were the only significant predictors for these three speech-recognition measures in subsequent multiple-regression analyses. The pool of predictor variables included age and several measures of cognitive function from these same elderly individuals, in addition to hearing loss. For the monotic and dichotic versions of the SSI, the significant negative correlations with average high-frequency hearing loss were -0.65 (SSI) and -0.55 (DSI). Interestingly, the multiple-regression analyses identified a second significant predictor variable for these two measures of speech-recognition, although each accounted for much less variance than average high-frequency hearing loss. Specifically, for the SSI, age was a significant predictor and accounted for an additional 12% of the total variance and, for the DSI, the Digit-Symbol score from the Wechsler Adult Intelligence Scale (WAIS-R; Wechsler, 1981) accounted for an additional 13% of the variance. Thus, for the two measures of speech-recognition in this study which included a single competing talker (SSI and DSI), additional variance in speech-recognition performance could be explained by individual differences in age or cognitive function. Nonetheless, for all five measures of speech-recognition performance comprising this battery of auditory processing measures, peripheral high-frequency hearing loss was a strong predictor of performance in these 200 older adults.

Historically, as noted previously, central auditory testing has frequently made use of degraded speech stimuli. The basic reasoning behind this, established in cases with known lesions in the auditory portions of the central nervous system (typically, not older adults), is that speech-recognition performance deteriorates in such cases only when both the intrinsic neural redundancy of the auditory pathways *and* the extrinsic redundancy of the speech stimulus have been reduced (Bocca & Calearo, 1963). The neural intrinsic redundancy presumably is reduced by the presence of the lesion in the auditory portions of the central nervous system. This reduction alone, however, is insufficient to produce a decline in performance for highly redundant speech stimuli. The extrinsic redundancy associated with the speech stimulus also must be reduced and this can be accomplished in a variety of ways, including the addition of competing stimuli (monaurally or dichotically), filtering of the speech stimulus, interruption of the speech stimulus, or time-compression of the speech stimulus, among others.

It has also been the case historically that most speech-based measures of (central) auditory processing in older adults have been administered at either relatively high sound pressure levels or at moderate sensation levels (32 to 50 dB SL) relative to speech-recognition threshold (SRT). This practice attempts to maximize performance and minimize or eliminate the influence of hearing loss on speech-recognition performance. As noted in the detailed review of the results of Jerger et al. (1991) from

200 older adults, use of a 50-dB sensation level for those five sets of speech stimuli clearly did not eliminate the strong, negative influence of high-frequency hearing loss on speech-recognition performance. This was also the case for many of the studies cited previously which found hearing loss to be the primary predictor of speech-recognition performance despite use of relatively high sound pressure levels (often 80–90 dB SPL) for the speech stimulus.

The primary reason for the continued influence of hearing loss on measures of suprathreshold speech recognition, despite use of moderate sensation levels or high sound pressure levels, has to do with the frequency-specific nature of the hearing loss in older adults. Whereas SRT (or babble-detection threshold as in Jerger et al. [1991]) is primarily determined by pure-tone threshold sensitivity at low and middle frequencies (500, 1000, and 2000 Hz), a frequency region of relatively good hearing in older adults, suprathreshold speech recognition is often more strongly correlated with mid to higher frequencies (1000, 2000, and 4000 Hz). The dashed lines in the top panel of Figure 8–1 illustrate the long-term average root-mean-square (rms) speech spectrum, as well as the peak and minimum amplitudes, for conversational speech and normal vocal effort. These values are from the ANSI standard on the Speech Intelligibility Index, SII (ANSI, 1997). Also shown are the average hearing thresholds for young, normal-hearing adults (solid line). Clearly, for normal-hearing young adults, the full 30-dB range of speech amplitudes from minimum to peak amplitudes is audible from 160 Hz to about 7000 Hz.

The lower panel of Figure 8–1, however, illustrates the corresponding situation for two different speech levels (rms level = 60 or 90 dB SPL; short dashed lines) and for the average hearing loss for 60-, 70-, and

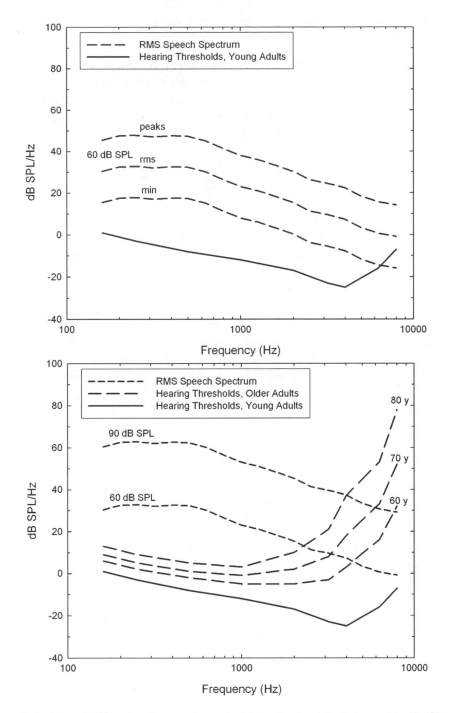

Figure 8–1. *Top:* RMS speech spectrum (*middle dashed line*) for a 60 dB SPL overall speech level. Upper and lower dashed lines represent momentary amplitude peaks and minima, respectively, for the speech stimulus and represent a 30-dB range of sound intensities. The solid line represents average hearing threshold for normal-hearing young adults. All values are from the ANSI standard for the SII (ANSI, 1997). *Bottom:* RMS speech spectra for speech levels of 60 (*lower dashed line*) and 90 dB SPL (*upper dashed line*). Three medium-dashed lines represent average hearing thresholds for males aged 60, 70, or 80 years (values from ISO, 2000).

80-year-old males who have been screened to eliminate other causes of hearing loss, such as chronic middle-ear disease or noise (ISO, 2000; long dashed lines). Whereas it is probably not too surprising to see the obvious influence of high-frequency hearing loss on the rms speech spectrum at 60 dB SPL, it is not often appreciated that this "typical" age-related hearing loss can have such an impact for the higher presentation level. Moreover, when considering the illustration in the bottom panel of Figure 8–1, there are several things to keep in mind. First, as noted, these age-related hearing thresholds are for a screened sample in which other causes of hearing loss have been eliminated. In that sense, it may not be "typical" of older adults in general or at least older adults seen at the audiology clinic. Second, also as noted, these threshold values are for males only and corresponding median thresholds for females will be about 5 to 7 dB better in the high frequencies for each age decade (ISO, 2000). Third, it should be kept in mind that these are average (median) thresholds. For a given age decade, the range for thresholds from the 10th to the 90th percentiles in the higher frequencies is about ±20 dB relative to the median. Thus, 50% of the older individuals in a given age decade will have thresholds worse than those shown here. Finally, notice that in terms of sensation level relative to mid-frequency hearing thresholds (500, 1000, and 2000 Hz), the 90 dB SPL stimulus is about 50 to 60 dB sensation level for the various age groups. Again, despite a high presentation level (90 dB SPL) and a moderately high sensation level (50–60 dB SL), much of the high-frequency portion of the speech spectrum is likely to be inaudible. Moreover, on average, progressively more of the speech spectrum would be rendered inaudible as age increased and performance would be expected to progressively decline with age as a result.

The top panel of Figure 8–2 shows a scatterplot of speech-recognition as a function of high-frequency (1000, 2000, and 4000 Hz) pure-tone average (HFPTA) for data from the Audiology Research Laboratory at Indiana University, an analysis of which was published by Humes (2005). In this case, the extrinsic redundancy of the speech stimulus was degraded by time compression, another common means of degrading the speech signal for tests administered to older adults. Speech stimuli were presented at 90 dB SPL in this study. The results for the 249 older adults shown here indicate clearly that speech-recognition performance for time-compressed monosyllables depends ($r = -0.74$, $p < .01$) on the amount of high-frequency hearing loss. One could imagine, however, that, given the general trend for high-frequency hearing loss to increase with age, the observed correlation was simply a manifestation of an age effect. In this particular sample of 249 older adults, however, the correlation of HFPTA with age was nonsignificant ($r = 0.16$, $p > .05$). Moreover, the strong negative correlation with HFPTA remained for partial correlations which controlled for the effects of age. The bottom panel of Figure 8–2 shows a subset of the data from the subjects in the top panel for whom the listener's SRT in the test ear was less than 30 dB HL. Given a 90 dB SPL (70 dB HL) presentation level, this corresponds to sensation levels of at least 40 dB for each subject in the lower panel. Clearly, even for these 78 more mildly impaired older adults, performance for the time-compressed monosyllabic words still depends critically on the average high-frequency hearing loss ($r = -0.62$, $p < .01$).

An interesting approach to minimizing the effects of high-frequency hearing loss on speech-recognition performance in older adults was used by Wiley et al. (1998). In this large-scale study of 3,189 adults between the

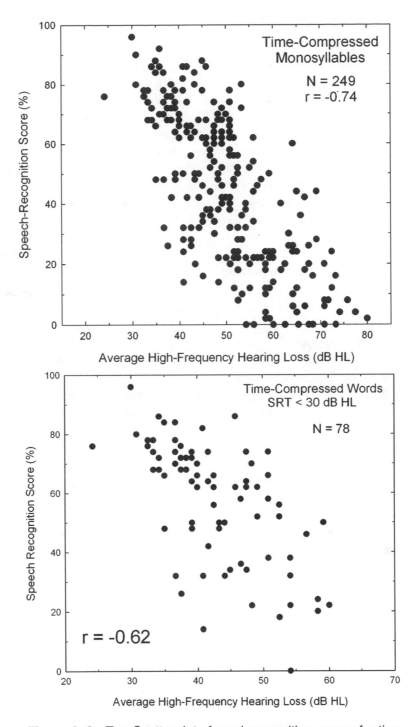

Figure 8–2. *Top:* Scatterplot of word-recognition scores for time-compressed speech as a function of average high-frequency hearing loss for 249 older adults between the ages of 60 and 90 years. *Bottom:* Same scatterplot as in top panel, but for only those older adults with mild hearing loss (SRT of 25 dB HL or less). All data are from Humes (2005).

ages of 48 and 92 years, word-recognition scores for a female talker were measured in the presence of speech produced by a competing male talker. To minimize the impact of high-frequency hearing loss, these investigators presented the speech materials at 36 dB SL *relative to hearing threshold at 2000 Hz*, rather than SRT as is typically the case. Unfortunately, even with this novel approach, pure-tone thresholds were the best predictor of individual differences in performance and suggest that this approach didn't fully minimize the loss of audibility. Perhaps a similar strategy based on hearing thresholds at 4000 Hz would have done so.

As noted, although time compression has been a common form of speech-signal degradation used with older adults to assess (central) auditory processing, many other forms of stimulus degradation have been used over the years. It has already been noted, for example, that a competing background has been another common approach to reducing the extrinsic redundancy of the speech stimulus. At least since the 1970s, word-recognition testing in a background of white noise has been suggested as a central auditory test, at least in patients with true central auditory lesions, such as 8th-nerve tumors or temporal-lobe damage (Olsen, Noffsinger, & Kurdziel, 1975). As noted, when this work was extended to older adults in subsequent years, the standard approach had been to present speech at a fixed sensation level or high sound pressure level, adjusting the background competition to a specified signal-to-noise ratio for all patients. As demonstrated, the use of fixed presentation levels, as well as fixed signal-to-noise ratios for a given presentation level, often yields results that are negatively impacted by the presence of high-frequency hearing loss. Essentially, it is as though the stimulus has been low-pass filtered by the presence of the high-frequency

hearing loss, thereby removing important high-frequency speech cues.

Since the work of Plomp (1978, 1986) in the Netherlands, however, there has been a shift in the approach to measuring speech-recognition performance in background noise. Rather than fixing the speech level and signal-to-noise ratio, the level of the noise background is varied over a range of levels and for each of these noise levels, SRT for sentence materials is measured. In the end, these measurements typically have been reduced to two values: (1) SRT in quiet; and (2) SRT in noise, the latter obtained in a background of steady-state noise of moderate intensity with the noise having an average spectrum identical to the long-term rms spectrum of the speech stimuli used. When results of older adults are compared to those of younger adults, a common pattern has often emerged. Specifically, older adults not only exhibit a hearing loss for speech in quiet, but also in noise, such that, for the same background noise level, a higher speech level is needed in the older adults to reach SRT. This has typically been interpreted as the older adults needing a "better than normal" speech-to-noise ratio to understand 50% of the sentences (i.e., to reach SRT).

Although Plomp originally attributed this need for an improved signal-to-noise ratio by older adults to some form of "distortion" above and beyond the loss of audibility, there is ample evidence to suggest that this is not the case. Instead, loss of audibility in the high frequencies can explain the need for a better-than-normal signal-to-noise ratio by older adults (Lee & Humes, 1993; Plomp, 1986). This is illustrated in Figure 8–3. The distortion, "SNR loss," or the amount that the signal-to-noise ratio has to be improved relative to that of young normal-hearing listeners listening with the full bandwidth available, measured in sev-

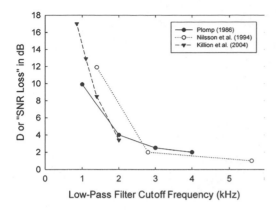

Figure 8–3. Plot of "SNR Loss" or "Distortion, D" in dB as a function of low-pass filter cut-off frequency from three studies of young, normal-hearing listeners using sentence-based SRT in noise measures.

eral studies is plotted in this figure along the *y*-axis. These data were obtained from young normal-hearing listeners. The *x*-axis illustrates the cutoff frequencies for various low-pass filters that were used to filter both the sentences and the spectrally shaped background noise. Results appear in Figure 8–3 for three sentence-in-noise tests: (1) the Dutch materials used by Plomp in the Netherlands (Plomp, 1986); (2) the American English equivalent of those materials, the HINT test (Nilsson, Soli, & Sullivan, 1994); and (3) the Quick-Speech In Noise (Quick SIN) test (Killion, Niquette, Gudmundsen, Revit, & Banerjee, 2004). Despite the use of different materials, subjects, languages, and cutoff frequencies, the results are fairly consistent across these three studies. The reader should keep in mind that a value of 0 dB on the ordinate in this graph indicates that the subjects, in this case all normal-hearing young adults, did not need a change in signal-to-noise relative to the unfiltered, full bandwidth condition. Also, in general, although this varies somewhat

across the three tests, a difference in signal-to-noise ratio of about 2 dB is considered a significant change given the test-retest variability of these measures.

Note that the general trend of the data across the three studies in Figure 8–3 is that when the stimulus (and competition) energy at or above 4000 Hz was removed by low-pass filtering, young normal-hearing adults required a 2-dB better signal-to-noise ratio. In similar fashion, the signal-to-noise ratio had to be increased about 3 dB for the low-pass cutoff frequency of 3000 Hz and 4 dB for the low-pass filter cutoff frequency of 2000 Hz. Thus, even though there has been a paradigm shift in terms of how speech recognition in noise is measured in older adults in the clinic and in the laboratory in recent years, it is still the case that the audibility of high frequencies is critically important to performance, even for young adults with normal hearing. In support of this peripheral audibility-based explanation for the observed need for a better than normal speech-to-noise ratio by older adults, Killion et al. (2004) reported a significant correlation of $r = 0.4$ between the signal-to-noise ratio and average hearing loss for 100 adults who were primarily older adults. Similarly, Walden and Walden (2004) reported correlations between pure-tone average hearing loss and either aided or unaided Q-SIN SRT values of about 0.55 for a group of 50 older adults. Unfortunately, the measure of average hearing loss used by Killion et al. (2004) and Walden and Walden (2004) was based on the pure-tone-average for frequencies of 500, 1000, and 2000 Hz. As noted previously, many studies have reported the strongest correlations between speech-recognition performance and pure-tone hearing loss for frequencies of 1000, 2000, and 4000 Hz for groups of older adults. Given the typical sloping high-frequency hearing loss in this population, it is not surprising that this higher frequency pure-tone average better captures the contributions of hearing loss to speech-recognition performance. It can only be surmised that the correlations reported by Killion et al. (2004) and Walden and Walden (2004) would have been even stronger if the high-frequency pure-tone average had been used in the correlations instead.

Clearly, loss of high-frequency hearing sensitivity can have a negative impact on the speech-recognition performance of older listeners. One strategy that some researchers have taken to minimize the apparent impact of the high-frequency hearing loss in older adults is to demonstrate that the older adults failed to exhibit much of a performance decrement relative to younger adults for some baseline condition. For example, it might be reported that the older group had a mean speech-recognition score in quiet of 90% and this was only 4 to 6% lower than that obtained by the younger subjects in the same test condition; a between-group difference that may or may not be statistically significant. Next, the speech stimulus is degraded in some way, as in noise masking or time compression, and large, statistically significant differences in performance are now observed between the two age groups. Thus, the high-frequency hearing loss present in the older adults was not enough to degrade performance in and of itself, so the observed group difference in performance for degraded speech must be due to age differences or, at a minimum, the interaction of the effects of hearing loss and aging.

That this may not necessarily be the case is illustrated nicely by the mean data from Lacroix, Harris, and Randolph (1979) shown in the top panel of Figure 8–4. The data shown in this figure represent means from groups of 20 young normal-hearing adults listening to sentence materials in various conditions. The results for three forms of speech degradation are shown in the top

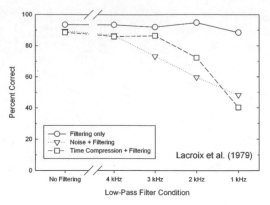

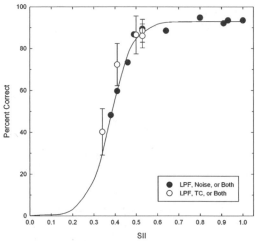

Figure 8–4. *Top:* Mean data from normal-hearing young adults from Lacroix et al. (1979) for three different listening conditions. *Bottom:* Transfer function relating percent-correct performance to SII derived from conditions represented by solid symbols (*noise and filtering*). Open symbols show fit of data to this same transfer function for a different set of listening conditions (*time compression and filtering*).

panel of Figure 8–4: low-pass filtering, speech-shaped noise at a +2 dB signal-to-noise ratio, and time compression. The data points to the far left in the top panel of Figure 8–4 illustrate the mean performance of the young normal-hearing listeners for broadband unfiltered stimuli (in quiet, in noise, or with time compression). The data points to the right of this illustrate the effects of progressively greater amounts of low-pass filtering, either in isolation (circles) or in combination with noise (triangles) or time compression (squares). Note that the impact of low-pass filtering on sentence comprehension is almost negligible in these young normal-hearing adults with the mean performance for unfiltered stimuli being approximately 94% and then dropping only to 89% with the extreme amount of low-pass filtering (1 kHz; far right circle). In this case, although this was a negligible drop in performance, it was a statistically significant decline (Lacroix, Harris, & Randolf, 1979). Note, however, the much more dramatic impact of this seemingly harmless cut of high-frequency stimulus energy when it has been combined with other forms of stimulus degradation. For example, when combined with either speech-shaped noise or time compression, speech-recognition performance dropped from about 90% without filtering to 40 to 50% with the extreme amount of low-pass filtering. Clearly, the missing high-frequency information as a result of low-pass filtering at 1000, 2000, or 3000 Hz, although not impacting performance in quiet when filtering was the only degradation, had a major impact on performance when combined with either of the other forms of distortion. Thus, by implication, demonstrating that the hearing loss of older adults failed to have much impact on speech-recognition in quiet does not mean that this will also be the case when this filtering effect is combined with other forms of speech degradation, such as background noise or time compression.

The basic concepts underlying the Speech Intelligibility Index (SII; ANSI, 1997) can help explain what is happening in such situations. Figure 8–5 illustrates the SII concept for low-pass filtered speech (top panel), speech in speech-shaped noise (middle

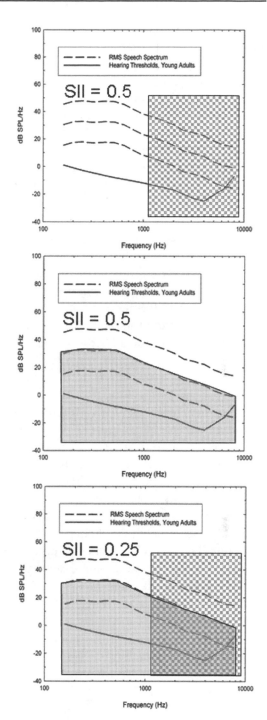

Figure 8–5. Schematic illustration of SII explanation of potential multiplicative effects of distortions. *Top:* low-pass filtering; *Center:* speech-shaped noise; *Bottom:* combined effects of low-pass filtering and speech-shaped noise.

panel), and the combination of both forms of degradation. The top panel is essentially a replication of the top panel of Figure 8–1, but with the addition of a checked rectangular region that schematically represents the elimination of the high frequencies via a low-pass filter. If the full 30-dB speech range (the region between the upper and lower dashed lines) in the top panel is audible across frequency (~160–7000 Hz), then the SII = 1.0. In the top panel, half of this area bounded by the upper and lower dashed lines has been removed by the low-pass filtering and, under a certain set of assumptions regarding the underlying importance of various frequency regions, we can assume that the SII has been cut in half to a value of 0.5 in the top panel. We can also slice this area (bounded by the upper and lower dashed lines) in half horizontally by introducing a spectrally shaped speech noise that masks the lower 15 dB of this 30-dB range. This is schematically illustrated in the middle panel of Figure 8–5 and also yields an SII value of 0.5 (no assumptions are needed here regarding the underlying importance of various frequencies to the speech-recognition score). In each of these two cases, low-pass filtering (top panel) and speech-noise masking (middle panel), the SII is the same and performance is therefore expected to be the same. The exact score predicted for an SII value of 0.5 depends on the performance-SII transfer function for the particular test materials.

Assume that a score of about 90% is obtained for the conditions represented in the top two panels of Figure 8–5. As neither form of degradation alone has much impact on speech-recognition performance, it might be conjectured that the combined effect would be negligible. This, however, is often not the case, as was shown in the data from Lacroix et al. (1979) for combined distortions (Figure 8–4, top panel). In fact, in

the simplified schematic representation of Figure 8–5, the result of both forms of distortion would be a multiplicative effect in terms of the SII value. That is, the SII for combined distortions, one confined exclusively to limiting the bandwidth (low-pass filtering or high-frequency hearing loss) and the other exclusively to a broadband impact on the 30-dB range of speech amplitudes at each frequency (speech-shaped noise), the SII from the combination of both forms of degradation is the product of each SII value. In the hypothetical example illustrated in Figure 8–5, the result is an expected SII value of 0.25 (0.5×0.5).

To examine the validity of this explanation and the consequences that would follow from it, SII values were calculated for the low-pass filtering, the noise only, and the noise + filtering conditions of Lacroix et al. (1979). Mean speech-recognition scores for these conditions from Lacroix et al. (1979) were then plotted as a function of SII and these appear as the filled circles in the bottom panel of Figure 8–4. A three-parameter sigmoidal function was then fit to these data ($r^2 = 0.99$) and appears in this same panel as the solid line. Next, using this derived transfer function and the mean score for the time-compression-only listening condition, the SII value corresponding to the effect of time-compression alone was determined. Here, it is only assumed that the impact of time compression is broadband and uniform across frequency, as in the case of the speech-shaped noise. Finally, the SII values calculated for each of the low-pass filter conditions used by Lacroix et al. (1979) were multiplied by the time-compression-alone SII value to yield SII values for the combined effects of time compression and low-pass filtering. The unfilled circles in the bottom panel of Figure 8–4 are the result of these calculations and reveal good agreement between observed speech-recognition performance and that predicted by this multiplicative SII-based approach. That is, the unfilled circles derived for time compression plus low-pass filtering are in close proximity to the best-fitting SII transfer function derived from the other data. Thus, these results for the combined effects of time compression and low-pass filtering validate the multiplicative effects of these two types of distortion on the SII.

What are the implications of these multiplicative effects on the SII? Applying the derived empirical transfer function to the hypothetical schematized scenario represented in Figure 8–5, if low-pass filtering (top panel) and speech-shaped noise (middle panel), or some other broadband, uniform degradation, each yielded an SII of 0.5, according to the transfer function in the bottom of Figure 8–4, this would correspond to a speech-recognition score for those sentences of about 85% for each form of degradation alone. When combined, however, the SII would decrease to 0.25 and, according to the transfer function in the bottom panel of Figure 8–4, performance would decrease to about 10%. Thus, it is possible for two seemingly innocuous degradations to combine to have a very significant negative impact on performance.

Of course, this is not always the case. For example, using the derived transfer function in the bottom panel of Figure 8–4, imagine that low-pass filtering alone produces an SII of 0.9 or 0.8 and so does speech-noise masking alone. When combined, the multiplicative effect would result in SII values for combined distortion of 0.81 (0.9 × 0.9) and 0.64 (0.8 × 0.8). Examination of the SII transfer function for these materials in the bottom panel of Figure 8–4 indicates that the predicted score would remain at about 93% for all values of the SII exceeding about 0.60. As a result, given this transfer function, scores for low-pass filtering alone,

noise alone, and the combination would all be expected to be about 93%. Thus, it is difficult to use speech-recognition scores from two or more forms of degradation alone to predict the combined influence of both forms of distortion when combined. If, as has been maintained here, one can use low-pass filtering by various degrees to approximate the effects of varying amounts of high-frequency hearing loss, at least for a fixed presentation level, then these notions apply to older adults with high-frequency hearing loss. Demonstrating that an older adult with high-frequency hearing loss has no difficulty with broadband speech in quiet (note that this is already one form of degradation for these listeners, but not for young, normal-hearing adults), does not mean that these same listeners will not show much larger effects for some other form of degradation, such as background noise or time compression, than observed in young normal-hearing listeners. In the older adults, the bandwidth-limiting high-frequency hearing loss can have a multiplicative impact on the SII when other stimulus degradation is introduced, such as background noise or time compression. As illustrated above, the consequences of these multiplicative SII effects can range from negligible to extreme depending on the specific SII values for each form of distortion alone and the SII transfer function of the materials used.

The point of emphasis in this section of the chapter is that the performance of older adults can be critically and negatively impacted by the presence of high-frequency hearing loss and these peripheral effects must be accounted for before one can attribute a central origin to the older adult's speech communication difficulties. Although we have been reviewing the impact of high-frequency hearing loss on speech-recognition in general, with emphasis on some tests and forms of degradation commonly used in test batteries for (central) auditory processing assessment in older adults, Jerger, Jerger, Oliver, and Pirozzolo (1989) provided some direct evidence on the impact of high-frequency hearing loss on the diagnosis of auditory processing disorder in older adults. In the study by Jerger, Jerger, Oliver, and Pirozzolo, (1989), a test battery composed of various speech-recognition measures was used to assess 130 older adults. Half of the group was ultimately diagnosed with central auditory processing disorder by Jerger et al. (1989). For the 65 older adults with speech-recognition scores deemed consistent with auditory processing disorder, 82% had average high-frequency sensorineural hearing loss exceeding 25 dB HL. On the other, only 38% of those determined not to have auditory processing disorders had average high-frequency hearing loss exceeding 25 dB HL. Thus, if one had average high-frequency hearing loss exceeding 25 dB HL, it was more than twice as likely that this person would be determined to have central auditory processing disorders on the basis of his or her speech-recognition performance.

Contributions of Cognitive Factors

In the overwhelming majority of the studies of individual differences in speech-recognition among older adults cited previously, the speech stimulus was presented at a fixed presentation level, either defined in terms of sensation level or sound pressure level. In the previous section, the important role played by high-frequency hearing thresholds in determining individual differences in speech-recognition performance was noted repeatedly, even for relatively high presentation levels. In fact, in several of these studies, the proportion of variance accounted

for by the listener's average high-frequency hearing loss is so great that there is little systematic variance left to account for by other predictor variables. This factor plays such a large role in determining individual differences in speech-recognition performance that the contributions of other factors may only be revealed when the issue of the audibility of the high frequencies has been negated or at least minimized.

There are at least two ways in which the role of high-frequency hearing loss in the speech-recognition performance of older adults can be minimized. One approach is to test only older adults with very little or no hearing loss in the high frequencies. Although this approach has been used for between-group comparisons in factorial designs with relatively small sample sizes and has proven extremely valuable in teasing apart effects attributable to hearing loss, aging, or the combination of these two factors (e.g., Dubno, Dirks, & Morgan, 1984; Gordon-Salant & Fitzgibbons, 1993, 1999, 2001), there have been few, if any, large-scale studies of individual differences in speech-recognition performance among so-called "elderly normal-hearing" individuals. This is undoubtedly due to the general difficulty in finding enough such individuals. Often, attempts to do so result in compromises as to how closely the high-frequency thresholds match those of young normal-hearing subjects such that, although the elderly normal-hearing subjects have very good hearing for their age and hearing thresholds that are better than conventional upper limits for normal hearing (i.e., 25 dB HL), hearing thresholds frequently remain significantly elevated relative to those of young normal-hearing adults, especially at frequencies of 3000, 4000, 6000, and 8000 Hz. In some cases, these seemingly minimal differences in hearing thresholds can again explain some of the differences observed in speech-recognition performance between young and elderly "normal hearing" groups (e.g., Halling & Humes, 2000).

Another general approach to minimizing the contributions of high-frequency hearing loss to speech-recognition measures in older adults is to incorporate some degree of spectral shaping for the speech stimuli (and competing stimuli, if used). Humes (2007) has reviewed several different variations of this approach that have been pursued in the Audiology Research Laboratory in recent years. The variations investigated to date have ranged from use of a high presentation level for the stimuli with additional gain provided in the high frequencies (at and above 1000 Hz, for example), on either a group or individual basis, to individually tailoring the stimuli to ensure that the rms amplitude spectrum of the stimulus is at least 15 dB SL from low frequencies through some specified high frequency (such as 4000, 5000, or 6000 Hz). Of course, in principle, the latter strategy could be implemented with conventional hearing aids. In reality, though, it has often been challenging to realize sufficient high-frequency gain with actual hearing aids, due primarily to feedback limitations, and this has resulted in a continuing influence of high-frequency hearing loss on the *aided* speech-recognition performance of older listeners (e.g., Humes, 2002). Even with the improved, but less than optimal (according to SII concepts) audibility resulting from the fitting of real hearing aids, however, Humes (2002) was able to identify significant contributions of cognitive function to individual differences in aided speech-recognition performance. Although audibility was again the primary predictor of performance, accounting for 53% of the total variance, individual differences in age and in cognitive function accounted for about 13% of additional variance in that study.

When spectrally shaped stimuli have been delivered to older adults via earphones to ensure audibility of the speech (and competing) stimuli through 4000 to 6000 Hz, a common pattern across several laboratory studies emerged: (1) average high-frequency hearing loss was no longer a predictor of "aided" speech-recognition performance; and (2) cognitive factors were significant predictors of individual differences in performance (Humes, 2007). That average high-frequency hearing loss no longer predicts individual differences in performance for spectrally shaped or "aided" stimuli may at first seem obvious as audibility limitations have been overcome. However, the degree of underlying pathology in the basal regions of the cochlea covaries with average high-frequency hearing loss (e.g., Bredberg, 1968). Thus, although it has been maintained in the preceding section that it was the inaudibility of the higher frequencies that was responsible for the correlations of average high-frequency hearing loss with speech-recognition performance in older adults, it is possible that the degree of hearing loss was simply a quantitative behavioral marker of the underlying cochlear pathology and this was the factor underlying the observed correlations. The fact that the correlations with average high-frequency hearing loss disappeared in most, but not all, studies reviewed by Humes (2007) suggests that the factor underlying the observed correlations was in fact inaudibility of the higher frequencies and not the degree of underlying pathology. As importantly, once the restricted inaudibility has been overcome, individual differences in speech-recognition among older adults were generally found to be correlated with cognitive factors, age, or both. The specific cognitive measurements investigated varied from study to study, however, such that there was no convergence on a specific cognitive variable that was predictive of individual differences in speech-recognition among older adults.

One of the studies reviewed briefly by Humes (2007) was an investigation of auditory selective and divided attention among older adults (Humes, Lee, & Coughlin, 2006). The measurement paradigm used in the study by Humes et al. (2006) enabled the measurement of selective and divided attention for monaural and dichotic stimulus presentations that were otherwise identical. In audiology, dichotic tasks are often considered to be a measure of (central) auditory processing and frequently reveal aspects of hemispheric dominance for speech when the dichotic paradigm makes use of speech stimuli. For example, in young normal-hearing adults, when temporally overlapping stimuli are presented simultaneously to both ears in a dichotic paradigm and ear-specific scores are computed, it is often the case that the score for the right ear is higher than that of the left ear, yielding the so-called "right ear advantage" (e.g., Berlin, Lowe-Bell, Cullen, & Thompsen, 1973; Kimura, 1967). It has been argued that the observed domination of the right ear for speech is due to the predominant innervation of the left temporal lobe by the right ear and the specialization of the left temporal lobe for speech processing. There certainly appears to be evidence for speech-specific (or, at least, linguistic-specific) processing that emerges from the dichotic speech-identification paradigm in the form of a right-ear advantage. In the study by Humes, Lee, and Coughlin (2006), there was evidence of a right-ear advantage of similar magnitude in both age groups, which has often been observed by others. Occasionally, a small percentage of older adults will show an enormous right-ear advantage on such tasks, so much so that it has often been labeled as a "left-ear disadvantage" in the elderly (Jerger & Jordan, 1992; Jerger, Chmiel, Allen, & Wilson, 1994;

Roup, Wiley & Wilson, 2005). When the individual ear-specific scores of both age groups are compared, it is apparent in these rare cases that the speech-recognition score for the right ear is close to an expected value, but the score for the left ear is much lower than expected. It has been suggested that older adults with extreme left-ear disadvantage may have poor interhemispheric transfer across temporal lobes, possibly at the corpus callosum (Martin & Jerger, 2005).

Dichotic processing, however, also has an attentional component to it. When competing speech stimuli are presented simultaneously to both ears and the signal to one ear is cued for the listener, performance can be determined, in part, by how well the listener can ignore the message at the noncued ear. Historically, this attentional aspect of dichotic listening has an even longer history than the aspect associated with linguistic-specific hemispheric processing (e.g., Broadbent, 1954; Cherry, 1953). Evidence for the contribution of cognitive (attentional) processing factors to performance on the dichotic task in Humes et al. (2006) was provided by comparing the listeners' performance for the identical task administered monaurally. When correlations were calculated for young and older adults across monaural and dichotic listening conditions, significant Pearson-r correlation coefficients of 0.94 and 0.87 were observed for the young and older adults, respectively. Thus, performance for the linguistic-specific interhemispheric dichotic conditions was strongly correlated to performance observed under monaural listening conditions; that is, without interhemispheric competition. Those who could better ignore the competing temporally overlapping stimulus when both were presented monaurally could also do so when each was presented to a separate ear. In addition, performance in the divided-attention condition, whether monaural or dichotic, was significantly, moderately, and positively correlated with digit-span scores for the older adults, further supporting common underlying cognitive processes for both monaural and dichotic presentation conditions. When older adults perform worse than young adults on dichotic speech-recognition measures, it may be difficult to attribute such deficits to modality-specific (central) auditory-processing problems rather than general cognitive-processing problems, such as attentional deficits. Relative ear advantages (or disadvantages) derived from dichotic paradigms, however, do appear to at least be linguistic-specific measures, rather than cognitive measures. Here, however, care must be taken to eliminate asymmetries in peripheral high-frequency hearing thresholds as a factor underlying individual differences in ear advantages observed among the elderly (e.g., Humes et al., 2006).

Further evidence that dichotic speech-identification performance in older adults may be determined to some degree by individual differences in cognitive processing can be found in analyses of individual differences in performance conducted in several studies. Recall from the discussion of the role of peripheral hearing loss in the previous section, for example, that Jerger et al. (1991) observed significant correlations between high-frequency pure-tone average and all five measures of speech-recognition performance included in that study. Although average high-frequency hearing loss was the primary predictor for all five measures, for the Dichotic Sentence Identification (DSI) test, 30% of the variance in dichotic speech-identification performance could be explained by average high-frequency hearing loss, but an additional 13% of the variance could be explained by scores on the Digit-Symbol test of the WAIS-R. The total explained variance of 43% for the DSI approximates the maximum possible variance

that one could expect to explain given the relatively low test-retest reliability of this test in older adults (Cokely & Humes, 1992; Humes, Coughlin, & Talley, 1996).

Figure 8–6 shows a scatterplot of percent-correct scores for a dichotic consonant-vowel (CV) identification task versus WAIS-R IQ score from 246 older adults (Humes, 2005). The Pearson-r correlation coefficient between these two measures is 0.36 (p <0.01) and represents the strongest correlation observed in these analyses among various predictors of dichotic speech-identification performance. Many other measures of auditory function (audiometric measures plus various measures from otoacoustic emissions and auditory brainstem responses) and cognitive function (various scales from the WAIS-R) were examined as possible predictors of performance, but IQ emerged as the best predictor. Hallgren, Larsby, Lyxell, and

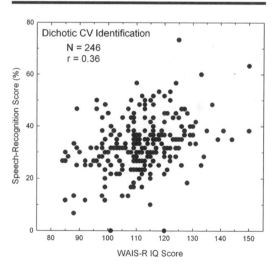

Figure 8–6. Scatterplot of speech-recognition scores versus WAIS-R IQ scores for 246 older adults between the ages of 60 and 90 years. Speech-recognition measure was the closed set identification of consonant-vowel (CV) syllables presented dichotically. Data are from Humes (2005).

Arlinger (2001) have noted similar correlations between various measures of cognitive function and performance on dichotic speech-identification tasks in older adults. Correlations such as these also suggest that clinical measures of dichotic speech identification may not represent pure measures of auditory processing and may be determined to a greater extent by individual differences in cognitive function.

Further concerns about the validity of the common test battery used to assess (central) auditory processing in older adults were provided by Jerger et al. (1989). In this study, 130 older adults completed the battery of (central) auditory processing tests described previously (DSI, SSI, SPIN-PL, SPIN-PH, and PB words). Participants also received a battery of cognitive measures as a part of a neurologic assessment. Based on criteria established by Jerger et al. (1989), each participant was classified as "normal" or "abnormal" for central auditory status and cognitive status. Using their criteria, Jerger et al. (1989) identified 65 of the 130 older adults as having abnormal central auditory status. Of these 65 older adults with abnormal central auditory status, 35 (54%) were also determined to have abnormal cognitive status. This compared to 18 of 65 (28%) in the "normal" central auditory status category who were determined to have abnormal cognitive status. This clearly demonstrates overlap between abnormal cognitive and abnormal central auditory status and suggests that in many cases, diagnosis of abnormal central auditory status may actually be manifestation of abnormal cognitive function when using sounds as the stimuli.

Interestingly, 38 (58%) of the 65 older adults categorized as having abnormal central auditory status failed either the DSI alone ($N = 12$) or the DSI plus any other measure in the auditory-processing battery ($N = 26$). For these two subgroups, as well as three

others with other patterns of results for the auditory-processing tests, Jerger et al. (1989) obtained control groups of older adults who were matched for age, gender, hearing loss, and general cognitive function. The performance of the control group and the corresponding subgroup with abnormal central auditory status was then compared on a variety of measures. Of the five sets of subgroup comparisons performed by Jerger et al. (1989), the only two subgroups which differed significantly from their matched controls on detailed measures of cognitive function were the two subgroups who had failed the DSI. Moreover, these two subgroups differed from their controls primarily on various memory tasks. As noted previously, Humes et al. (2006) found correlations between digit-span measures of memory and measures of divided attention for dichotic and monaural presentation conditions. Thus, this pattern of subgroup differences reported by Jerger et al. (1989) suggests further that individual differences in cognitive function (memory or attention) may underlie individual differences observed in measures of (central) auditory processing, especially tasks involving dichotic processing.

Another approach to establishing the validity of modality-specific auditory-processing deficits is to examine performance for parallel tasks in other modalities (Cacace & McFarland, 1998, 2005; Humes, Christopherson, & Cokely, 1992; McFarland & Cacace, 1995). The notion here is that, if the deficit is unique to the auditory processing of sounds, then individuals assessed on identical tasks in the auditory and a nonauditory sensory modality should demonstrate impaired performance only for the auditory modality. If the problem is an amodal cognitive deficit, on the other hand, then performance on parallel tasks should be correlated across modalities (e.g., Watson, Qiu, Chamberlain, & Li, 1996).

Two recent studies have examined correlations across the auditory and visual modalities for similar speech-in-noise tasks in older adults (George et al., 2007; Humes, Burk, Coughlin, Busey, & Strauser, 2007). George et al. (2007) made use of an adaptive SRT-based sentence test developed by Plomp and Mimpen (1979) for auditory testing. (The subsequent development of the Hearing In Noise Test [HINT; Nilsson et al., 1994] in the United States is the American English equivalent of the Dutch SRT measure.) George et al. (2007) administered this test in the typical background of steady-state speech-shaped noise, as well as in a background of amplitude-modulated speech-shaped noise. These investigators then measured the text reception threshold (TRT) from a visual analog of the modulated-noise SRT task developed by Zekveld, George, Kramer, Goverts, and Houtgast (2007). In this task, the text of an entire sentence is displayed momentarily and in a word-by-word sequence on a computer screen in the presence of a horizontal array of vertical black bars that obscured portions of the text. The horizontal widths of the black bars were adjusted adaptively from trial to trial to converge on the 50% threshold or TRT. Although additional data were obtained in this study, the focus here is on the relationship observed between the auditory SRT and the visual TRT in the 13 elderly normal-hearing and 21 elderly hearing-impaired adults assessed. For the auditory presentations, the speech and noise stimuli were spectrally shaped for each subject to minimize the contributions of inaudibility of the higher frequencies. For the 13 elderly normal-hearing listeners, the correlations between TRT and SRT were positive, moderate, and significant. Pearson-r correlation coefficients were 0.61 and 0.80 for the SRT in steady-state and the SRT in modulated noise, respectively. The results for modulated noise

background are similar to those observed by Zekveld et al. (2007) for a group of normal-hearing adults with an wider range of ages than used in George et al. (2007). For the 21 older adults with impaired hearing, however, the correlations between TRT and SRT were somewhat weaker ($r = 0.34$ and 0.42 for steady-state and modulated noise, respectively) and not significant statistically. Even for this group, however, TRT was a significant secondary predictor of individual differences in SRT for modulated noise, accounting for 9% of the variance. A psychophysical measure of auditory temporal resolution was the primary predictor in this case, however, and accounted for 48% of the variance in SRT for modulated noise. In summary, this study supports contributions of both modality-specific and amodal, possibly cognitive, factors to the understanding of speech in noise by older adults, especially when the audibility restrictions from hearing loss have been removed, either through assessment of older adults with normal hearing or through spectral shaping of the speech and noise stimuli. The correlations across modalities are generally stronger for parallel tasks; that is, modulated speech noise and "modulated visual noise."

Humes et al. (2007) chose to focus on two types of speech-recognition measure used in the assessment of (central) auditory function in older adults. As noted previously, the general framework for the development of speech-based measures of auditory processing requires that the extrinsic redundancy of the speech stimulus be degraded in some way. Two very common approaches have been to speed up the auditory speech stimulus, typically via time compression, or to degrade the stimulus through the addition of background noise. Humes et al. (2007) employed both forms of signal degradation using two measures of speeded speech and one measure of speech in noise. Performance was measured in 13 young normal-hearing adults, 10 elderly normal-hearing adults, and 16 older adults with impaired hearing. In particular, one measure was the use of uncompressed and 45% time-compressed NU-6 monosyllables developed by Wilson et al. (1994). For these speech-recognition measures and all others used in this study, a high overall presentation level (≥90 dB SPL) and additional spectral shaping to boost the high frequencies was used. Because it was not clear how to implement time compression in the visual domain, a second speeded-speech measure, referred to as "speeded spelling," was developed for use in the study by Humes et al. (2007). In this measure, each of the 26 letters of the alphabet was recorded in isolation for a female talker. The talker was instructed to produce three brief repetitions of each letter in succession with short pauses between each. The clearest of the three productions was then retained and used in the speeded-spelling task. In the actual task, monosyllabic words composed of three to five letters were spelled out auditorily by concatenating the WAV files for each letter and inserting a fixed duration silent period between each successive letter in the string. For example, if the word was "dog," the digital WAV files for "d," "o," and "g" were concatenated with silent intervals of fixed duration inserted between the "d" and "o" and be-tween the "o" and "g." The spelling of the word could then be varied in rate by varying the interval of silence between successive letters, leaving the actual letters intact. Two rates of presentation were used by Humes et al. (2007) and the listener's ability to identify each of the 26 letters in isolation when presented in random order was also assessed. The visual analogue of this task was created by presenting black letters against a gray background with the durations of the visual letters approximating the average duration of the spoken letters and blank intervals between the visual presentation of letters on the screen matched to those used in the auditory task. As with the auditory speeded-spelling task, the visual task also had a control condition for the identification of each of the 26 letters of the alphabet in isolation.

The speech-in-noise test used by Humes et al. (2007) was the SPIN test, both PL and PH items, completed in a background of multitalker babble at several signal-to-noise ratios. For the visual analog of this task, each word of the PL or PH sentence was flashed on the computer screen in front of the participant with the duration and rate of presentation approximating the average word and silence durations measured for the auditory SPIN tests. Each word was presented individually in sequence, rather than presenting the entire sentence at once, as Speranza, Daneman, and Schneider (2000) found no differences in performance for these two presentation modes for young or older adults. The background was composed of a randomly varying pixelated rectangular area surrounding the text (i.e., "visual noise").

Analyses were performed by Humes et al. (2007) on both the group and individual data. Group differences emerged such that older adults did worse than young adults on all tasks, but most of these differences disappeared when baseline differences based on peripheral processing were partialed out. Consider, for example, the SPIN test in each modality. Older adults generally had lower scores on both the PL and PH items, but when the differences for the high-context PH items were reanalyzed with PL scores as a covariate, group differences disappeared in each modality. In other words, the relative benefit from context (PH-PL) was the same for all groups. The Pearson-*r* correlation coefficient for SPIN scores across modalities, moreover, was approximately 0.6 across conditions. Thus, there was a substantial amount of shared variance across the auditory and visual versions of these two tasks suggesting a common amodal (cognitive) underlying mechanism.

A somewhat different pattern emerged, however, for the speeded-speech measures in each modality. Again, there was a moderate correlation across modalities, as with the SPIN test, but using (peripheral) baseline measures as covariates had differential effects across modalities. For the visual speeded-spelling task, for example, using the visual alphabet identification scores as a covariate eliminated differences in performance across age groups. Doing so for the auditory speeded-spelling task, however, did not yield the same results. There were still significant differences between age groups when baseline auditory alphabet scores were used as a covariate. Both elderly groups again performed worse than the young adults. The same was true for the time-compressed auditory materials. The older adults performed worse than young adults on the time-compressed NU-6 words whether or not the baseline uncompressed NU-6 scores were included as a covariate in the analyses. Thus, for the speeded-speech or speeded-text recognition tests, there was evidence of both a common shared amodal mechanism operating and a modality-specific auditory mechanism impacting the performance on the auditory speeded-speech measures. The general amodal factor observed could be associated with the common observation of general age-related "cognitive slowing" that has been observed frequently in a variety of contexts (e.g., Salthouse, 1985, 1991, 2000), including the recognition of time-compressed speech (e.g., Wingfield, Poon, Lombardi, & Lowe, 1985, Wingfield, Tun, Koh, & Rosen, 1999; Wingfield & Tun, 2001). The auditory-specific deficit may very well be an additional deficit in auditory temporal resolution experienced by elderly listeners, as suggested by several others previously (e.g., 2002; George et al., 2006, 2007; Gordon-Salant & Fitzgibbons, 1993, 1997, 2000, 2004; Konkle, Beasley, & Bess, 1977; Schneider, Pichora-Fuller, Kowalchuk, & Lamb, 1994; Schneider & Pichora-Fuller; Schneider, Speranza, & Pichora-Fuller, 1998; Snell, 1997; Snell & Frisina, 2000; Strouse, Ashmead, Ohde, & Granthan, 1998). It should be noted that Schneider, Daneman, and Murphy (2005) have recently questioned whether the typical means of implementing time compression results in speech that is only temporally distorted or also involves spectral distortion of the speech signal. Nonetheless, because there may be both amodal cognitive and modality-specific temporal or temporal plus spectral distortions contributing to a particular older adult's performance on speeded speech materials, it is imperative that the audiologist have some means of teasing apart these contributions prior to establishing a diagnosis as an auditory-processing disorder. Tests parallel to those used to measure auditory processing, but in a different sensory modality, offer one possible means of doing so.

Other Issues in the Diagnostic Assessment of Auditory Processing in Older Adults

The foregoing sections of this chapter offered evidence that challenged the validity of several speech-recognition measures used frequently to assess (central) auditory processing in older adults. The two primary challenges were in the form of contributions of peripheral hearing loss or amodal cognitive processing to individual differences in performance for these measures of presumed (central) auditory processing in older adults.

As noted previously by Humes, Christopherson, and Cokely (1992), however, these issues regarding the validity of the measurements, as well as the diagnosis that follows from them, are not the only issues of concern in the assessment of auditory processing in older adults. Two other problem areas concern the test-retest reliability of the measures used frequently to assess auditory processing in older adults and the design of the test battery incorporating these measures. Each of these issues is addressed below.

Test Reliability

As was noted by Humes et al. (1992), the criteria used with various speech-recognition measures to establish the presence of auditory processing disorders are difficult to reconcile with known characteristics of the test scores comprising these criteria. For example, one common criterion applied to the interpretation of differences between PB word scores and SSI scores is that differences exceeding 20% are consistent with the presence of a (central) auditory processing disorder (e.g., Jerger et al., 1989). This same 20% difference-score criterion is applied to interpret significant declines in speech-recognition performance at high intensities, so-called "rollover," for either PB word scores or SSI scores (e.g., Cooper & Gates, 1991; Jerger et al., 1989). A given SSI score, however, is typically based on a single set of 10 sentences and, in this context, a given PB-word score is typically based on a set of 25 sentences. It is well established (e.g., Thornton & Raffin, 1978) that there is considerable variability to be expected around scores based on tests composed of only 10 or 25 items. For example, 95% critical differences for a score of 50%-correct on a test composed of 10 items range from 10% to 90%. In other words, it is very likely that an

initial SSI score of 50% will yield significant "rollover" of at least 20% on retest alone. Although the situation is improved for PB-word scores based on 25 items, the 95% critical difference bounds still exceed the 20% rollover criterion by 3 to 4% for a wide range of initial PB-word scores (~20–80%).

There is no need to rely on abstract discussion of 95% critical differences for percent-correct scores, however, to evaluate the reliability of many of these measures. Some studies have directly assessed the reliability of several of the tests of (central) auditory processing used with older adults. Dubno and Dirks (1983), for example, found the SSI to be unreliable when based on a single 10-item test and suggested that each score be based on 30 sentence presentations to ensure reliable results. Feeney and Hallowell (2000) found that older adults required at least three practice lists prior to uses of the SSI in order to obtain reliable scores. They also found significant differences across several of the randomized lists of the SSI and suggested that only six of the lists be used for reliable results. Finally, Pugh, Crandell, and Griffiths (1998) obtained data challenging the reliability of the SSI and suggested the addition of supplemental background noise to the competing speech stimulus as a means of improving test reliability.

With regard to the DSI and the SPIN test, Cokely and Humes (1992) assessed test-retest reliability of these measures in 17 older adults. Neither test was found to be reliable as typically used and it was recommended that test length be expanded to increase reliability. Cokely and Humes (1992) noted, moreover, that the variability of these measures was sufficient to result in changes in diagnostic disposition from test to retest.

Although many of the measures that have been used historically to perform (central) auditory assessments in older adults have significant test reliability short-comings, this is not the case for all such measures. One set of tests available for such applications, but not yet in widespread use for this purpose in older adults, is the Test of Basic Auditory Capabilities (TBAC; Surprenant & Watson, 2001; Watson, 1987; Watson, Jensen, Foyle, Leek, & Goldgar, 1982). A nice feature of this test for use with older adults, many of whom have high-frequency hearing loss, is the use of tonal stimuli confined to frequencies below 3000 Hz on many of the tests. Christopherson and Humes (1992) found most of the eight tests comprising the original test battery to be reliable in young normal-hearing adults, older normal-hearing adults, and older adults with impaired hearing. Moreover, only the two tests making use of speech stimuli revealed any impact of peripheral high-frequency hearing loss on performance. The original TBAC evaluated by Christopherson and Humes (1992) has been updated (Surprenant & Watson, 2001) and the reliability of the tests added to the newer version has yet to be evaluated in older adults.

Humes, Coughlin, and Talley (1996) evaluated 10 of the 15 auditory processing tasks included on a compact disk developed by the Department of Veterans Affairs (VA-CD; Noffsinger, Wilson, & Musiek, 1994) in 40 young normal-hearing adults and 38 older adults. The 10 measures of auditory processing were well represented by three underlying factors and at least one measure associated with each of these factors was found to be reliable. Eight of the ten measures evaluated by Humes et al. (1996), however, made use of speech stimuli and six of the eight were found to be significantly correlated with average high-frequency hearing loss. Nonetheless, with regard to reliability alone, many of these measures on the VA-CD were found to be reliable when used with older adults.

Test Battery Design

When one administers a battery of diagnostic tests there are a variety of ways in which the tests can be administered and the results interpreted. Consider, for example, a test battery composed of three diagnostic tests: A, B, and C. One strategy for test administration is to only administer Test B, if Test A has been failed, and Test C, if both Test A and B have been failed. This sequential administration of tests comprising the battery is referred to as a serial test battery. Another approach is to always administer all three tests to every patient, regardless of the outcome on any particular test. This is referred to as a parallel test battery. To the author's knowledge, all test batteries designed to date for assessment of (central) auditory processing disorder in older adults have been of a parallel structure.

In addition to the way in which the tests are administered within the battery, the clinician has choices as to how the results will be interpreted with regard to the presence or absence of the disorder. That is, the clinician or researcher can establish the criterion for failing (or passing) the test battery. Assuming a parallel test battery comprised of three tests, for example, a very loose criterion is to identify the presence of the disorder when any one of the three tests has been failed. On the other hand, the strictest criterion for test-battery failure and presence of the disorder would be failure of all three tests. Again, to the author's knowledge, all such test-battery approaches for (central) auditory processing disorders in older adults have made use of the most loose criterion possible: failure of one of the tests in the battery is all that is required for identification of the presence of the disorder.

Cooper and Gates (1991) applied a parallel test battery composed of three measures of (central) auditory processing to a sample of 1,018 older adults. The top panel of Figure 8–7 illustrates the results from that study using various criteria for the presence of (central) auditory processing disorder. The three vertical bars to the left in this panel show the percentage of older adults in this sample who failed each of the three measures in the test battery. The lowest percentage of failures was for rollover of the performance-intensity (PI) function for PB words at high presentation levels (PI-PB RO), with only 1% of the older adults exhibiting rollover, whereas the highest failure percentage (18%) was observed for the PB-SSI difference score. If one applies the loosest possible criterion to this battery

of three tests (i.e., failing any of the three tests), 23% of the elderly individuals would be considered to have (central) auditory processing disorder. On the other hand, if the most conservative criterion was applied (i.e., failing all three tests), then 0% of the sample manifested (central) auditory processing disorders (far right vertical bar). Thus, the clinician's or researcher's decision as to the criterion used in interpreting the test battery results has a strong impact on the observed prevalence of (central) auditory processing disorders in older adults.

This is illustrated further in the bottom panel of Figure 8–7. In this case, the data from 130 older adults tested by Jerger et al. (1989) are plotted in a manner similar to that in the upper panel of this figure. Jerger et al. (1989) reported that the prevalence of (central) auditory processing disorders among this sample of older adults was 50%, based on failure of any of the three measures administered. Note from the data in Figure 8–7, however, that this could be as low as 5% if the criterion for failure was failing the two tests other than the DSI (i.e., PB-SSI difference and SPIN PH-PL difference) or 20% for failing the DSI plus anything else. Again, this illustrates the dependence of prevalence estimates for (central) auditory processing disorder in older adults on the criterion used by the clinician or researcher. The use of the loosest possible criterion when interpreting the results of parallel test batteries yields the highest possible prevalence estimates. Of course, the assumption throughout this discussion of test batteries is that the measures comprising the batteries are themselves reliable. This is an assumption that was called into question earlier. When the criterion for failure for a given test is basically within the test-retest reliability of the measures themselves, the prevalence estimates will be inflated further by the use of a parallel test battery with

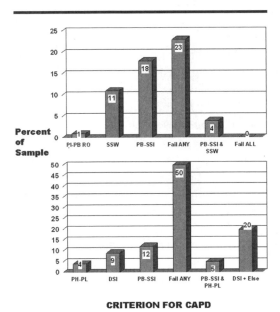

CRITERION FOR CAPD

Figure 8–7. Percentages of individuals identified as having (central) auditory processing disorders in Cooper and Gates (1990; *top panel*) and Jerger et al. (1989; *bottom panel*). Vertical bars represent percentages labeled as having auditory processing disorders based on individual tests comprising the test battery or various combinations of measures.

loose criterion. These two factors, poor test reliability and the use of the loosest criterion in a parallel test battery, can combine to yield unrealistically high estimates of the prevalence of (central) auditory processing disorders among older adults (e.g., Stach, Spretnjak, & Jerger, 1990).

It is unclear why the test-battery strategy in this area of research universally has been the use a parallel test battery with the loosest possible criterion. Such a strategy could be feasible if it was clearly established that each test was tapping a distinct and independent aspect of (central) auditory processing. As noted previously, there are some measures of (central) auditory processing that have been found to be reliable in older adults (Christopherson & Humes, 1992; Humes et al., 1996). Humes et al. (1996) also performed a factor analysis on the results from 10 of the 15 tests of the VA-CD and found that three independent factors emerged: (1) a general speech-recognition performance factor; (2) a temporal sequencing factor; and (3) a dichotic competition factor. With this structure confirmed, it would then be possible to select one or two reliable tests from each domain and combine these tests into a parallel battery. In this case, failure of a particular test would be sufficient to fail the battery and would identify the specific type of auditory-processing problem experienced by the individual. The validity of this approach, however, depends on the use of reliable measures within each of several potential domains of auditory processing and then confirmation of the independence of each domain in large samples of older adult through analyses such as factor analysis. Even then, it may not be appropriate to conclude that failure of a given test in the battery establishes the presence of (central) auditory processing disorder. For example, in the factor analysis by Humes et al. (1996),

the general speech-recognition performance factor was found to be strongly negatively correlated with average high-frequency hearing loss. Thus, it is important that the tests comprising the parallel battery not only be reliable and tap independent domains, but also that the domains being tapped are, in fact, domains of (central) auditory processing and not aspects of peripheral hearing loss (or cognitive function), as noted previously in this chapter.

References

American National Standards Institute. (1997). ANSI S3.5-1997. *American National Standard methods for the calculation of the Speech Intelligibility Index*. New York: Author.

Berlin, C. I., Lowe-Bell, S. S., Cullen, J. K., Jr., & Thompson, C. L. (1973). Dichotic speech perception: an interpretation of right-ear advantage and temporal offset effects. *Journal of the Acoustical Society of America, 53,* 699–709.

Bilger, R. C., Nuetzel, M. J., Rabinowitz, W. M., & Rzeckowski, C. (1984). Standardization of a test of speech perception in noise. *Journal of Speech and Hearing Research, 27,* 32–48.

Bocca, E., & Calearo, C. (1963). Central hearing processes. In J. Jerger (Ed.), *Modern developments in audiology* (pp.337–370). New York: Academic Press.

Bredberg, G. (1968). Cellular pattern and nerve supply of the human organ of Corti. *Acta Otolaryngologica, Supplement, 236,* 1–135.

Broadbent, D. E. (1954). The role of auditory localization in attention and memory span. *Journal of Experimental Psychology, 47,* 191–196.

Cacace, A. T., & McFarland, D. J. (1998). Central auditory processing disorder in school-aged children: A critical review. *Journal of Speech, Language, and Hearing Research, 41,* 335–373.

Cacace, A. T., & McFarland, D. J. (2005). The importance of modality specificity in diagnosing central auditory processing disorder. *American Journal of Audiology, 14*, 112-123.

Cherry, E. C. (1953). Some experiments of on the recognition of speech, with one and with two ears. *Journal of the Acoustical Society of America, 25*, 975-979.

Christopherson, L. A., & Humes, L. E. (1992). Some psychometric properties of the Test of Basic Auditory Capabilities (TBAC). *Journal of Speech and Hearing Research, 35*, 929-935.

Cokely, C. G., & Humes, L. E. (1992). Reliability of two measures of speech recognition in elderly people. *Journal of Speech and Hearing Research, 35*, 654-660.

Committee on Hearing and Bioacoustics and Biomechanics (CHABA). (1988). Speech understanding and aging. *Journal of the Acoustical Society of America, 83*, 859-895.

Cooper, J. C., Jr., & Gates, G. A. (1991). Hearing in the elderly—the Framingham cohort, 1983-1985: Part II. Prevalence of central auditory processing disorders. *Ear and Hearing, 12*, 304-311.

Cruickshanks, K. J., Wiley, T. L., Tweed, T. S., Klein, B. E. K., Klein, R., Mares-Perlman, J. A., et al. (1998). Prevalence of hearing loss in older adults in Beaver Dam, Wisconsin: The epidemiology of hearing loss study. *American Journal of Epidemiology, 148*, 879-886.

Divenyi, P. L., & Haupt, K. M. (1997a). Audiological correlates of speech understanding under non-optimal conditions in elderly listeners with mild-to-moderate hearing loss. I. Age and laterality effects. *Ear and Hearing, 18*, 42-61.

Divenyi, P. L., & Haupt, K. M. (1997b). Audiological correlates of speech understanding under non-optimal conditions in elderly listeners with mild-to-moderate hearing loss. II. Correlational analysis. *Ear and Hearing, 18*, 100-113.

Divenyi, P. L., & Haupt, K. M. (1997c). Audiological correlates of speech understanding under non-optimal conditions in elderly listeners with mild-to-moderate hearing loss. III. Factor representation. *Ear and Hearing, 18*, 189-201.

Dubno, J., Ahlstrom, J., & Horwitz, A. (2000). Use of context by young and aged persons with normal hearing. *Journal of the Acoustical Society of America, 107*, 538-546.

Dubno, J. R., & Dirks, D. D. (1983). Suggestions for optimizing reliability with the Synthetic Sentence Identification test. *Journal of Speech and Hearing Disorders, 48*, 98-103.

Dubno, J. R., Dirks, D. D., & Morgan, D. E. (1984). Effects of age and mild hearing loss on speech recognition. *Journal of the Acoustical Society of America, 76*, 87-96.

Dubno, J., Lee, Matthews, F., & L., Mills, J. (1997). Age-related and gender-related changes in monaural speech recognition. *Journal of Speech and Hearing Research, 40*, 444-452.

Feeney, M. P., & Hallowell, B. (2000). Practice and list effects on the Synthetic Sentence Identification test in young and elderly listeners. *Journal of Speech, Language, and Hearing Research, 43*, 1160-1167.

Fifer, R., Jerger, J., Berlin, C., Tobey, E., & Campbell, J. (1983). Development of a dichotic sentence identification test for hearing-impaired adults. *Ear and Hearing, 4*, 300-305.

Gates, G. A., Cooper, J. C., Jr., Kannel, W. B., & Miller, N. J. (1990). Hearing in the elderly: The Framingham cohort, 1983-1985. Part I. Basic audiometric test results. *Ear and Hearing, 11*, 247-256.

George, E. L. J., Festen, J. M., & Houtgast, T. (2006). Factors affecting masking release for speech in modulated noise for normal-hearing and hearing-impaired listeners. *Journal of the Acoustical Society of America, 120*, 2295-2311.

George, E. L. J., Zekveld, A. A., Kramer, S. E., Goverts, S. T., Festen, J. M., & Houtgast, T. (2007). Auditory and nonauditory factors affecting speech reception in noise by older listeners. *Journal of the Acoustical Society of America, 121*, 2362-2375.

Gordon-Salant, S., & Fitzgibbons, P. J. (1993). Temporal factors and speech recognition performance in young and elderly listeners. *Journal of Speech and Hearing Research, 36*, 1276-1285.

Gordon-Salant, S., & Fitzgibbons, P. J. (1999). Profile of auditory temporal processing in older listeners. *Journal of Speech, Language and Hearing Research, 42*, 300-311.

Gordon-Salant, S., & Fitzgibbons, P. J. (2001). Sources of age-related recognition difficulty for time-compressed speech. *Journal of Speech, Language, and Hearing Research, 44,* 709-719.

Gordon-Salant, S., & Fitzgibbons, P. J. (2004). Effects of stimulus and noise rate variability on speech perception by younger and older adults. *Journal of the Acoustical Society of America, 115,* 1808-1817.

Hallgren, M., Larsby, B., Lyxell, B., & Arlinger, S. (2001). Cognitive effects in dichotic speech testing in elderly persons. *Ear and Hearing, 22,* 120-129.

Halling, D. C., & Humes, L. E. (2000). Factors affecting the recognition of reverberant speech by elderly listeners. *Journal of Speech, Language, and Hearing Research, 43,* 414-431.

Helfer, K. S. (1992). Aging and the binaural advantage in reverberation and noise. *Journal of Speech and Hearing Research, 35,* 1394-1401.

Helfer, K. S., & Wilber, L. A. (1990). Hearing loss, aging, and speech perception in reverberation and noise. *Journal of Speech and Hearing Research, 33,* 149-155.

Humes, L. E. (1996). Speech understanding in the elderly. *Journal of the American Academy of Audiology, 7,* 161-167.

Humes, L. E. (2002). Factors underlying the speech-recognition performance of elderly hearing-aid wearers. *Journal of the Acoustical Society of America, 112,* 1112-1132.

Humes, L. E. (2005). Do "auditory processing" tests measure auditory processing in the elderly? *Ear and Hearing, 26,* 109-119.

Humes, L. E. (2007). The contributions of audibility and cognitive factors to the benefit provided by amplified speech to older adults. *Journal of the American Academy of Audiology, 18,* 590-603.

Humes, L. E., Burk, M. H., Coughlin, M. P., Busey, T. A. & Strauser, L. E. (2007). Auditory speech recognition and visual text recognition in younger and older adults: Similarities and differences between modalities and the effects of presentation rate. *Journal of Speech, Hearing Research, 50,* 283-303.

Humes, L. E., & Christopherson, L (1991). Speech-identification difficulties of the hearing-impaired elderly: The contributions of auditory-processing deficits. *Journal of Speech and Hearing Research, 34,* 686-693.

Humes, L. E., Christopherson, L. A., & Cokely, C. G. (1992). Central auditory processing disorders in the elderly: fact or fiction? In J. Katz, N. Stecker, & D. Henderson (Eds.), *Central auditory processing: A transdisciplinary view* (pp. 141-150). Philadelphia: B. C. Decker.

Humes, L. E., Coughlin, M., & Talley, L. (1996). Evaluation of the use of a new compact disc for auditory perceptual assessment in the elderly. *Journal of the American Academy of Audiology, 7,* 419-427.

Humes, L. E., Lee, J. H., & Coughlin, M. P. (2006). Auditory measures of selective and divided attention in young and older adults using single-talker competition. *Journal of the Acoustical Society of America, 120,* 2926-2937.

Humes, L. E., & Roberts, L. (1990). Speech-recognition difficulties of hearing-impaired elderly: The contributions of audibility. *Journal of Speech and Hearing Research, 33,* 726-735.

Humes, L. E, Watson, B. U, Christensen, L. A., Cokely, C. A., Halling, D. A., & Lee, L. (1994). Factors associated with individual differences in clinical measures of speech recognition among the elderly. *Journal of Speech and Hearing Research, 37,* 465-474.

International Standards Organization (ISO). (2000). *Acoustics-Statistical distribution of hearing thresholds as a function of age, ISO-7029.* Basel, Switzerland: Author.

Jerger, J., & Chmiel, R. (1997). Factor analytic structure of auditory impairment in elderly persons. *Journal of the American Academy of Audiology, 8,* 269-276.

Jerger, J., Chmiel, R., Allen, J., & Wilson, A. (1994). Effects of age and gender on dichotic sentence identification. *Ear and Hearing, 15,* 274-286.

Jerger, J., Jerger, S., Oliver, T., & Pirozzolo, F. (1989). Speech understanding in the elderly. *Ear and Hearing, 10,* 79-89.

Jerger, J., Jerger, S., & Pirozzolo, F. (1991). Correlational analysis of speech audiometric scores, hearing loss, age and cognitive abilities in the elderly. *Ear and Hearing, 12,* 103-109.

Jerger, J., & Jordan, C. (1992). Age-related asymmetry on a cued-listening task. *Ear and Hearing, 13,* 272–277.

Kalikow, D., Stevens, K., & Elliott, L. (1977). Development of a test of speech intelligibility in noise using test material with controlled word predictability. *Journal of the Acoustical Society of America, 61,* 1337–1351.

Killion, M. C., Niquette, P. A., Gudmundsen, G. I., Revit, L. J., & Banerjee, S. (2004). Development of a quick speech-in-noise test for measuring signal-to-noise ratio loss in normal-hearing and hearing-impaired listeners. *Journal of the Acoustical Society of America, 116,* 2395–2405.

Kimura, D. (1967). Functional assymetry of the brain in dichotic listening. *Cortex, 3,* 163–178.

Konkle, D., Beasley, D., & Bess, F. (1977). Intelligibility of time-altered speech in relation to chronological aging. *Journal of Speech and Hearing Research, 20,* 108–115.

Lacroix, P. G., Harris, J. D., & Randolph, K. J. (1979). Multiplicative effects on sentence comprehension for combined acoustic distortions. *Journal of Speech and Hearing Research, 22,* 259–269.

Lee, L. W., & Humes, L. E. (1993). Evaluating a speech-reception threshold model for hearing-impaired listeners. *Journal of the Acoustical Society of America, 93,* 2879–2885.

Lopez, O. L., Jagust, W. J., DeKosky, S. T., Becker, J. T., Fitzpatrick, A., Dulberg, C., et al. (2003). Prevalence and classification of mild cognitive impairment I the Cardiovascular Health Study Cognition Study. *Archives of Neurology, 60,* 1385–1389.

Martin, J. S., & Jerger, J. F. (2005). Some effects of aging on central auditory processing. *Journal of Rehabilitative Research and Development, 42,* 25–44.

McFarland, D. J., & Cacace, A. T. (1995). Modality specificity as a criterion for diagnosing central auditory processing disorders. *American Journal of Audiology, 4,* 36–48.

Nilsson, M., Soli, S., & Sullivan, J.A. (1994). Development of the Hearing In Noise Test for the measurement of speech reception thresholds in quiet and in noise. *Journal of the Acoustical Society of America, 94,* 1085–1099.

Noffsinger, D., Wilson, R. H., & Musiek, F. E. (1994). Department of Veterans Affairs Compact Disc (VA-CD) recording for auditory perceptual assessment: Background and introduction. *Journal of the American Academy of Audiology, 5,* 231–235.

Olsen, W. O., Noffsinger, D., & Kurdziel, S. (1975). Speech discrimination in quiet and in white noise by patients with peripheral and central lesions. *Acta Otolaryngologica, 80,* 375–382.

Pichora-Fuller, M. K., Schneider, B. A., & Daneman, M. (1995). How young and old listen to and remember speech in noise. *Journal of the Acoustical Society of America, 97,* 593–608.

Plomp, R. (1978). Auditory handicap of hearing impairment and the limited benefit of hearing aids. *Journal of the Acoustical Society of America, 63,* 533–549.

Plomp, R. (1986). A signal-to-noise ratio model for the speech-reception threshold of the hearing impaired. *Journal of Speech and Hearing Research, 29,* 146–154.

Plomp, R., & Mimpen, A. M. (1979). Improving the reliability of testing the speech reception threshold for sentences. *Audiology, 18,* 43–52.

Portet, F., Ousset, P. J., Visser, P. J., Frisoni, G. B., Nobili, F., Scheltens, P., et al. Mild cognitive impairment (MCI) in medical practice: a critical review of the concept and new diagnostic procedure. Report of the MCI Working Group of the European Consortium on Alzheimer's Disease. *Journal of Neurology, Neurosurgery, and Psychiatry, 77,* 714–718.

Pugh, K. C., Crandell, C. C., & Griffiths, S. K. (1998). Reliability issues with the Synthetic Sentence Identification test. *Journal of the American Academy of Audiology, 9,* 227–233.

Rabbitt, P. (1968). Channel capacity, intelligibility and immediate memory. *Quarterly Journal of Experimental Psychology, 20,* 241–248.

Roup, C., Wiley, T., & Wilson, R. (2006). Dichotic word recognition in young and older adults. *Journal of the American Academy of Audiology, 17,* 230–240.

Salthouse, T. A. (1985). *A theory of cognitive aging.* Amsterdam: North-Holland.

Salthouse, T. A. (1991). *Theoretical perspectives on cognitive aging*. Hillsdale, NJ: Lawrence Erlbaum Associates.

Salthouse, T. A. (2000). Aging and measures of processing speed. *Biological Psychology, 54*, 35–54.

Schneider, B. A., Daneman, M., & Murphy, D. R. (2005). Speech comprehension difficulties in older adults: Cognitive slowing or age-related changes in hearing? *Psychology and Aging, 20*, 261–271.

Schneider, B. A., & Pichora-Fuller, M. K. (2000). Implications of perceptual processing for cognitive aging research. In F. I. M. Craik & T. A. Salthouse (Eds.), *The handbook of aging and cognition* (2nd ed.). Mahwah, NJ: Lawrence Erlbaum Associates.

Schneider, B. A., Pichora-Fuller, M. K., Kowalchuk, D., & Lamb, M. (1994). Gap detection and the precedence effect in young and old adults. *Journal of the Acoustical Society of America, 95*, 980–991.

Schneider, B. A., Speranza, F., & Pichora-Fuller, M. K. (1998). Age-related changes in temporal resolution: envelope and intensity effects. *Canadian Journal of Experimental Psychology, 52*, 184–191.

Snell, K. B. (1997). Age-related changes in temporal gap detection. *Journal of the Acoustical Society of America, 101*, 2214–2220.

Snell, K. B., & Frisina, D. R. (2000). Relationships among age-related differences in gap detection and word recognition. *Journal of the Acoustical Society of America, 107*, 1615–1626.

Souza, P. E., & Turner, C. W. (1994). Masking of speech in young and elderly listeners with hearing loss. *Journal of Speech and Hearing Research, 37*, 655–661.

Speaks, C., & Jerger, J. (1965). Method for measurement of speech identification. *Journal of Speech and Hearing Research, 8*, 185–194.

Speranza, F., Daneman, M., & Schneider, B.A. (2000). How aging affects the reading of words in noisy backgrounds. *Psychology and Aging, 15*, 253–258.

Stach, B., Spretnjak, M., & Jerger, J. (1990). The prevalence of central presbycusis in a clinical population. *Journal of the American Academy of Audiology, 1*, 109–115.

Strouse, A., Ashmead, D. H., Ohde, R. N., & Granthan, D. W. (1998). Temporal processing in the aging auditory system. *Journal of the Acoustical Society of America, 104*, 2385–2399.

Surprenant, A. M. (2007). Effects of noise on identification and serial recall of nonsense syllables in older and younger adults. *Aging, Neuropsychology and Cognition, 14*, 126–.143.

Surprenant, A. M., & Watson, C. S. (2001). Individual differences in the processing of speech and non-speech sounds by normal-hearing listeners. *Journal of the Acoustical Society of America, 110*, 2086–2095.

Thornton, A. R., & Raffin, M. J. M. (1978). Speech-discrimination scores modeled as a binomial variable. *Journal of Speech and Hearing Research, 21*, 507–518.

van Rooij, J. C. G. M., & Plomp, R. (1990). Auditive and cognitive factors in speech perception by elderly listeners. II. Multivariate analyses. *Journal of the Acoustical Society of America, 88*, 2611–2624.

van Rooij, J. C. G. M., & Plomp, R. (1992). Auditive and cognitive factors in speech perception by elderly listeners. III. Additional data and final discussion. *Journal of the Acoustical Society of America, 91*, 1028–1033.

van Rooij, J. C. G. M., Plomp, R., & Orlebeke, J. F. (1989). Auditive and cognitive factors in speech perception by elderly listeners. I. Development of test battery. *Journal of the Acoustical Society of America, 86*, 1294–1309.

Wake, M., Tobin, S., Cone-Wesson, B., Dahl, H. H., Gillam, L., McCormick, L., et al. (2006). Slight/mild sensorineural hearing loss in children. *Pediatrics, 118*, 1842–1851.

Walden, T. C., & Walden, B. E. (2004). Predicting success with hearing aids in everyday living. *Journal of the American Academy of Audiology, 15*, 342–352.

Watson, C. S. (1987). Uncertainty, informational masking, and the capacity of immediate auditory memory. In W. A. Yost & C. S. Watson (Eds.), *Auditory processing of complex sounds* (pp. 267–277). Hillsdale, NJ: Lawrence Erlbaum.

Watson, C. S., Jensen, J. K., Foyle, D. C., Leek, M. R., & Goldgar, D. E. (1982). Performance of 146 normal adult listeners on a battery of auditory discrimination tests. *Journal of the Acoustical Society of America, 71,* S73.

Watson, C. S., Qiu, W. W., Chamberlain, M. M., & Li, X. (1996). Auditory and visual speech perception: Confirmation of a modality-independent source of individual differences in speech recognition. *Journal of the Acoustical Society of America, 100,* 1153–1162.

Wechsler, D. (1981). *The Wechsler Adult Intelligence Scale-Revised.* New York: Psychological Corporation.

Wiley, T. L., Cruickshanks, K. J., Nondahl, D. M., Tweed, T. S., Klein, R., & Klein, B. E. K. (1998). Aging and word recognition in competing message. *Journal of the American Academy of Audiology, 9,* 191–198.

Willott, J. F. (1991). *Aging and the auditory system: Anatomy, physiology, and psychophysics.* San Diego, CA: Singular.

Wilson, R. H., Preece, J. P., Salmon, D. L., Sperry, J. L., & Bornstein, S. P. (1994). Effects of time compression and time compression plus reverberation on the intelligibility of Northwestern University Auditory Test No. 6. *Journal of the American Academy of Audiology, 5,* 269–277.

Wingfield, A., Poon, L. W., Lombardi, L., & Lowe, D. (1985). Speed of processing in normal aging: Effects of speech rate, linguistic structure, and processing time. *Journal of Gerontology, 40,* 579–585.

Wingfield, A., & Tun, P. A. (2001). Spoken language comprehension in older adults: Interactions between sensory and cognitive change in normal aging. *Seminars in Hearing, 22,* 287–301.

Wingfield, A., Tun, P. A., Koh, C. K., & Rosen, M. J. (1999). Regaining lost time: Adult aging and the effect of time restoration on recall of time-compressed speech. *Psychology and Aging, 14,* 380–389.

Zekveld, A. A., George, E. L. J., Kramer, S. E., Goverts, S. T., & Houtgast, T. (2007). The development of the Text Reception Threshold test: A visual analogue of the Speech Reception Threshold test. *Journal of Speech, Language and Hearing Research, 50,* 576–584.

CHAPTER 9

Speech-in-Noise Measures as Necessary Components of Routine Audiologic Evaluations and Auditory Processing Disorder Evaluations

RICHARD H. WILSON AND RACHEL McARDLE

Basic human communication involves a source, a transmission medium, and a receiver. The source is regarded generally as the person speaking a message, the medium is the acoustic (and other) environment through which the message travels, and the receiver is the listener for whom the message is intended. In the simplest communication link a high-fidelity utterance of a word or sentence is produced by the speaker. The message is transmitted through an acoustic medium that is void of noise and received by a listener with normal hearing. This idealized communication link, more often than not, is degraded in the transmission medium or in the receiver. In the transmission medium the signal can be distorted by a variety of variables, the most common of which is noise. At the receiver, peripheral hearing loss and/or auditory processing disorders (APD) can contribute to the degradation of the signal. Of particular interest to this chapter are the older adults with hearing loss and younger individuals with APD who have an auditory commonality, in that typically both groups of listeners have more difficulty understanding speech when the medium is contaminated with background noise than do young adults with normal hearing. The question, therefore, is: does the difficulty understanding speech in background noise reflect the same auditory mechanism(s) for these two groups of listeners? For example, perhaps with the young listeners with APD, the speech intelligibility deficit in noise can be attributed to immature neuronal development and neuronal organization. Similarly, in older adults with hearing loss there may be neuronal deterioration that in many ways mimics the immature neuronal development and organization that may be associated with the young listeners with APD (Berlin, personal communication, March 12, 2007). Alternatively, there may be little or no similarities between the two groups of listeners in the mechanisms that account for the deficit in understanding speech-in-noise. Differences between the older adults with hearing loss and the younger individuals with APD start at the auditory periphery. Pure-tone threshold data indicate that the majority of older listeners with hearing loss in effect low-pass filter the incoming speech signal whereas the younger listeners with APD have little or no peripheral filtering effects applied to the incoming speech signal. What happens to the encoded auditory speech signal beyond the auditory periphery for both groups of listeners is at best speculative but deserving of experimental probing.

This chapter presents a discussion of speech-in-noise paradigms that are considered in the degraded speech domain. First, the chapter reviews an informational framework that considers redundancy (extrinsic and intrinsic) and uncertainty as viewed by Miller (1951) and Bocca and Calearo (1963). Second, the effects of hearing loss on speech intelligibility are presented in the context of two components of hearing loss, "acuity" or attenuation and "clarity" or distortion (Carhart, 1951; Plomp, 1978; Stephens, 1976). Next, the different information gained from

speech-in-quiet and speech-in-noise tasks are considered and why it is important in the course of a routine audiologic evaluation to access the ability of the patient, adult or child, to understand speech in background noise. The chapter concludes with a presentation of several speech-in-noise tasks/materials followed by a brief discussion of three common types of noise and their differential effect on older listeners with hearing loss and listeners with auditory processing disorders. The authors have recently reviewed and discussed these topics in a review article (Wilson & McArdle, 2005).

Dual Processing

Historically, language has been viewed by many speech perceptionists as hierarchically organized with the acoustic properties of an utterance as the foundation (e.g., Jusczyk & Luce, 2002). For spoken word recognition, stimulus-driven perception is located at the bottom of the hierarchy, whereas complex cognitive systems (e.g., memory) are located at the top of the hierarchy (Lindgren & Lindblom, 1983). Information can flow both from the bottom of the system to the top of the system (bottom-up processing) and from the top of the system to the bottom of the system (top-down processing). Bottom-up processing involves the encoding of incoming perceptual information for utilization by higher level cognitive processing. Top-down processing uses information already stored in the cognitive system to influence or shape the perception of the incoming information. A hierarchal view often is used to describe the active process of recognizing speech in adverse listening situations. Bottom-up processing refers to the use of the available acoustic information at the "bottom" of the hierarchy to aid in recognition of an utterance. Top-down processing refers to use of higher level cognitive information such as word frequency or familiarity found towards the "top" of the hierarchy to assist with recognition.

Another way of describing the processes involved in speech recognition is by discussing the redundancy and uncertainty of the message. The information contained in the message is redundant in that there are more informational cues available in the message than the informational face value that is contained in the message (Miller, 1951). From the point of view of the listener, the acoustic cues and aforementioned bottom-up information are termed *extrinsic redundancies* (Bocca & Calearo, 1963). To complement the extrinsic redundancies, Bocca and Calearo proposed that the listener had certain *intrinsic redundancies* that enabled the interpretation of the message. These intrinsic redundancies, which are based on the collective experiences of the listener, take the form of vocabulary, syntactic, semantic, linguistic, and other types of language rules and are similar to that discussed as top-down processing. One additional condition must be attached to this redundancy scheme, the extrinsic and intrinsic redundancies must reflect the same language, otherwise there is a mismatch and the two redundancy types are not complementary.

The combination of the extrinsic and intrinsic redundancies provides substantially more than enough combined redundancy for (theoretically) greater than 100% of the message to be understood. Using the communication sequence of a high-fidelity source, a quiet medium, and a listener with normal hearing, the simplest way to reduce

the redundancies in the message is by attenuating the message at the source, as the message passes through the medium, and/or at the receiver in the form of hearing loss. As the level of the message progressively is reduced, the amount of information correctly understood (e.g., the percent correct recognition) likewise will decrease until a level is reached at which zero information is received by the listener. If the redundancies or informational cues of a message were reduced at any point(s) between (and including) the source and the receiver, then *uncertainty* for the listener occurs regarding their ability to understand the message. A graphic example of this phenomenon in the form of a psychometric function is shown in Figure 9–1, in which percent correct recognition is plotted on the ordinate and the presentation level is plotted on the abscissa. When the presentation level is high, redundancies abound, uncertainty is nil, and recognition performance is very

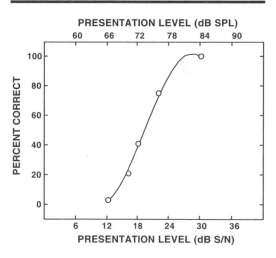

Figure 9–1. A psychometric function depicted as percent correct on the ordinate and presentation level in both dB S/N (*bottom abscissa*) and dB SPL (*top abscissa*).

good. As the presentation level is reduced, the redundancies likewise are reduced, uncertainty is increased, and performance deteriorates. Another way that the inherent extrinsic redundancy in the message can be reduced is through the introduction of noise into the transmission medium. As the level of the noise increases and the signal-to-noise ratio (SNR or S/N) is reduced, the extrinsic redundancies available in the message progressively are reduced (via interference or masking) and recognition performance by the listener decreases to 0%. As an aside, but within the context of the current discussion, the goal of audiologic rehabilitation should be to maximize redundancies and minimize uncertainties in the communication stream.

Top-down processing or intrinsic redundancies, which range from probabilistic phonotactics to semantic, syntactic, and pragmatic rules of a language, help to convey a degraded message. As indicated above, a highly redundant language such as English employs more information or linguistic cues in the structure of the language than necessary to convey a specific meaning. The redundancy of the English language is easily explained through the relative frequencies of verbal elements. For example, English can be transcribed using approximately 40 phonemes; however, nine of these 40 phonemes make up more than half of our vocal behavior. Similarly, 12 syllables of the over 1370 syllables that can be found in the English language make up 25% of our verbal behavior (Miller, 1951). Another example of redundancies is the work of Boothroyd and Nittrouer (1988) who derived mathematical constants related to the constraints imposed at the phonemic level (j factor) and contextual constraints imposed at the sentence level (k factor). Successive words in English are not unrelated. The j and k factors represent numerically the interdependencies among successive items in a message whether it is successive phonemes (probabilistic phonotactics) or successive words (linguistic context). Redundant languages are more dependable under adverse conditions such as listening to speech in a background of noise (Miller, 1951). Thus, young adult listeners with normal hearing are able to recognize degraded speech given the limited or distorted bottom-up information.

Psychometric validation has been limited for the plethora of objective instruments used in assessing APD. This is especially concerning for the degraded speech tests given that the speech-recognition abilities of young children are not as fine grained or segmental as those abilities are with an adult (Walley, 2005). Not only is speech recognition more holistic in early and middle childhood but the redundancies of the language are still being developed as the child has continued exposure to their native language. In addition, during early and middle childhood there is a considerable increase in the size of the lexicon. In keeping with the aforementioned framework, the increase in vocabulary size raises the level of uncertainty prior to the development of the necessary redundancies that aid in speech recognition in adverse listening situations most likely affecting recognition performance. Degraded speech tests such as filtered or compressed speech measures that are difficult for an adult would pose even greater strain on the not yet fully developed perceptual system of a child. For these reasons, with children, it is imperative to have well-founded normative data that can be used to interpret psychometric data. Although there are other procedures that can be used to "degrade" the information in the speech message (e.g., frequency filtering and time compressing), the focus of this chapter is on speech recognition as related to masking and SNR.

Two-Component Framework of Hearing Loss

In his 1951 seminal paper, Carhart recognized that there were two predominant components to hearing loss—acuity and clarity. The acuity component, which we now would term sensitivity (Ward, 1964), referred to the change in pure-tone or speech thresholds that are the gold standard used to describe hearing loss. Carhart considered the clarity component in terms of the inability of the listener to understand speech. Carhart further recognized that with some individuals this inability to understand speech could be overcome by presenting the speech at increasingly higher presentation levels. With other individuals, however, the deficit in understanding speech could not be overcome regardless of the presentation level. Twenty-five years later, Stephens (1976) referred to the two components of hearing loss as attenuation and distortion. Shortly thereafter, Plomp (1978) formally described a framework of hearing loss in those two terms, attenuation (audibility) and distortion.

The attenuation component of hearing loss, which was *acuity* in the Carhart terminology (1951), is relatively linear and for the most part predictable regarding the relation between pure-tone thresholds and speech intelligibility. Threshold measures for pure tones and, to some degree, speech signals are used to quantify the attenuation component of hearing loss. Conductive hearing loss is the purest type of attenuation hearing loss followed by a mild sensorineural hearing loss, especially in a young adult. Because of its nature, the attenuation component of hearing loss is corrected easily with amplification. The distortion component of hearing loss, which was *clarity* in the Carhart terminology, is actually a "catchall" term that includes the many aspects of hearing loss that are little understood. Lutman (1987) suggests that the distortion category includes such auditory phenomenon as frequency resolution, temporal resolution, suppression, and amplitude discrimination, all of which are often adversely affected in individuals with sensorineural hearing loss. Interestingly, these auditory phenomena have often been linked to individuals with APDs. Clinically, the distortion component is best focused on with a speech-in-noise task. Data are accumulating that indicate that although two individuals can have the same attenuation hearing loss, that is, pure-tone thresholds, and the same word-recognition performance in quiet, their performance on a word-recognition task in background noise can be substantially different. The disparity in performances on the word-recognition task in noise is interpreted as different reflections of the distortion component. Unlike the attenuation component of hearing loss that was described as linear and for the most part predictable, the distortion component is nonlinear and is difficult to predict regarding the relations between pure-tone thresholds, speech intelligibility in quiet, and speech intelligibility in noise. Carhart realized that the distortion component of hearing loss is difficult to remediate with amplification. He contended that for many individuals with hearing loss merely increasing the presentation level of the signal did not improve their ability to understand speech.

As Plomp and Duquesnoy (1982) stated, "a hearing loss for speech in noise of 3 dB is more disturbing than a hearing loss for speech in quiet of 21 dB" (p. 101). The 3-dB hearing loss for speech in noise is a reflection of the distortion component of hearing loss, whereas the 21-dB hearing loss for speech in quiet is a reflection of the attenuation component of hearing loss. Finally, the attenuation and distortion components of hearing loss coexist to different degrees in most individuals, especially older individuals. For adults, it would appear that in the early stages of hearing loss, especially in the younger years, the attenuation component is the major factor, but as the hearing loss progresses, especially into the later years of life, the distortion component becomes the major factor. In contrast, for children with APD and similar disorders, the distortion component of hearing loss appears to be the major factor with the attenuation component reserved as a compounding issue for children with some peripheral hearing loss.

Recognition Performance of Speech-in-Quiet Versus Speech-in-Noise

The involvement of both the attenuation and distortion components compound hearing loss can make the prediction of word-recognition performance in quiet from pure-tone sensitivity data difficult. Another prediction that is perhaps more difficult to make is word-recognition performance in background noise from recognition performance in quiet. The data in Figure 9–2 from 387 listeners with sensorineural hearing loss illustrate this point using the Words-in-Noise (WIN) test developed in our laboratories (Wilson, 2003; Wilson & Burks, 2005, Wilson & McArdle, 2007). The WIN incorporates in a multitalker babble paradigm either 5 or 10 Northwestern University Auditory Test No. 6 (NU No. 6; Tillman & Carhart, 1966) words at each of 7 SNRs from 24- to 0-dB S/N in 4-dB decrements. The level of the babble is fixed and the words are taken

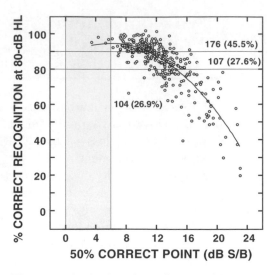

Figure 9–2. A plot of word-recognition performance in quiet in percent correct (*ordinate*) versus the 50% point of recognition performance in multitalker babble on the WIN (*abscissa*). The shaded area represents the 10th and 90th percentiles for individuals with normal hearing on the WIN. The numbers represent the number of listeners who had word recognition in quiet ≥90%, ≥80%, and ≤70% correct on the words in quiet. The data are combined from McArdle et al, 2005a, 2005b. (Taken from Wilson and McArdle, 2005).

from the VA compact disc (Department of Veterans Affairs, 2006), thereby providing assessment in quiet and in babble by the same materials spoken by the same speaker. The data in Figure 9–2, which were jittered (offset) for graphic clarity using a multiplicative algorithm between 0.975 and 1.025, were compiled from two studies (McArdle, Wilson, & Burks, 2005; McArdle, Chisolm, Abrams, Wilson, & Doyle, 2005b). In the figure, the percent correct word-recognition performance in quiet at 80-dB HL (ordinate) is shown as a function of the 50% point (dB S/N) obtained with the words-in-noise list (WIN), which are the same words spoken by the same speaker used for the words in quiet (Wilson, 2003). The 80-dB HL presentation level in quiet corresponds to the presentation level of the words-in-noise at 20-dB S/N. The mean correct word-recognition in quiet for the 387 listeners with hearing loss was 84.6% (SD = 14.0%). The shaded region of the figure defines the range of performances obtained by listeners with normal hearing on the WIN task (Wilson, Abrams, & Pillion, 2003). The 90th percentile for the listeners with normal hearing was 6-dB S/N.

Four relations among the data in Figure 9–2 deserve mention. First, five of the listeners with sensorineural hearing loss performed in the normal range on both the quiet and noise tasks. The remaining 383 listeners had a mean performance on the WIN of 12.5-dB S/N, which with reference to 90th percentile for listeners with normal hearing (6.0-dB S/N) yields a mean 6.5-dB S/N hearing loss (the range was from 6.8- to 23.6-dB S/N). With the W-22 words, Beattie (1989) reported a 5-dB S/N difference between performances by listeners with normal hearing and listeners with hearing loss, which is in good agreement with the data in Figure 9–2 considering the different lists, different speakers, and so forth, that were used in the two studies. Interestingly, the mean 50% point of 12.5-dB S/N is almost identical to the 50% points obtained under similar conditions by Dirks et al. (12-dB S/N; [1982]) and Beattie (11.3-dB S/N). Second, 45.5% of the listeners had word-recognition performances in quiet at 80-dB HL that were ≥90% correct. Third, all of the 107 listeners who had word-recognition performances in quiet between 80 and 90% correct had poorer than normal performances on the WIN. Fourth, 26.9% of the listeners had word recognition in quiet that was <80% correct. Two conclusions can be drawn from the data in Figure 9–2. Although the majority of listeners with sensorineural hearing loss

operate in the normal range on word recognition in quiet (i.e., ≥80% correct), the vast majority of listeners with hearing loss have abnormal performance on word recognition in background noise. Finally, the data in Figure 9–2 emphasize that good word recognition in quiet is not an indicator of good word recognition in background noise. One can safely say, however, that poor word recognition in quiet only produces poor(er) word recognition in noise.

Importance of Speech-in-Noise Testing

Although no gold standard exists for the identification of APD, four main types of tests have been recommended when screening for APD: binaural integration, binaural separation, monaural separation, and temporal ordering (ASHA, 1996; Bellis, 2006; Bellis & Ferre, 1999; Schow et al., 2000). Test batteries such as the SCAN Screening Test for Auditory Processing Disorders (SCAN; Keith, 1986) were developed to assess the ability of an individual to process auditory stimuli and to identify individuals with APD. For children and adolescents the necessity of multiple degraded speech tests may be necessary for the development of individualized education plans, especially if the child is displaying academic difficulties. For older adults, however, the need for multiple tests may be unnecessary if a single measure like speech-in-noise were able to identify those with abnormal processing difficulties. Schow and Chermak (1999) used factor analysis to examine the data for the SCAN (Keith, 1986) and the Staggered Spondaic Word test (SSW; Katz, 1968) from 331 school children. The analysis identified two factors for which performances on the SCAN and the SSW were related. The first factor was termed binaural separation/competition factor, which is more commonly described as dichotic listening. The second factor was monaural low-redundancy degradation and was loaded on by the filtered words subtest and the auditory-figure ground subtest of the SCAN. The task in the auditory-figure ground subtest is a monosyllabic word-in-noise task presented at a single SNR.

The Schow and Chermak (1999) data suggest that a measure of both dichotic listening ability and speech recognition in noise ability would be sufficient to identify an APD. Furthermore, Putter-Katz and colleagues (2002) recently looked at performance pre- and post-training for 20 children 7 to 14 years old who were referred for APD evaluations. Preliminary testing found that 11 of the children showed mainly poor speech-recognition performance in noise whereas the remaining nine children showed a deficit both in speech-recognition performance in noise and in dichotic listening. Of importance is that all 20 children were characterized by a subjective deficiency for recognizing speech in a competing background by an APD assessment. Thus, the question arises that if poor speech recognition in noise is a primary sign of APD, then why do audiologists refrain from using a speech-in-noise recognition task routinely during a basic audiologic assessment? This question is applicable for both children and adults.

The majority of audiologists acknowledge that the most common complaint that adult patients have about their hearing loss is their inability to understand speech in the presence of background noise, especially background noise that is composed of multiple speech sources. Generalizing from a previous section, patient complaints of difficulty understanding speech in background noise are a characteristic manifestation of the "clarity" or "distortion" component of hearing loss (Carhart, 1951; Plomp, 1978; Stephens,

1976). Thirty-eight years ago, Carhart and Tillman (1970) suggested that the communication handicap imposed by sensorineural hearing loss was not only characterized by a hearing loss in terms of the threshold for speech and a "discrimination" loss in terms of listening to speech in quiet but additionally the handicap should be specified in terms of "the masking efficiency of competing speech and other background sounds that plague the patient when he is in complex listening environments" (p. 279), that is, the ability of the listener to understand speech in background noise. This observation was precipitated by experimental evidence in which listeners with sensorineural hearing loss functioned at a 10 to 15 dB disadvantage compared to listeners with normal hearing when listening in a competing background noise (Carhart & Tillman, 1970; Groen, 1969; Olsen & Carhart, 1967). Carhart and Tillman urged the inclusion in the audiologic evaluation of an instrument that quantified the ability (or inability) of listeners to understand speech in a background of speech noise.

Individual 50% points from the WIN are plotted in Figure 9–3 for 315 listeners with hearing loss (open circles) as well as 24 listeners with normal hearing (open squares). The shaded area represents the 10th to 90th percentile recognition performances for the listeners with normal hearing and the dashed line represents the mean performance of the 315 listeners with hearing loss. As can be seen in Figure 9–3, the WIN data are very heterogeneous with a random distribution among the listeners with hearing loss. The lack of homogeneity among listeners with hearing loss exemplifies that the WIN is sensitive to individual differences in speech-recognition performance in noise that may be unidentified during routine pure-tone testing and speech recognition testing in quiet. Thus, the high performance variability

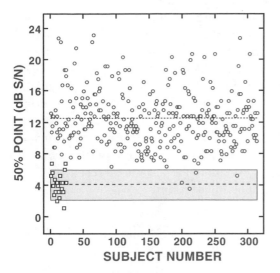

Figure 9–3. The 50% points calculated with the Spearman-Kärber equation for the individual WIN data obtained from the 315 listeners with hearing loss during Session 1 (*circles*) in the Wilson and McArdle (2007) study. The squares depict similar data obtained from 24 listeners with normal hearing (Wilson et al., 2003). The shaded region defines normal performance on the WIN task. The dotted line represents the mean performance by the listeners with hearing loss and the dashed line represents the mean performance by the listeners with normal hearing. (Taken from Wilson & McArdle, 2007).

for listeners with hearing loss supports the need for routine clinical measurement of speech-recognition performance in noise to quantify and validate the complaint of difficulty understanding speech in noise.

In a recent survey, Strom (2006) indicated that fewer than half of "dispensing professionals" use some type of speech-in-noise task to evaluate the abilities of their patients to understand speech in background noise. There are several reasons a speech-in-noise task typically has not been included in audiologic evaluations. First, unlike the tests of word-recognition abilities in quiet for

which there is a plethora of normative data, there have been no standardized tests of word-recognition ability in background noise that are readily available. Sentence materials presented in background noise have been developed, particularly for research purposes, but have not been implemented clinically. Second, educational programs emphasize assessing the ability of patients to understand speech, usually monosyllabic words, presented in quiet. Third, audiologists, like everyone, are resistant to changes. The evaluation of the ability of a listener to understand speech in background noise is a big change (addition) in most audiology settings. Finally, time spent with the patient is a major issue. Adding a speech-recognition task in noise adds to the length of an evaluation.

Why should a speech-in-noise task be included in an audiologic evaluation? First, the metric addresses the most common complaint of the patient, that is, her or his inability to understand speech in background noise. This complaint is expressed by most older adults and by many children when the question is posed and pursued. Second, the data from a speech-in-noise task can be used to screen for APD in children and possibly adults and the distortion component of sensorineural hearing loss so often associated with adults. Third, speech-in-noise data can provide insight into the amplification strategy that would be most appropriate for the patient. Fourth, and equally important, speech-in-noise results can be used when counseling the patient, especially with regard to the expectations the patient has about the benefits received from a hearing aid when listening in background noise. For the most part the speech-in-noise instrument has been dormant in audiology clinics for the past 35 years. Only recently has there been a revival of sorts of protocols that evaluate the ability of patients to understand speech in background noise.

Speech-in-Noise Tests

To date, several sentence materials in competing noise paradigms have been developed to assess speech recognition in noise performance. Some of the most are common sentence-in-noise tests are the Connected Sentence Test (CST; Cox, Alexander, & Gilmore, 1987), the Hearing-in-Noise Test (HINT; Nilsson, Soli, & Sullivan, 1994), the Quick Speech-in-Noise Test (QuickSIN™; Killion, Niquette, Gundmundsen, Revit, & Banerjee, 2004), and the BKB-Speech in Noise Test (Bamford-Kowal-Bench, BKB-SIN™, Niquette et al., 2003; Etymōtic Research, 2005). The sentence tests are constructed differently varying on many dimensions such as type of target stimuli, speaker gender, types of background noises, physical paradigms, and scoring metrics. In addition to sentence materials, digits-in-noise (Smits et al., 2004; Wilson & Weakley, 2004) as well as the already discussed monosyllabic words-in-noise (WIN; Wilson, 2003; Wilson & Burks, 2005) materials also have been developed to assess the ability of listeners of all ages to understand speech in background noise.

The aforementioned speech-in-noise tests (digits, words, and sentences) measure recognition performance in terms of the SNR needed to obtain 50% correct performance (an exception is the CST that measures recognition performance in terms of percent correct at a single SNR). The interpretation of 50% points in terms of decibels SNR is not as familiar to clinicians as is describing speech-recognition abilities in the traditional terms of percent correct recognition. The HINT (Nilsson et al., 1994) uses a modified adaptive paradigm to bracket the 50% point on the psychometric function. The QuickSIN, BKB-SIN, WIN, and digits-in-noise were all developed using a descending presentation level paradigm (modified method of constants) that measures recognition performance at multiple SNRs and yields the 50% point using the Spearman-Kärber equation (Finney, 1952; Wilson et al., 1973). The benefit of the descending paradigm is the assessment of recognition performance at multiple SNRs thereby providing a broader view of overall recognition performance. Descriptions of several of the common speech-in-noise tests are presented in the following sections.

Hearing-in-Noise Test (HINT) and BKB-SIN

The HINT (Nilsson et al., 1994) and the BKB-SIN (Etymōtic Research, 2005) utilize Americanized BKB sentences (Bench & Bamford, 1979) that are short, highly redundant sentences rich with semantic and syntactic context and were designed for a first-grade reading level. For background noise, the BKB-SIN uses multitalker babble, whereas the HINT uses speech-spectrum noise (recent data from Wilson et al. [2007b] indicate that these two noises produce similar 50% points [±2 dB]). Each list of the BKB-SIN is composed of 10 sentences with each sentence administered at a different SNR from 21- to −6-dB in 3-dB decrements. Each sentence has three target words except for the sentence presented at 21-dB S/N, which has four words. To maintain the appropriate SNRs, the first eight sentences of the BKB-SIN materials are at a constant level with the level of the 9th sentence attenuated 3 dB and the level of the 10th sentence attenuated 6 dB. The level of the multitalker babble with the BKB-SIN materials is incremented 3 dB through the 8th sentence with the babble levels of the 8th, 9th, and 10th sentences constant. Each list of the HINT also has 10 sentences. The level of the speech-spectrum noise is held constant whereas the level of the sentences is varied. The first sentence is presented repeatedly at increased levels until the listener is able to repeat back the entire sentence correctly. The presentation level is then dropped 4 dB and the rest of the sentences are presented. If the listener repeats the sentence correctly, then the presentation level is decreased 4 dB until the fourth sentence beyond which the decrement changes to 2 dB. Depending on whether the listener repeats the 10th sentence correctly or incorrectly, a presentation level is recorded for the anticipated 11th sentence although no 11th sentence is presented. To score the HINT the presentation levels for the 4th through the 11th sentence are averaged and that value is compared to the level of the speech-spectrum noise to determine the SNR for the 50% point.

QuickSIN

The QuickSIN has 12 lists of sentences and three sets of list pairs (Killion et al, 2004; McArdle & Wilson, 2006). Each list consists of six sentences with five target words each. The level of the sentences is fixed whereas the level of the multitalker babble, which is continuous throughout the list of sentences, varies in 5-dB increments from 25 to 0 dB. The sentences are 2.5 to 3.0 sec with a 5- to 6-sec interval between. Each list of sentences is ~55 sec.

Digits-in-Noise and Monosyllabic Words-in-Noise (WIN)

The digits-in-noise test, which is modeled after a similar test developed by Smits et al. (2004) in Dutch, employs nine random digit triplets in multitalker babble at each of seven SNRs (S/N) that range from 4 to −20 dB in 4-dB decrements (Wilson & Weakley, 2005). The level of the multitalker babble is fixed and the level of the digits varies. The approximately 3.5-sec digit triplets are sep-

arated by a 4-sec quiet interstimulus interval (ISI). Each track of 72 digit triplets is 2 minutes and 55 sec. As previously mentioned, the WIN (Wilson, 2003) is composed of 70 monosyllabic words from the NU No. 6 presented in multitalker babble at each of 7 SNRs from 24 to 0 dB S/N (Wilson & Burks, 2005). As with the digit materials, the level of the babble, which is present continuously throughout the list of words, is fixed, the level of the words varied, and an ~2.7-sec ISI is used. The WIN can be used either as a 70-word list or as two, 35-word lists of 2 minutes and 23 sec (Wilson & Burks, 2005).

Performance Comparisons Among Speech-in-Noise Materials

Two recent studies examined recognition performance differences as a function of the type of test material used to assess SNR hearing loss (McArdle et al., 2005; Wilson et al., 2007b). McArdle et al. examined the differences among three speech-in-noise tasks (i.e., digits-in-noise, WIN, and QuickSIN) for listeners with normal hearing and listeners with hearing loss and found that all three materials provided the same ~8-dB separation between mean recognition performances by listeners with normal hearing and mean recognition performances by listeners with hearing loss. In addition, the QuickSIN and WIN produced recognition performances by listeners with hearing loss that were equivalent, that is, mean 50% points of approximately 12 dB S/N. The results from a similar study (Wilson et al., 2007b) are depicted in Figure 9–4 in which functions for the BKB-SIN, QuickSIN, and WIN are shown for listeners with normal hearing (top) and listeners with hearing loss (bottom). Within the two groups of listeners at the 50% point, the QuickSIN and WIN

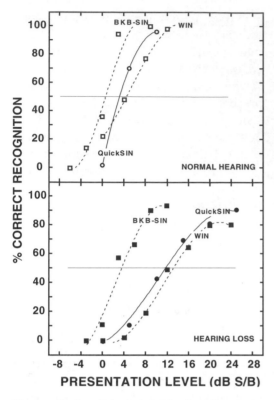

Figure 9–4. Psychometric functions are shown for the BKB-SIN, the QuickSIN, and the WIN materials obtained from 24 listeners with normal hearing (*top*) and from 72 listeners with sensorineural hearing loss (*bottom*). (Derived from Wilson, McArdle, & Smith, 2007b.)

terms of 50% point, which permits comparisons of performance between these materials. The monosyllabic words used in the WIN provide a good measure of basic auditory function because the effects of working memory and linguistic context on recognition performance are minimized, thereby forcing individuals to rely on the acoustic cues of the target to facilitate recognition. Monosyllabic word targets recorded in isolation enhance the role of acoustic cues by decreasing the blurring of phoneme boundaries that occurs with coarticulation. The IEEE sentences (IEEE, 1969) used in the QuickSIN provide mainly syntactic cues with only subtle semantic cues to aid in recognition. Because the IEEE sentences are constructed with proper syntax yet lack strong semantic cues, the use of IEEE sentences as target stimuli increases the contextual cues available to the listener as compared to monosyllabic words. The increase in context decreases the reliance of the listener on acoustic cues and allows the probability of a correct target word to be influenced by the surrounding syntactical context along with the acoustic cues. Equivalent 50% points obtained with the QuickSIN and the WIN suggest that the additional benefit from the limited context provided by the IEEE sentences does not significantly improve the recognition performances of listeners with hearing loss. It is possible that the additional cognitive load related to the listeners required to repeat the entire sentence, which can range from 6 to 12 syllables, versus a single word recorded in isolation can counteract to some degree the recognition improvement that would be expected from the additional context. Other differences like speaker differences probably contribute to the relation.

Given that recognition performances were similar for the QuickSIN and the WIN, Wilson et al. (2007b) subsequently exam-

exhibit similar performances with the WIN requiring about a 1.5 dB better SNR for equal performance. Interestingly, the differences between the two groups of listeners were about 8.5 dB for the QuickSIN and WIN, decreasing to about 3.5 dB for the BKB-SIN. Again, the materials with the least amount of information or fewest redundancies are the most difficult for the listeners with hearing loss.

The McArdle et al. (2005a) data suggest that the WIN and QuickSIN provide comparable recognition performances in

ined in listeners with normal hearing and listeners with hearing loss the within and between group differences obtained with four commonly available speech-in-noise protocols (*viz.*, BKB-SIN, HINT, QuickSIN, and WIN). Figure 9–5 is a four-panel bivariate plot of the individual data for the listeners with normal hearing (circles) and the listeners with hearing loss (squares) in which the percent correct word-recognition score on the NU No. 6 materials presented in quiet at 104-dB SPL is shown on the ordinate and the level (dB S/N) at which the 50% correct point occurred for the four materials is shown on the abscissa. The larger filled symbols depict the mean data and the lines through the data points are second degree polynomials used to describe the data from the listeners with hearing loss. The vertical dashed line in each panel is the 95th percentile for performance by the 24 listeners with normal hearing, which were 2.5-, 5.9-, 6.9-, and 5.5-dB S/N for the BKB-SIN, HINT, QuickSIN, and WIN, respectively. The numbers listed beside the dashed lines are the percent of the 72 listeners with hearing loss whose performance was in the normal range (to the left of the dashed line) and whose performance was outside of the normal range (to the right of the dashed line). The percentage data in the figure indicate that the materials on which performance was based were more dependent on acoustic cues than on contextual cues (QuickSIN and WIN) and provided better separation between recognition performances by the listeners with normal hearing and the listeners with hearing loss than did the materials that had more contextual cues (BKB-SIN and HINT). With the BKB-SIN and HINT materials, substantially more listeners with hearing loss (22 to 28%) had performances in the normal range. As the QuickSIN and the WIN appear more sensitive to subtle differences in auditory func-

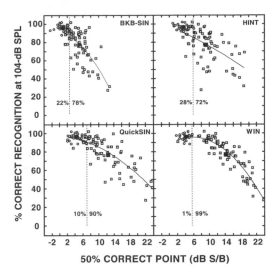

Figure 9–5. Bivariate plots of the percent correct recognition on the NU No. 6 materials presented at 104-dB SPL in quiet on the ordinate and the 50% correct points (in dB S/B) on the abscissa. Datum points for the listeners with normal hearing (*circles*) and the listeners with hearing loss (*squares*) are listed with the larger, filled symbols representing the mean data points. The curvilinear line in each panel represents the best-fit, second-degree polynomial used to describe the data for the listeners with hearing loss. The vertical dotted lines represent the 95th percentile in recognition performance by the listeners with normal hearing. The numbers listed by the dotted lines indicate the percent of listeners with hearing loss who performed in the normal range (*left of the line*) and in the abnormal range (*right of the line*). To avoid overlapping data points, a jittered algorithm was used that randomly multiplied the *x* and *y* values by 1.025 to 0.975 in 0.05-steps. (Taken from Wilson, McArdle, & Smith, 2007b).

tion, these two instruments should be the preferable choice to use in the course of a routine audiologic evaluation and to use as a degraded speech measure when screening for APD.

Masking

As mentioned above, recognizing speech in a background of noise creates a degraded speech task by decreasing the redundancies available acoustically through the use of noise. The question is what is noise and how are noise and masking related? We recognize the philosophical discussions that are ongoing in the psychoacoustic arena (e.g., Carhart et al., 1969; Watson, 2005; Yost, 2006), but for the purposes here the focus on noise and masking is maintained within the traditional audiologic framework. That being said, noise takes many forms but in the audiology community noises used to degrade speech signals are resricted basically to three types. First, is random or white noise that is either broadband (i.e., limited by the frequency response of the transducer) or filtered to mimic, usually the long-term spectrum of ongoing speech, which is the so-called speech-spectrum noise. Typically, the amplitude waveform of these noises is fairly constant with only minor amplitude modulations. The second type of noise is multitalker babble that is composed usually of six or more speakers simultaneously reading selected passages. Although multiple speakers are involved, the waveform is characterized by obvious amplitude modulations. A visual comparison of the waveform envelops of speech-spectrum noise and multitalker babble is provided by Wilson et al. (2007a, Figure 1). The third type of noise is a competing message that is produced by a single speaker reading isolated sentences. Because only one speaker is involved, the amplitude modulation characteristics of the waveform are exaggerated in comparison to the amplitude modulations associated with multitalker babble. Thus, across these three types of noises or maskers, the amplitude modulation characteristics form a continuum from minimal as with speech-spectrum noise to substantial as with a single-speaker competing message. Collectively, the results from two recent studies from our laboratories indicate that young adult listeners with normal hearing progressively are less affected as the noise sequences along the continuum from speech-spectrum noise to the competing message (Smith et al., 2007; Wilson et al., 2007a). Using speech-spectrum noise as the reference listening condition, this lessening of the masking effects observed with young adults with normal hearing is referred to as an *escape from masking* or *release from masking*, which simply means that masking by multitalker babble and single-speaker competing messages are not as effective as the masking accomplished with speech-spectrum noise. The escape from masking is attributed to the ability of the listener to perceive speech cues during the "valleys" of the amplitude modulations, which in other terms are "listening windows of opportunity." In sharp contrast, older listeners with hearing loss (and perhaps individuals with APD) obtain little escape or release from masking with the latter two noises. Although there are individual exceptions, to the older listener with hearing loss the three types of noises produce in effect about the same amount of masking. Somehow, with these listeners with hearing loss, perhaps through forward and backward masking or other mechanisms, the listening windows of opportunity created by the valleys in the amplitude modulations of the noise are obscured as if the noise envelope were void of the valleys in the modulations. This phenomenon can be equated to the reduced ability of older adults to detect gaps in the various gap detection experiments (Gordon-Salant & Fitzgibbons, 1999; Lister et al., 2000). In the following paragraph, data from the Wilson et al. study illustrate this behavior.

Wilson et al. (2007a) examined the differential effects of masking using a speech spectrum noise (SSN) and a multitalker babble noise (MTB) on recognition performance for listeners with normal hearing and listeners with hearing loss. The two maskers were expected to produce similar overall masking because the rms levels were equivalent and because the spectra of the two maskers were similar (Miller, 1947). The results, however, showed that the listeners with normal hearing obtained some release from masking in the MTB condition, re: SSN, that was not obtained from the listeners with hearing loss. The data displayed in Figure 9–6 show the psychometric functions for recognition performance of monosylla-

bles in noise using SSN (dotted line) and MTB (solid line) as the masking noise with the listeners with normal hearing drawn in the top panel and the listeners with hearing loss in the lower panel. Examination of the 50% points in each panel of Figure 9–6 show that for the listeners with normal hearing, less signal-to-noise was needed for the MTB condition as compared to the SSN condition. This was not seen for the listeners with hearing loss who achieved 50% at the same SNR for both MTB and SSN. Thus, it was concluded that listeners with normal hearing take advantage of the amplitude "valleys" in the noise allowing for glimpses of the target acoustic information in the reduced SNRs that occur during the amplitude modulations of the MTB, whereas listeners with hearing loss as a group are not able to take advantage of the reduced SNR afforded by the amplitude fluctuations.

Speech-in-Noise Tests to Screen for APD

Degraded speech tests vary the amount of bottom-up information available to the listener by changing the spectral or temporal characteristics of the signal. By varying the bottom-up information, degraded speech tests increase uncertainty and decrease extrinsic redundancies available to the listener. Many variations of degraded speech tests are used in a typical APD battery; however, data to support the need for multiple measures, at least in the adult population, are lacking.

With adults, the identification of those listeners who have difficulty understanding speech in background noise can be accomplished efficiently with a number of instruments ranging from sentences-in-noise to words-in-noise to digits-in-noise. Psychometric properties such as normative data,

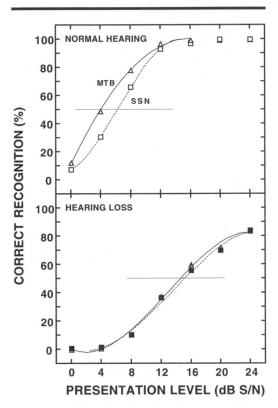

Figure 9–6. The mean functions for the multitalker babble (MTB) and speech-spectrum noise (SSN) maskers are shown for the 24 listeners with normal hearing (*top panel*) and the 48 listeners with hearing loss (*bottom panel*). (Taken from Wilson et al., 2007b).

test-retest differences, as well as critical differences for both the WIN (Wilson et al, 2003; Wilson & McArdle, 2007) and the QuickSIN (Killion et al, 2004, McArdle et al, 2005a) have been reported for the adult population. The same techniques need to be applied to children, but first some basic questions need to be answered. For example, developmentally, at what age can we expect children with normal hearing sensitivity to perform on a given speech-in-noise task in a manner that is similar to a young adult listener with normal hearing sensitivity? For maximum performances, different ages may be required for different speech-in-noise tasks. Once this age range is established, there is no reason for children not to be evaluated with a speech-in-noise instrument. Additionally, what types of modifications can be made to speech-in-noise materials that would make them suitable for children below the above mentioned age range? Finally, comparisons among the various degraded speech tasks need to be made on substantial-sized populations of children across a representative age range to determine the necessity of evaluating the ability of a child to perform on several degraded speech tasks.

References

American Speech-Language-Hearing Association. (1996). Central auditory processing: Current status of research and implications for clinical practice. *American Journal of Audiology*, *5*, 41–54.

Beattie, R. C. (1989). Word recognition functions for the CID W-22 Test in multitalker noise for normally hearing and hearing-impaired subjects. *Journal of Speech and Hearing Disorders*, *54*, 20–32.

Bellis, T. J. (2006). Audiologic behavioral assessment of APD. In T. K. Parthasarathy (Ed.), *An introduction to auditory processing disorders in children.* (pp. 63–80). Mahwah, NJ: Lawrence Erlbaum Associates.

Bellis, T. J., & Ferre, J. M. (1999). Multidimensional approach to the differential diagnosis of auditory processing disorders in children. *Journal of the American Academy of Audiology*, *10*, 319–328.

Bench, J., & Bamford, J. (1979). *Speech-hearing tests and the spoken language of hearing-impaired children.* London: Academic Press.

Bocca E., & Calearo C. (1963). Central hearing processes. In J. Jerger (Ed.), *Modern developments in audiology* (pp. 337–370). New York: Academic Press.

Boothroyd A., & Nittrouer S. (1988). Mathematical treatment of context effects in phoneme and word recognition. *Journal of the Acoustical Society of America*, *84*, 101–114.

Carhart, R. (1951). Basic principles of speech audiometry. *Acta Otolaryngologica*, *40*, 62–71.

Carhart, R., & Tillman, T. W. (1970). Interaction of competing speech signals with hearing losses. *Archives of Otolaryngology*, *91*, 273–279.

Carhart, R., Tillman, T. W., & Greetis, E. S. (1969). Perceptual masking in multiple sound backgrounds. *Journal of the Acoustical Society of America*, *45*, 694–703.

Cox, R. M., Alexander, G. C., & Gilmore, C. (1987). Development of the Connected Speech Test (CST). *Ear and Hearing*, *8*, 119S–125S.

Dirks, D. D., Morgan, D. E., & Dubno, J. R. (1982). A procedure for quantifying the effects of noise on speech recognition. *Journal of Speech and Hearing Disorders*, *47*, 114–123.

Etymōtic Research. (2001). QuickSIN™ [Compact disk]. 61 Martin Lane, Elk Grove Village, IL 60007.

Finney, D.J. (1952). *Statistical method in biological essay.* London: C. Griffen.

Gordon-Salant, S., & Fitzgibbons, P. (1999). Profile of auditory temporal processing in older adults. *Journal of Speech, Language, and Hearing Research*, *42*, 300–311.

Groen, J. J. (1969). Social hearing handicap: Its measurement by speech audiometry in noise. *International Audiology*; *8*, 182–183.

IEEE. (1969). IEEE recommended practice for speech quality measurements. *IEEE Transactions on Audio and Electroacoustics, 17,* 227–246.

Jusczyk, P. W., & Luce, P. A. (2002). Speech perception and spoken word recognition: Past and present. *Ear and Hearing, 23,* 2–40.

Katz, J. (1968). The SSW test: An interim report. *Journal of Speech Hearing Disorders, 33,* 132–146.

Keith, R. W. (1986). *SCAN: A screening test for auditory processing disorders: Manual.* San Diego, CA: The Psychology Corporation.

Killion, M. C., Niquette, P. A., Gudmundsen, G. I., Revit, L. J., & Banerjee, S. (2004). Development of a quick speech-in-noise test for measuring signal-to-noise ratio loss in normal-hearing and hearing-impaired listeners. *Journal of the Acoustical Society of America, 116,* 2395–2405.

Lindgren, R., & Lindblom, B. (1983). Speech perception processing. *Scandinavian Audiology Supplement, 18,* 57–70.

Lister, J. J., Koehnke, J. D., & Besing, J. M. (2000). Binaural gap duration discrimination in listeners with impaired hearing and normal hearing. *Ear and Hearing, 21,* 141–150.

Lutman, M. E. (1987). Speech tests in quiet and noise as a measure of auditory processing. In M. Martin (Ed.), *Speech audiometry* (pp. 63–73). London: Taylor and Francis.

McArdle, R., Chisolm, T. H., Abrams, H. B., Wilson, R. H., & Doyle, P. (2005b). The WHO-DAS II: Measuring outcomes of hearing aid intervention for adults. *Trends in Amplification, 9,* 127–143.

McArdle, R. A., & Wilson, R. H. (2006). Homogeneity of the 18 QuickSIN Lists. *Journal of the American Academy of Audiology, 17,* 157–167.

McArdle, R., Wilson, R. H., & Burks, C. A. (2005a). Speech recognition in multitalker babble using digits, words, and sentences. *Journal of the American Academy of Audiology, 16,* 726–739.

Miller, G. A. (1947). The masking of speech. *Psychological Bulletin, 44,* 105–129.

Miller, G. A. (1951). *Language and communication.* New York: McGraw-Hill.

Nilsson, M., Soli, S., & Sullivan J. (1994). Development of the Hearing in Noise Test for the measurement of speech reception thresholds in quiet and in noise. *Journal of the Acoustical Society of America, 95,* 1085–1099.

Niquette, P., Arcaroli, J., Revit, L., Parkinson, A., Staller, S., Skinner, M., & Killion, M. (2003, March). *Development of the BKB-SIN Test.* Paper presented at the Annual Meeting of the American Auditory Society, Scottsdale. http://www.amauditorysoc.org/pages/abstracts/2003/2003-pp-1.html

Olsen, W. O., & Carhart, R. (1967). Development of test procedures for evaluation of binaural hearing aids. *Bull Prosthetics Research, 10,* 22–49.

Plomp, R. (1978). Auditory handicap of hearing impairment and the limited benefit of hearing aids. *Journal of the Acoustical Society of America. 63,* 533–549.

Plomp, R., & Duquesnoy, A. J. (1982). A model for the speech-reception threshold in noise without and with a hearing aid. *Scandinavian Audiology Supplement, 15,* 95–111.

Putter-Katz, H., Said, L. A., Feldman, I., Miran, D., Kushnir, D., Muchnik, C., & Hildesheimer, M. (2002). Treatment and evaluation indices of auditory processing disorders. *Seminars in Hearing, 23,* 357–364.

Schow, R. L., & Chermak, G. (1999). Implications from factor analysis for central auditory processing disorders. *American Journal of Audiology, 8,* 137–142.

Schow, R. L., Seikel, J. A., Chermak, G. D., & Berent, M. (2000). Central auditory processes and test measures: ASHA 1996 revisited. *American Journal of Audiology, 9,* 63–68.

Smith, S. L., Wilson, R. H., & McArdle, R. A. (2007). Word recognition performance in competing sentence and multitalker babble paradigms in listeners with hearing loss. *Proceedings of the International Symposium on Auditory and Audiological Research,* Helsingør, Denmark.

Smits, C., Kapteyn, T. S., & Houtgast, T. (2004). Development and validation of an automatic SRT screening test by telephone. *International Journal of Audiology, 43,* 15–28.

Stephens, S. D. G. (1976). The input for a damaged cochlea—A brief review. *British Journal of Audiology, 10,* 97–101.

Strom, K. E. (2006). The Hearing Review 2006 dispenser survey. *The Hearing Review, 13,* 16–39.

Tillman, T. W., & Carhart, R. (1966). *An extended test for speech discrimination utilizing CNC monosyllabic words: University Auditory Test No. 6.* [Technical Report Number SAM-TR-66-55]. Brooks Air Force Base, TX: USAF School of Aerospace Medicine.

Walley, A. C. (2005). Speech perception in childhood. In D. B. Pisoni & R. E. Remez (Eds.), *The handbook of speech perception* (pp. 449–468). Oxford, UK: Blackwell.

Ward, D. W. (1964). "Sensitivity" versus "acuity." *Journal of Speech and Hearing Research, 7,* 291–303.

Watson, C. S. (2005). Some comments on informational masking. *Acta Acoustica, 91,* 502–512.

Wilson, R. H. (2003). Development of a speech in multitalker babble paradigm to assess word-recognition performance. *Journal of the American Academy of Audiology, 14,* 453–470.

Wilson, R. H., Abrams, H. B., & Pillion, A. L. (2003). A word-recognition task in multitalker babble using a descending presentation mode from 24 dB to 0 dB in signal to babble. *Journal of Rehabilitative Research and Development, 40,* 321–328.

Wilson, R. H., & Burks, C. A. (2005). Use of 35 words for evaluation of hearing loss in signal-to-babble ratio: a clinic protocol. *Journal of Rehabilitation Research and Development, 42,* 839–852.

Wilson, R. H., Carnell, C. S., & Cleghorn, A. L. (2007a). The Words-in-Noise (WIN) test with multitalker babble and speech-spectrum noise maskers. *Journal of the American Academy of Audiology, 18,* 522–530.

Wilson, R. H., & McArdle, R. (2005). Speech signals used to evaluate functional status of the auditory system. *Journal of Rehabilitation Research & Development, 42,* 79–94.

Wilson, R. H., & McArdle, R. (2007). Intra- and intersession test retest reliability of the Words-in-Noise (WIN) Test. *Journal of the American Academy of Audiology, 18*(10), 813–825.

Wilson, R. H., McArdle, R., & Smith, S. L. (2007b). An Evaluation of the BKB-SIN, HINT, QuickSIN, and WIN materials on listeners with normal hearing and listeners with hearing loss. *Journal of Speech, Language, and Hearing Research. 50,* 844–856.

Wilson, R. H., Morgan, D. E., & Dirks, D. D. (1973). A proposed SRT procedure and its statistical precedent. *Journal of Speech and Hearing Disorders. 38,* 184–191.

Wilson, R. H., & Weakley, D. G. (2004). The use of digit triplets to evaluate word-recognition abilities in multitalker babble. *Seminars in Hearing, 25,* 93–111.

Yost, W. (2006). Informational masking: What is it? Message posted to: http://www.isr.umd.edu/Labs/NSL/Cosyne/Yost.htm

CHAPTER 10

Controversies in Standardization of Auditory Processing Tests

ROBERT W. KEITH

Introduction

The field of audiology is generally considered to be a scientific profession that conforms to the highest standards of objective measurement. For example, early research at the Bell Laboratories into auditory function defined equal loudness curves and the specifics of the articulation gain function that forms the basis of clinical speech recognition testing in use today. Many other examples of basic science investigation into frequency ranges required for understanding of the speech signal, differential thresholds for frequency and intensity, pitch matching, and a myriad of other details regarding the psychoacoustics of hearing are reported in the early audiology literature (Hirsh, 1952; Stephens, 1951). More recently, there are

detailed studies on a wide range of behavioral and electrophysiologic aspects of audition. Those studies lead us to a precise understanding of the range of intensities required for an acoustic reflex threshold, the latency of various waves of the auditory brainstem response, and the frequency response and signal-to-noise ratio of the normal otoacoustic emission. In view of this rich heritage, it is surprising to consider the current status of "normative" data used in the interpretation of tests of central auditory function. While the spirit of this textbook is to explore issues of contention and unresolved questions pertaining to various topics in auditory processing disorder (APD), the purposes of this chapter are:

1. To describe the current status of normative data used in tests for the evaluation of APD

2. To discuss the clinical value of well-normed tests of APD

3. To describe standardized norm-referenced tests

4. To give, by comparison, examples of tests used in speech-language pathology, and

5. To recommend future goals.

Review of Consensus Statements Regarding Use of Test Norms

ASHA Task Force on Central Auditory Processing (ASHA, 1996)

The first national consensus conference was hosted by the American Speech-Language Hearing Association. The panel in that conference consisted of 18 individuals and participants from a wide range of professional backgrounds in communication sciences and disorders. In addition to publishing background information and expressing opinions about a number of issues related to APDs, the conference dealt briefly with the topic of normative data in APD testing. Specifically, the panel reported that some measures of auditory processing that were available for clinical use at that time suffered from inadequate normative data, and had questionable validity and test-retest reliability. They noted that clinicians should consider availability of age-appropriate norms, test sensitivity and specificity, test reliability and validity, and age appropriateness when selecting assessment procedures. There was no suggestion for the need to obtain better normative data on tests that measure auditory processes in the final statement of research priorities. To their credit, the task force noted that they were impressed at the gulf between science and practice that seemed evident at the consensus conference.

Callier Center Conference (Jerger & Musiek, 2000)

A subsequent consensus conference on the diagnosis of auditory processing disorders in school-age children convened 13 audiologists from academic or medical center environments and one speech-language pathologist. The consensus panel noted that acceptable psychometric standards should be met by any screening instrument, including concepts of sensitivity and specificity, predictive values of positive and negative results, interobserver reliability, intertest consistency, and validity (Jerger & Musiek, 2000). There is no other statement in the document on the status of, or need for, improvement in the availability of normative data on current or future tests of auditory processing.

Clinical and Research Concerns (Katz, Johnson, Brandner, et al., 2002)

A following statement of concerns about the recommendations made by Jerger and Musiek (2000) was published by a group of audiologists representing a wide range of work environments, although many came from educational audiology. Katz et al. (2002) noted the statement by Jerger and Musiek that screening tests should meet, "acceptable psychometric standards ... " (p. 469). However, Katz et al. stated the belief that *none* of the tests specifically recommended by Jerger and Musiek meet these criteria. They went on to declare their concern with the dichotic digits test norms because of instructions to users of that test are advised as follows: "We strongly recommend that you collect your own norms in your own area" (p. 2). They commented that when norms are collected by the author of the test, it poses a serious limitation and is inappropriate for a test that is proposed as a standard test for all APD cases. Furthermore, Katz et al. note that if clinicians are expected to collect their own norms, then they would also need to gather the sensitivity-specificity data that Jerger and Musiek indicate are necessary to determine if the test meets acceptable psychometric standards. Regarding the dichotic digits test, Katz et al. point out that although it has some positive features, it does not have (a) strong literature support, (b) national norms, (c) "acceptable psychometric standards," and (d) no norms, of any sort, are reported below 7 years-of-age. There are many potential problems created by clinics collecting their own norms. Different clinics may use a variety of methodologies that produce fundamentally different results; there may be lack of quality control, different subject inclusion/exclusion criteria may be used, and so forth. All of these examples add further confusion to the ability of audiologists to directly compare findings across clinics. Finally, any comparison of results from different researchers and research studies is difficult, if not impossible.

Katz et al. expressed other concerns about the status of normative data when testing for APD. For example, they state that, at a minimum, any recommended procedure must be validated on children with APD and have age-appropriate norms. In a summary, after a detailed study of the tests recommended by Jerger and Musiek (2000) for evaluation of APD in children, Katz et al. found (a) almost no literature using these tests with the target population, (b) absence of normative data for these tests,

(c) lack of sensitivity and specificity data, and (d) no evidence that the physiologic tests are useful or appropriate as part of a minimal test battery. A summary of their review of available norms is shown on Table 10–1 (with permission).

ASHA Technical Report on (Central) Auditory Processing Disorder (ASHA, 2005)

According to the ASHA technical report (ASHA, 2005), tests with good reliability and validity that also demonstrate high sensitivity, specificity, and efficiency should be selected when administering a central auditory test battery. In addition, audiologists were advised to review the test normative information and background carefully to be sure that the test is appropriate for the individual to be evaluated. The document also states that absolute or norm-based interpretation is probably the most commonly used approach that involves judging an individual's performance relative to group data from normal controls. The authors of the document go on to state that relative or patient-based interpretation refers to judging an individual's performance on a given test relative to his or her own baseline. Patient-based interpretation is said to include intratest analysis that compares patterns observed with a given test, for example, ear differences scores and interhemispheric differences. Intertest analysis is said to be the comparison of trends observed across the diagnostic test battery, for example, patterns consistent with neuroscience principles, anatomic site of dysfunction, and comorbid clinical profiles. Finally, the document states that cross-discipline analysis compares results observed across disciplines including, for example, audiology, speech-language pathology, psychology, multimodality sensory function,

TABLE 10–1. Information and Support for Various Specific Tests in Jerger and Musiek's (2000) Minimal Test Battery and Screening Tests

Specified Minimal Test Battery Procedures	AP Literature Through 2000	Strong Support for Routing AP Use	AP Norms Available	APD Sensitivity Specificity Data	Listed By Martin et al. (1998) for CAP Test	Additional Comments
Performance-Intensity Function	None found	No	No	No	Yes 26%	Not generally thought of as APD test but audiologists used it for APD evaluations
Dichotic Digits	1 found	Mild	Recommend get own norms	14 hits of 22 S^s	No	No information found on how to interpret a failure
Temporal Noise Gap Detection	None found	No	No	No	No	No such noise test found commercially available
Duration Pattern Sequence	None found	No	No	No	No	No support for its use in the Minimal Test Battery
Otoacoustic Emissions—Inner ear	None found	No	Same criteria as inner ear?	No	No	No support for routine APD cases
Auditory Brainstem Response	None found	No	Same as VIII N. brainstem?	No	No	No support for routine APD use found
Middle Latency Responses	1 found	No	Same as for CNS?	No	No	Likely not appropriate below 10 years. No support for routine use for APD cases

Note: More general procedures (e.g., dichotic words) were mentioned in their article but not reviewed here because we did not know which specific tests the authors had in mind.

and so forth. According to the ASHA document, diagnosis of CAPD requires performance deficits that are two or more standard deviations below normal on two or more tests of central auditory function.

So What Is the Problem?

The problem with all of the consensus statements is that they make statements about availability of normative data on tests of central auditory function that do not mirror reality. In fact, as pointed out by Katz et al. (2002), few of the most popular tests of auditory processing used in the evaluation of subjects have adequate normative data. Many do not. For example, Table 10–2 indicates that instructions and/or manuals on several popular tests used to identify APD fail to provide any information on the number and demographics of the subjects, methods used in obtaining data, and any information about test reliability. In addition, some tests do not provide any information beyond a percentage cutoff score. When interpreting the results, therefore, it is impossible to know where subjects stand in relation to other subjects of the same age level, the variability of the measure, when a test-retest score is the same— or different, and how results of one test relate to others.

In contrast, the Test of Auditory-Perceptual Skills-Revised (TAPS-R) (Gardner, 1996) provides normative data for subjects 4 years through 12 years, 11 months, and norms for each subtest, such as: standard scores, scaled scores, percentile ranks, and stanines. Norms for the complete battery are provided in addition to norms for each subtest. Normative data were acquired on 1038 subjects with known demographics on subject age, grade, gender, and race. Finally,

normative data are provided in 2-month intervals for each age group. It is unfortunate that the TAPS-R is named a test of "auditory-perceptual skills" because it is not an auditory-specific test. It is fundamentally a language-based measure of auditory memory, discrimination, understanding, and interpretation of a linguistic message. Nevertheless, the test serves as an example of a test battery for which normative data are provided in the manual that allow interpretation of performance and comparison of results to a wide range of other psychological, educational, and language measures similarly standardized.

It is interesting to contemplate that such measures as the Frequency Pattern Test have no published norms in spite of being developed nearly 40 years ago by Ptacek and Pinheiro (Ptacek & Pinheiro, 1971). The same is true for dichotic digits testing that was described as early as 1983 (Musiek, 1983). Audiologists have to wonder why tests that are so popular have so few available norms, raising the question about the basis upon which clinical decisions are made. And so, what is an appropriate approach to this dilemma?

Interpreting Norm-Referenced Scores—or What Are the Advantages of Norm-Referenced Standardized Tests?

Standardized tests have many advantages over simple raw scores, cutoff scores, or mean scores and standard deviations. Standardized test scores enable the examiner to compare a subject's performance on a test with individuals of similar age across the country. Comparison can be made of a

TABLE 10–2. What Normative Data Are Available for Some Popular Tests of Auditory Processing?
Summary of tests of auditory processing disorders

Test Name	Type of Test	AP Norms Available	Number and Demographics of Subjects on Which Normative Data Were Gathered	Additional Comments
Dichotic Digits Test (Musiek, 1983)	Dichotic digits	Cutoff scores for each ear provided for children between 7 and 12 years	Unknown	Examiners are encouraged to collect their own norms
SCAN-C test of auditory processing disorders in children (Keith, 2000)	Filtered words, auditory figure-ground, dichotic words and sentences	SS, CI, PR*, and ear advantage provided for children from 6 through 11 years	650 normal hearing children between 5 years, 0 months and 11 years, 11 months. 144 6-0 to 11-11 y/o with CAPD tested for validity. Norms reported at 1-year intervals. Results compared to 1025 subjects in original SCAN (Keith, 1986)	Data were collected by 115 audiologists.
SCAN-A test of auditory processing disorders in adolescents and adults (Keith, 1994)	Filtered words, auditory figure-ground, dichotic words and sentences	SS, CI, PR* and ear advantage for subjects between 12 and 50 years.	125 normal hearing subjects, 12–50 years, equal male and female, with 38 subjects in a test-retest study and 25 matched subjects with APD	Data were gathered in 23 sites by 52 audiologists.

Test Name	Type of Test	AP Norms Available	Number and Demographics of Subjects on Which Normative Data Were Gathered	Additional Comments
Staggered Spondee Words Test (Katz, 1962)	Dichotic spondee word test	Number of errors and cutoff scores by age from 6 years through adults; 1 SD used for determining normal limits	183 normal-hearing subjects age 5 to 11 years, half male and female.	Data were collected by 40 examiners trained to admin and score the SSW
Time-Compressed Sentence Test (Keith, 2002)	Degraded speech test	Cutoff scores, SS, PR*	78 normal hearing 6 to 11 year old children; 34 male, 44 female	Data were collected by 13 audiologists.
Duration Patterns Test (Musiek, Baran, & Pinheiro ML. 1990)	Pattern recognition test	% cutoff scores on 4 age groups from 8 through 12 years	Unknown	
Frequency Patterns Test (Musiek,& Pinheiro, 1987)	Pattern recognition test	% cutoff scores on 4 age groups from 8 through 12 years	Unknown	
BKB-SIN™ (Nyquette, 2005)	Speech-in-noise test with variable signal-to-noise ratio	Mean and SD of signal-to-noise ratio for 50% correct for adults and children age 5 to 14 years	Norms developed from 84 normal children between ages 5 to 13 years	Data were collected in two sites.

continues

TABLE 10–2. *continued*

Test Name	Type of Test	AP Norms Available	Number and Demographics of Subjects on Which Normative Data Were Gathered	Additional Comments
QuickSIN™ (Nyquette, Gudmunsen, & Killion, 2001)	Speech-in-noise test with variable signal-to-noise ratio	Descriptive interpretation of various SNR loss from 0 to >15 dB	Following pre Beta-site testing Norms developed from 26 normal-hearing and 18 hearing-impaired subjects	Specific descriptions of development of the test items are available in the manual. Subsequent normative data were published by Bentler (2000)
Selective Auditory Attention Test (SAAT) (Cherry, 1980)	Speech-in-noise test at 0 dB S/N ratio.	Norms available for children age 4 to 9 years.	Norms collected on 385 children from preK–2nd grade (4 to 9 y/o)	
Department of Veterans Affairs Compact Disk Recording for Auditory Perceptual Assessment (Noffsinger, Wilson, & Musiek, 1994)	Several tests including dichotic digits and synthetic sentences, high and low-pass filtered words, frequency and duration tonal patterns, 45% and 65% time-compressed speech	Data, error statistics, and confidence ranges are provided but the authors emphasize that the results were not intended for use as absolute standards. The object was to produce a set of good test materials.	120 young adults with self-described normal hearing. Data collected at 9 major universities and/or medical centers. Twenty-one males and 99 females participated, 107 of them right handers.	No data are provided for subjects who are younger or older than the cohort described in column 4.

*SS = standard score, CI = confidence interval, % = percentile rank.

child's score to a previous score obtained in the past on the same test ito determine whether or not there was real change in performance. With standardized scores, the examiner can compare a child's performance on one test to another standardized test. For example, the audiologist can compare a child's performance on a standardized auditory test directly to a speech language measure, for example, the standard score of the Clinical Evaluation of Language Function (CELF-4) (Semel, Wiig, & Secord, 2003) or any IQ measure. Finally, standard scores can be used to help clients receive services, and help parents understand relationships that exist among various measures.

In most educational and psychological tests, the mean is 100 and the standard deviation is 15 (mean = 100, standard deviation = 15). In most subtests, the mean is 10 and the standard deviation is 3 (mean = 10, standard deviation = 3). A standard score of 100 represents the 50th percentile of the population. As a standard score of 115 is 1 standard deviation above the mean, it is always at the 84th percentile level. As a standard score of 85 is 1 standard deviation below the mean, it is always at the 16th percentile level. A standard score of 130 (2 standard deviations above the mean) is always at the 98th percentile level and a standard score of 70 (2 standard deviations below the mean) is always at the 2nd percentile level (Wright & Wright, 2000). Those relationships are shown on a bell-shaped curve (Figure 10-1).

Percentile Ranks

A percentile rank indicates the percentage of individuals who earned either the same or lower score on a test. For example, an individual with a percentile rank of 35, scores the same as or higher than 35% of individuals his or her age. The percentile

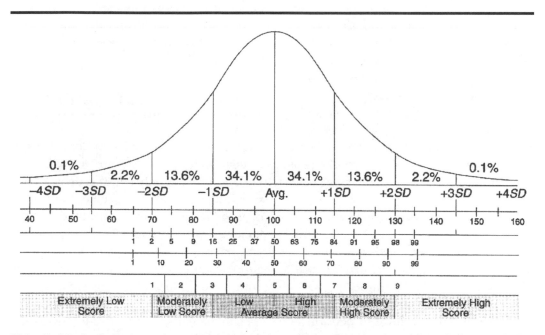

Figure 10-1. Bell-shaped curve showing the relationships among descriptive statistics (mean and standard deviation), and standard scores.

rank also indicates that 65% of individuals earned higher scores. Percentile rank should not be confused with the percent of correct answers on a test. In a standardized test, a standard score has a corresponding percentile rank as shown on the bell-shaped curve in Figure 10–1.

Confidence Intervals

Another issue in testing is to know when a score is actually different from another. In a general semantics sense the question is, "When does a difference make a difference?" Rather than using only the individuals obtained score to evaluate his or her performance, it is important to establish a "true score" confidence interval around the obtained score. The confidence interval around the obtained scores is a range of scores within which the examiner can be highly confident that the "true score" actually lies, taking measurement error into account. For example, suppose an 8-year-old child obtained a composite standard score of 120 on a particular test and that the norms on the test indicate that the 95% confidence interval is between 110 and 130. Those two scores represent the lower and upper bound of the confidence interval for the child's obtained composite standard score. In this case, the examiner can be 95% confident that this child's true composite standard score falls within the range of 110 and 130.

Because confidence intervals reflect the measurement error associated with a test, they should be used in cases where a child's normative ranking may be used in classification or placement decisions. Confidence intervals are also necessary to determine when a true change in performance has occurred. For example, when test-retest is conducted to determine whether a remediation program is effective, it is necessary

to know the range of error in the test score. Use of percent correct on a test cannot be used to determine effectiveness.

Without clearly established confidence intervals, use of "relative or patient-based interpretation refers to judging an individual's performance on a given test relative to his or her own baseline" (ASHA, 2005) has no meaning. Specifically, it is impossible to know whether a change in percent correct (or error) of items on a test is a meaningful change without knowing the measurement error associated with a test. Without that information it is possible to claim that the individual's performance is better or worse over time, or as a result of treatment, when the change is not actually meaningful.

In summary, the lack of confidence intervals makes it difficult to determine whether or not intervention programs lead to successful outcomes. For example, if a child obtains a raw score of X on a test and X plus some value on a retest, performance may seem to improve. However, the confidence interval may indicate that no true change has occurred, and that the second score is within measurement error.

Here Is an Example

Here is an illustration of the problems of evaluation tests that have no normative values and provide only cutoff scores. A child was evaluated with a documented history of language and learning problems, and a lifelong history of middle-ear disease. He was referred for auditory processing evaluation when he was 8 years, 7 months old with the question, "Does this child have an APD, and what strategies/activities can be used in the school setting to address his academic needs?" The child was tested for APD and a recommendation was made that he return for testing in a year to evaluate changes in his auditory system. He returned to the clinic when he was 9 years, 11 months. On both visits, the dichotic digits test was administered under two conditions; free recall with all digits repeated in any sequence and under divided-attention with precued report, with two numbers presented to each ear, using directed ear listening instructions. That is, in the Right Ear First (REF) condition he was instructed to repeat all the digits heard starting with the right ear first and then repeat from the left ear, and in the Left Ear First (LEF) condition he was instructed to repeat all the digits starting with the left ear first and then repeat from the right ear. Results of the dichotic digits test are shown in Table 10–3.

The questions to ask about these results are, did this child pass or fail, are the ear advantages normal or abnormal, are the changes from the first to the second test significant or not, are they within the confidence interval, and are they real improvements or not? The findings indicate that the child was below the cutoff score for both ears on both tests, with a slight left-ear advantage. On the second test, there was overall improvement in the test findings and the left-ear advantage decreased. What is not known is where this child stands relative to his peers. Is he lower than one or two standard deviations below the average child? Is he disordered? Does the retest indicate a "real" improvement? Because no confidence interval is available it is impossible to know whether the change from 64% to 70% is a real change or within test error. Finally, is the ear advantage truly significant—or not? All of these questions are essential because of the importance placed on interpretation of left-ear advantages, and the need to understand the rate of maturation when interpreting the test.

Here Is Another Example

A child was administered the SCAN-C Auditory Figure-Ground Test (Keith, 2000) at the age of age 6 years, 6 months and again when he was 8 years, 7 months. His test results are as shown in Table 10–4.

Review of the raw score data indicates that in 2 years this child's raw score improved from 19 to 28, an "impressive" gain. However, the raw score provides no insight into his performance relative to his peers. The addition of mean and standard deviations

TABLE 10–3. Test-Retest Dichotic Test Scores Obtained from a Child with Suspected APD*

	Right Ear	Left Ear	Norms
8 years, 7 months			
Total of divided-attention test results	54%	64%	RE = 70% LE = 55%
9 years, 11 months			
Total of divided-attention test results	64%	70%	RE = 80% LE = 75%

*Results were obtained using divided-attention with precued report, asking the child to repeat all digits starting with the REF, and then repeating the test from the LEF. Only the total ear scores are reported here.

TABLE 10–4. Test-Retest SCAN-C Auditory-Figure Ground Test Scores Obtained in a Child with a Confirmed Auditory Processing Disorder

Age	Right Ear	Left Ear	Total	Normal mean (± SD)	SS	%ile	Std Score 95% Confidence Interval
6 yrs, 6 mos	9* (%)	10	19	31.9 (9.6)	4	2	1 to 7
8 yrs, 7 mos	16* (%)	12	28	37.6 (8.4)	6	9	2 to 10

*Number correct out of 20 items.

allows the examiner to determine that the child is just below 1 standard deviation from the mean on both the first and second test, with little actual gain. In addition, although this child appears to be improving slightly in his auditory figure-ground abilities, as the standard score improved from 2 to 6 and the percentile rank from the 2nd to the 9th, the confidence interval indicates that there is no real improvement as the 95% confidence interval indicates there is a wide range of scores in which the "true" score lies. It would appear that this child continues to need classroom management and other intervention. Additional testing in the future will document whether true change is occurring or whether this child will have a long-term need for management. In this example, the addition of mean and standard deviations, percentiles, standard scores, and confidence intervals allows the examiner to more accurately analyze and interpret the findings.

What Is a Criterion-Referenced Test?

One additional way to standardize tests is to use criterion-referenced scores. Criterion-referenced testing, unlike norm-referenced testing, uses an objective standard or achievement level. The person being tested is required to demonstrate ability at a particular level by performing tasks at that degree of difficulty. Scores on criterion-referenced tests indicate what individuals *can* do—not how they have scored in relation to the scores of particular groups of persons, as in norm-referenced tests. Audiologists typically use criterion-reference scores as cutoff levels in screening tests. For example, a cutoff score is chosen that indicates performance is sufficiently "good" to pass, with performance below the cutoff score a fail. In order to establish a criterion-referenced score, it is necessary to know, for the test being studied, the raw score means and standard deviation by age for subjects with normal auditory processing abilities. The same data are required for a population of subjects with an APD. Using that data, the raw score point that maximizes the sensitivity and specificity of the test is selected as the criterion score for that age. The problem, again, for most screening tests is that there is not adequate documentation of the normal and abnormal performance on the auditory tests used for screening purposes.

Criterion for Abnormality When Testing for APD

One of the dilemmas faced by audiologists who are attempting to decide if a subject's performance is normal or not, and whether services should be recommended or not is determined by the cutoff score deemed to be appropriate. For example, Bellis, (2002) states that the vast majority of central auditory tests have not undergone national standardization and therefore the adoption of specific criteria for determining abnormality is difficult. Bellis' statement, although correct, has been ignored in ensuing discussions of central auditory testing. Bellis points out that, when general guidelines using norm-referenced criterion are used, the choice of greater than 1 standard deviation below the mean versus greater than 2 standard deviations below the mean will result in varying percentages of false positives for any test. Bellis is correct, as less than 1 standard deviation below the mean is the 16th percentile and below, whereas less than 2 standard deviations below the mean includes those individuals below the 3rd percentile; a difference that is substantial. For example, as students learn in an introductory statistics class, a type I error includes rejecting a hypothesis that is actually true and type II errors include retaining a hypothesis that is actually false. That is, the consequences of a type I error are to say a child has an APD when the child does not, and a type II error is to say a child has no APD when the child actually does. These errors have substantial consequence for the affected child who is administered either a screening or a diagnostic test battery. The implication is that, because so many tests commonly used in the assessment of APD have inadequate normative data, it is not possible to make informed decisions about the child's true status and whether to recommend or withhold remediation.

As an example of a state recommendation for establishing diagnostic criteria, the Florida technical assistance paper on APDs (Author, 2001) recommends that students must meet two criteria to be identified as having an educationally significant APD (p. 8). They include; scores that are below the age-corrected normal region (1.5 standard deviations below the mean for one or both ears on at least two different procedures) and evidence of difficulty in the academic setting based on observation, multidisciplinary assessment, and academic performance. On the other hand, the ASHA (2005) document states that diagnosis of CAPD requires performance deficits that are two or more standard deviations below normal on two or more tests of central auditory function.

Bellis also discusses the possibility of interpreting results using the child as his or her own control. She states that it is particularly true when dichotic test interaural asymmetries are greater than expected for age they provide strong evidence of abnormality. The same statement is echoed in the ASHA (2005) technical paper when the authors write "Patient-based interpretation is said to include intratest analysis which compares patterns observed with a given test, for example, ear differences scores and interhemispheric differences" (p. 10). Having said that, the problem remains of knowing what is greater than expected for age without having gathered sufficient normative data. Although these basic recommendations for interpretation of test battery (and in this case dichotic test) results are intuitively appropriate, the lack of normative data blunts the effectiveness of that approach.

Calculating the Standard Score and Percentile Rank

It is possible to calculate a standard score on any test if the population mean and standard deviation for a test, and the subject's obtained scores are known. The formula to calculate a Z-score is the population mean score minus the obtained subject score divided by the population standard deviation. When the Z-score is known, it is possible to view a standardization bell-shaped curve to determine what percentile coincides with that score, or look in a Z-table in any statistics book. The Z-table provides the percentile rank. Knowing the percentile rank it is possible to estimate the standard score as shown on the bell-shaped curve (see Figure 10–1). For example, the 16th percentile is 1 standard deviation below the mean (same as −1 Z-score) or a standard score of 85.

Here is an example from the SSW test. Assume a left competing score of 36 errors on a 7-year-old. The mean and standard deviation of the SSW score reported in the test manual for this condition are 18 and 11. The calculation is therefore:

$$Z = \frac{18-36}{11} \text{ equals } -1.63$$

In a statistical table of normal curve areas, $Z = -1.63$, placing this child at the 5.2nd percentile for a standard score of approximately 5. Given this calculation it is possible to compare the SSW score to any test that provides a standardized measure.

Construct Validity

One concept that is controversial, and sometimes poorly understood, is the concept of test validity. It is important to understand the importance of the controversy regarding test validity because entire test battery approaches are based (knowingly or not) on arguments about this belief. There is an often repeated phrase in the audiology literature that test efficiency must be validated on proven lesions involving the CANS and that there is no other way to determine the validity of a central auditory test (ASHA, 2005; Beck, 2000; Moncrieff, 2006; Musiek,

Baran, & Pinheiro, 1990) and many others. It is clear that assessment of patients with identified brain lesions is immensely helpful to our understanding of APD, but that approach is not the only way to validate tests of auditory processing.

The thinking that tests can be validated only on subjects with lesions is simplistic. Although it is true that not all children with learning disabilities have APD, that statement misses other ways of validating tests. That is, if you test, with a new measure, children who have APD by some agreed criterion and with certain other findings on an agreed test battery, and if the new measure identifies the same children as having APD, that new measure has test validity. In 1999 the American Educational Research Association (Author, 1999) re-defined validation of a test as follows:

> . . . test designers present information that they have available to demonstrated validity, and users decide if the test is actually valid or not. One should not focus too directly on "concurrent validity," since under the newly released testing guidelines; validity is now a unitary concept integrating all of the evidence.

This point is important because many tests of APD are valid even though test results on a series of patients with identified lesions are unavailable. For one thing, adults with confirmed lesions bear no relationship to findings that may be obtained on children who may have suffered similar lesions but have a different auditory system through plasticity. There is not always a direct relationship between structure and function in the auditory system, which can make it difficult to attribute auditory processing abnormalities to a specific lesion (Chermak & Musiek, 1997). Sometimes brain plasticity will permit normal performance even with a lesion present. That fact is implied in the ASHA technical report (ASHA, 2005) when the authors state that "because of the individuality of brain organization and the conditions that affect such organization, (C)APD can affect individuals differently."

In addition, as McFarland and Cacace (1997) point out, if subjects with lesions to the auditory nervous system are used to validate tests of APD, then it is important to ensure that damage is limited to areas exclusively involved in auditory processing. They cite their own review and discussion of the literature (McFarland & Cacace, 1995) that indicated most clinical cases involving lesions of the brain do not have localized damage (p. 40). Their interpretation is that as a result, human lesion studies have not been entirely effective in validating APD. The implication is that claims of test validation through auditory processing tests on individuals with brain lesions have inherent flaws because of the inability to state with any degree of certainty the precise site of lesion within the auditory system.

The ASHA (2005) document also states that validity of a particular test cannot be obtained by testing children with learning disabilities, primarily because not all children with LD have APD. (It is not clear how the authors determined that validation would be attempted with subjects who have LD, nor was it clear whether LD was intended to mean learning disabled or language disorders.) Contrary to this statement, there are two methods of validating central auditory tests. One is to compare "clinically identified" subjects with "control" samples as recommended by Katz et al. (2002) who stated that any recommended procedure must be validated on children with APD. The second method for validating an auditory processing test is to take a

"population-based" approach and seek evidence of specific aberrant auditory processing in stratified samples of the general public (Moore, 2006). The approach followed by Moore and his colleagues is to assume a certain percentage of the population will have APD (e.g., 5%), comprehensively test a large group of subjects and look for "outliers" in auditory processing and correlated performance in speech-in-noise and cognitive tests. Having identified tests that are sensitive and specific to those outliers, a large population study (e.g., 2000 subjects) is necessary to normalize those tests.

Summary: Why Is This Discussion of Normative Data Important to Audiologists?

In spite of all the discussion in consensus documents, it seems to this author that, in the main, audiologists have paid only lip-service to the need for well-standardized tests of auditory processing. In addition, there has been perpetuated the notion that norm-referenced tests and by implication even normative data are unnecessary in order to adequately interpret auditory processing test results, including the interpretation of ear differences in dichotic tests. Also, each of the consensus documents comments on the need to identify tests with appropriate sensitivity and specificity. However, there appears to be no recognition of the impossibility of determining sensitivity and specificity of tests when there is no agreed definition of APD. Without an agreed definition, it is not possible to determine when a test appropriately identifies an individual who has APD, or appropriately withholds a diagnosis of APD. Finally, there is a substantial difference in opinion that exists whether validation of tests of auditory processing is accomplished only by testing patients with verified lesions, or whether test validation can be accomplished by other methods. Most of these controversies have not been discussed in the available literature on auditory processing, in spite of their importance to the profession.

What Can We Do About This Situation?

At this point in time, there are several major needs in the area of APDs. They include the determination of which of the available tests and which of many possible future tests provide appropriate test sensitivity, specificity, and validity (ASHA, 1996). Furthermore, how can we develop age-appropriate norms? It would appear that there are several possible solutions to the problem of inadequate normative data. One specific example is provided by the work of Wilson and his colleagues. In 1994 a series of articles were published that included data on a variety of monotic, diotic, and dichotic tests used in a central auditory test battery (Noffsinger, Wilson, & Musiek, 1994). The tests were recorded on the Department of Veterans Affairs compact disk (VA-CD) known as Tonal and Speech Materials for Auditory Perceptual Assessment, Disc 1.0. Each of a series of articles reporting data from "compact disk trials" that involved 120 young adults with self-described normal hearing. Nine major universities and/or medical centers in the United States participated in the collection of normative data. The purposes of the studies were to gather data on average performance by young listeners with normal hearing and provide illustrations on the degree

of confidence examiners could use in differentiating normal from abnormal listeners. The authors emphasized that the data were not intended for use as absolute standards. Their intent was to create a set of good materials that would last and to provide a framework within which the work of defining what is and what is not normal auditory behavior.

Similarly, in 1986, Keith collaborated with five different individuals across the United States to gather normative data on 1034 children who were between the ages of 3 and 13 years; and in the year 2000 collaborated with 115 persons who volunteered to gather normative data on 650 children between 5 years and 11 years, 11 months in the standardization of SCAN-C Test for Auditory Processing Disorders–Revised (Keith, 2000). Those studies were conducted with corporate support from The Psychological Corporation® who provided incentives to cooperating investigators, a method common with large-scale studies of commercially available tests in audiology, speech-language pathology, and psychology. At the time of this writing, Moore and his colleagues (Moore, 2006) are in the process of gathering data on 1,600 to 2,000 children in order to norm a new central auditory test battery designed for use in the United Kingdom. Their multicenter/multi-investigator study will be used to normalize the data, develop sub profiles of auditory processing disorders, and estimate the prevalence of APD. That research is funded by the Medical Research Council, Institute of Hearing Research.

The idea of collaborative studies on a variety of central auditory tests, as modeled by Wilson, Keith, and Moore serve as an example of methods investigators can use to gather normative data on a large number of subjects in a relatively short time. In view of the enormous need for standardized tests of auditory processing abilities, it would be helpful for one of the major professional associations to organize such an endeavor. For example, the American Speech-Language and Hearing Association, through one of its special interest groups, could design and fund an investigator or group of investigators who could organize and coordinate such an effort. The same could be true of the American Academy of Audiology, or the Educational Audiology Association. Finally, the amount of educational costs associated with diagnosis, failure to diagnose, or the overdiagnosis of APDs is tremendous. The provision of funding through a service organization, private foundation, or one of the funding agencies of the federal government is in order and would allow for appropriate diagnosis and placement of individuals with APD. In short, there are many possible ways to organize and conduct needed studies, though the effort is not trivial.

References

ASHA. (1996). Central auditory processing: Current status of research and implications for clinical practice. *American Journal of Audiology, 5*(2), 41–54.

ASHA. (2005). *(Central) auditory processing disorders—The role of the audiologist* [Position statement]. Washington, DC: Working Group on Auditory Processing Disorders, ASHA.

Author. (1999). *Standards for educational and psychological testing.* Washington, DC: American Educational Research Association.

Author. (2001). *Auditory processing disorders. Technical assistance paper* (pp. 1–74). Washington, DC: Federal Department of Education, Bureau of Instructional Support.

Beck, B. (2000). CAPD intervention: Strategies that work. *The Hearing Review*, August, 30–34.

Bellis, T. J. (2002). Perspectives on hearing and hearing disorders in childhood. ASHA special interest Division 9, *Hearing and Hearing Disorders in Childhood, 12*, 3–9.

Bentler, R. A. (2000). List equivalency and test-retest reliability of the Speech-in-Noise test. *American Journal of Audiology, 9*, 84–100.

Chermak, G. D., & Musiek, F. (1997). *Central auditory processing disorders: New perspectives.* San Diego, CA: Singular.

Cherry, R. (1980). *Selective Auditory Attention Test (SAAT).* St. Louis, MO: Auditec.

Gardner, M. F. (1996). *Test of Auditory-Perceptual Skills-Revised.* Hydesville, CA: Psychological and Educational Publications.

Hirsh, I. J. (1952). *The Measurement of Hearing.* New York: McGraw-Hill.

Jerger, J., & Musiek, F. (2000). Report of Consensus Conference on the Diagnosis of Auditory Processing Disorders in School-Aged Children. *Journal of the American Academy of Audiology, 11*, 467–474.

Katz, J. (1962). The use of staggered spondaic words for assessing the integrity of the central auditory nervous system. *Journal of Auditory Research, 2*, 327–337.

Katz, J., Johnson, C., Brandner, C., Delagrange, T., Ferre, J., King, J., et al. (2002). Clinical and research concerns regarding the 2000 APD consensus report and recommendations. *Audiology Today*, 13–19.

Keith, R. W. (1986). *SCAN: A Screening Test for Auditory Processing Disorders.* San Antonio, TX: The Psychological Corporation.

Keith, R. W. (2000). Development and standardization of SCAN-C: Test for Auditory Processing Disorders in Children-Revised. *Journal of the American Academy of Audiology 11*, 438–445.

Keith, R. W. (2000). *SCAN-C: Test for Auditory Processing Disorders in Children-Revised.* San Antonio, TX: The Psychological Corporation.

Keith, R. W. (2002). Standardization of the Time Compressed Sentence Test. *Journal of Educational Audiology, 10*, 15–20.

McFarland, D. J., & Cacace, A. T. (1995). Modality specificity as a criterion for diagnosing central auditory processing disorders. *American Journal of Audiology, 4*, 36–48.

McFarland, D. J., & Cacace, A. T. (1997). Modality specificity of auditory and visual pattern recognition: implications for the assessment of central auditory processing disorders. *Audiology, 36,* 249–260.

Moncrieff, D. (2006). Identification of binaural integration deficits in children with the Competing Words Subtest: Standard score versus interaural asymmetry. *International Journal of Audiology, 45,* 200–210.

Moore, D. R. (2006). Auditory processing disorder (APD): Definition, diagnosis, neural basis, and intervention. *Audiological Medicine, 4,* 4–11.

Musiek, F. E. (1983). Assessment of central auditory dysfunction: The dichotic digit test revisited. *Ear and Hearing 4,* 79–83.

Musiek, F. E., & Pinheiro, M. L. (1987). Frequency patterns in cochlear, brainstem and cerebral lesions. *Audiology, 26,* 79–88.

Musiek. F. E., Baran, J. A., & Pinheiro, M. L. (1990). Duration pattern recognition in normal subjects and patients with cerebral and cochlear lesions. *Audiology, 29,* 304–313.

Noffsinger, D., Wilson, R. H., & Musiek, F. E. (1994). Department of Veterans Affairs Compact disc recording for auditory perceptual assessment: Background and introduction. *Journal of the American Academy of Audiology, 5,* 231–235.

Nyquette, P. A. (2005). *BKB-SIN Speech-in-Noise Test* (pp. 2–20). Elk Grove Village, IL: Etymotic Research.

Nyquette, P., Gudmunsen, G., & Killion, M. (2001). *QuickSIN Speech-in-Noise Test* (pp. 2–23). Elk Grove Village, IL: Etymotic Research.

Ptacek, P. H., & Pinheiro, M. (1971). Pattern reversal in auditory perception. *Journal of the Acoustic Society of America, 49,* 493–498.

Semel, E., Wiig, E., & Secord, W. (2003). *Clinical Evaluation of Language Function Fourth Edition.* San Antonio, TX: The Psychological Corporation.

Stephens, S. S. (1951). *Handbook of experimental psychology.* New York: John Wilkey & Sons.

Wright, W. D., & Wright, P. D. (2000). Understanding tests and measurements for the parent and advocate. LD OnLine: /http/:www.ldonline.org/article/6026.

CHAPTER 11

Putting the Auditory Processing Back into Auditory Processing Disorder in Children

JUSTIN COWAN, STUART ROSEN, AND DAVID R. MOORE

Recent clinical and research efforts have reinvigorated the field of auditory processing disorder (APD) research with developments that pose important challenges to popular understandings of APD, the current practice of clinicians, and the directions of future research. This chapter highlights recent developments which have been led by the Medical Research Council's Institute of Hearing Research and the "APD working party" set up by the British Society of Audiology. Both of these bodies have produced novel definitions of APD that have provided the impetus to research employing a variety of methodological approaches.

The confusion that many experience when first encountering the term APD is understandable, given the imprecision of the term, as the word "disorder" itself is unwarranted. *Impairment* is a term used to describe loss or abnormality of body struc-

ture or of a physiologic or psychological function. A *disorder* describes a clinically significant syndrome or pattern of disturbance of function, structure, or both, resulting from failure in development or from exogenous factors. The important distinction is that the existence of an impairment does not necessarily result in the existence of an allied disorder. To date, auditory processing impairments have not been demonstrated to contribute in a unique way to a clearly defined condition so as to warrant the inclusion of APD in either of the established nosologic systems such as the American Psychiatric Association's Diagnostic and Statistical Manual of Mental Disorders (APA, 1995) or the World Health Organisation International Classification of Diseases (ICD-10, WHO, 1980). It may be that the term APD, implying a discrete clinical entity, is a misnomer.

A clearer description of what APD may entail is crucial for developing our understanding of the possible nature of APD, whether an impairment or a disorder, and also the relationship of APD to other clinical conditions. With this in mind, we propose a novel working definition of APD with the aim of injecting new scientific rigor into a field of research that was stagnating, at least partly due to imprecise terminology. This definition does not necessarily imply validity but has been laid out to provide a working framework of APD to guide further research. The key differentiating features from other definitions (e.g., ASHA, 2006) are intended to permit the investigation of the central tenets of APD and to establish the validity of APD as a construct in its own right (Table 11–1). The aims of this chapter are to describe how the features of this working definition have significant consequences for how APD is characterized. These features include: the role of the peripheral auditory system, distinguishing between auditory versus linguistic abilities, the fractionation of auditory processing, and accounting for the role of other cognitive abilities in assessing auditory processing abilities. The importance of conducting a holistic assessment of children with suspected APD and establishing the psychometric robustness of measures used in characterizing auditory processing are discussed before outlining the different research methodologies that are likely to be fruitful for the field of APD research.

TABLE 11–1. Criteria for APD

1. APD should be suspected (i.e., referred) following (a) complaints about listening difficulties, *and* (b) normal audiometry (PTA ≤20 dB HL), *and* (c) impaired speech reception thresholds.

2. APD appears as deficits in the localization, detection, or discrimination of temporal or spectral aspects of nonspeech sounds.

3. Performance on tasks measuring the abilities listed in Criterion 2 involves both task-specific and procedural demands. Task-specific demands tap perceptual abilities (e.g., frequency selectivity) whereas procedural demands tap nonsensory abilities (e.g., general attention and memory). In understanding APD it is necessary to distinguish perceptual from nonsensory factors so as to identify the primary auditory nature of the deficit.

4. There should be a clear demarcation between the stimuli used in auditory processing tests and linguistic processing. Individuals with language problems may also have APD, but APD and language problems can only be separately diagnosed by a performance mismatch between auditory and language tests.

5. The individual's test performance profile should show relative discrepancies between auditory processing abilities and other perceptual and cognitive abilities, such as visual processing and more general aspects of memory and attention. The deficits should be primarily, though not necessarily solely, of an auditory nature.

6. APD should be diagnosed solely on the basis of behavioral evidence. Although known neurologic deficits may contribute to APD, they are not a necessary component. The neural basis of APD is presently unknown.

The Role of the Peripheral Auditory System

The functioning of the peripheral auditory system is widely thought to be uncompromised in APD. However, the simple division between the periphery and more central auditory processing is under revision with recent evidence of a dynamic interplay between peripheral structures and more central auditory processing.

A distinction between pure-tone sensitivity and the performance of more complex auditory tasks has been long recognized (Gatehouse, Naylor, & Elberling, 2003). For convenience of expression, these different abilities have been referred to as "hearing" (sensitivity) and "listening" (complex). The two are closely linked, as both are adversely affected by outer hair cell dysfunction, which is commonly the first recognizable sign of sensorineural hearing loss (Dallos, 1992). This causes both an elevation of pure-tone threshold and a decline in temporal and spectral resolution (see Oxenham & Bacon, 2003). These effects may be subclinical for hearing loss (i.e., PTA = 20 dB HL), but nevertheless impair speech reception and, hence, result in practical "listening" difficulties. For this reason, it is presently inappropriate to refer to APD as "central" APD (abbreviated as CAPD or ([C]APD). Nevertheless, we recognize that central contributions to listening (and, in fact, hearing) difficulties may also occur. This point is taken up below.

It is sometimes imagined that gradual changes in auditory function of the sort that may underlie APD must be produced in the central auditory system because the peripheral auditory system does not change in response to auditory experience. However, that idea is being turned around as the number of new findings of peripherally mediated functional dynamics multiplies.

Aside from the influence of the efferent auditory system (see below), other recently described phenomena that may be relevant to APD include experience dependent membrane cycling in stereocilia (Grati, Scheider, Lipkow, Stehler, Wenthold, & Kachar, 2006), and supporting cell transdifferentiation in the cochlea (Kelley, 2006). It therefore appears that auditory processing impairments may arise from the dynamic interplay of multiple factors, both peripheral and central.

Auditory Processing and Language Abilities

It is widely considered that the primary presenting complaint of individuals with APD is poor listening abilities; difficulties that are particularly noticeable in noisy environments. Yet it is well known that language abilities in themselves can have an impact on speech perception, and deficits in speech perception in the absence of auditory deficits have even been claimed to be characteristic of specific language impairments (Ziegler, Pech-Georgel, George, Alario, & Lorenzi, 2005).

It is important to make explicit that our working definition posits that it is the *auditory processing* deficits that are the primary etiologic factors in these impairments. Therefore, a core distinction of the current definitions of APD driving recent research is that auditory processing deficits reside primarily in the processing of non-speech sounds rather than with higher level linguistic abilities (for a further example of this approach see BSA, 2005). This distinction is shown in criteria 2 and 4 in Table 11–1.

This focus on auditory processing has significant implications for the approach to assessing individuals with suspected APD, as a common approach is to use test materials laden with speech (Keith, 1995; Neijenhuis, 2003). For example, all the subtests of the SCAN (Keith, 1995) use linguistic stimuli, resulting in a test that is highly associated with measures of receptive and expressive language (Keith, Rudy, Donahue, & Katbamna, 1989), culturally dependent (Marriage, King, Briggs, & Lutman, 2001), and highly susceptible to learning effects (Domitz & Schow, 2000). The demands these measures place on linguistic processing make them unsuitable for the evaluation of distinct auditory processing components relative to receptive and expressive language ability.

However, the assessment of children with APD requires traditional speech-in-noise measures as an appropriate first step. Having obtained speech reception thresholds indicative of significantly impaired performance, measures should then be administered that are capable of identifying deficits in "pure" auditory processing abilities.

Fractionation of Auditory Processing

Given that auditory processing abilities are the feature of interest, and are a departure from the popular screening tests used to assess for APD, exactly how we are conceptualizing these abilities needs to be described. We ascribe to the now widely accepted view that the functional architecture of the human brain is modular (Fodor, 1983; Shallice, 1988). Support for the organization of cognitive processes being modular has been found across different fields in developmental cognitive neuroscience. Such evidence includes dissociations that have been found, for example, for semantic and episodic memory (Gadian et al., 2000; Temple & Richardson, 2004; Vargha-Khadem et al., 1997) and developmental surface and phonological dyslexia (Temple, 1986; Tem-

ple & Marshall, 1983). Within the field of auditory processing, a growing body of evidence suggests functionally different auditory processing streams, with a dorsal pathway for the processing of sound location (De Santis, Clarke, & Murray, 2007) and a ventral pathway for the processing of auditory objects (Griffiths et al., 2007). Further evidence shows additional auditory areas sharing functions (i.e., analysis of location and motion) with visual areas (Bushara et al., 1999; Poremba et al., 2003).

The trend in cognitive neuroscience over the last two decades has been to pursue deficits in specific components. However, it is unlikely that a single system theory will be able to account for all the symptoms associated with APD. Nevertheless, our understanding of several known, neurologic disorders of auditory processing, cortical deafness, auditory agnosia, pure word deafness, and phonagnosia, suggests that, together with a modular conceptualization of auditory processing, it will be the associations between the various components that will define the disorder (Bishop, 1997; Polster & Rose, 1998). Thus, it is likely that the pattern of associated impairments will be the focus of future research rather than a specific deficit of any one component, a perspective that is particularly important in developmental research, where a far more flexible view of modularity is necessary. Moreover, it is likely that disparate patterns of impairments will have differing developmental trajectories (Karmiloff-Smith et al., 2004). However, the fractionation of any hypothetical system necessarily precedes any investigation (cross-sectional or longitudinal) of the potential interactions between the components.

Fractionation of AP, where selective components underpin discrete functions, can be used to build a model of auditory processing. With the assumption that APD is a neurodevelopmental disorder, a typology of auditory processing components based on normal developmental trajectories of low-level auditory processing abilities (Griffiths, Warren, Scott, Nelken, & King, 2004) has been developed by the MRC Institute of Hearing Research (MRC-IHR) group who have subsequently explored the possible fractionation of auditory processing into distinct subcomponents (Cowan, 2007). With the lack of a consensual theoretical framework of the components of auditory processing, and informed by developmental studies of the normal auditory system and clinical studies of language impaired children, we identified a range of candidate auditory processes that, if impaired, may have serious consequences for normal development and were therefore worthy of further attention.

Developmental normative data on a battery of auditory processing measures were obtained for typically developing children aged 6 to 11 years old with normal audiometric thresholds, tympanometry, and acoustic reflexes. The auditory processing battery contained seven measures chosen to capture different temporal and spectral aspects of auditory processing: masking level difference, backward masking, temporal integration, frequency selectivity, frequency discrimination, and frequency and amplitude modulation detection. Auditory processing tests were embedded within a suite of computer games, each employing a three-interval, three-alternative forced-choice response paradigm with a staircase adaptive method. Auditory processing measures generally showed lower thresholds and/or reduced variance with increasing age. Adultlike thresholds were generally attained by 10 to 11 years.

Pertinent for the issue of fractionation is whether auditory processing can be fractionated along several different dimensions or whether it is a unitary measure. A popular statistical technique for exploring construct validity is factor analysis. This technique was employed by the MRC-IHR group who found that the battery of tests were capturing distinct and different aspects of auditory functioning with two components being identified (Cowan, 2007). Of interest was that the two components did not follow the expected temporal and spectral divisions, but grouped along different lines. The two-factor solution produced was notable as the first component contained both a derived measure (frequency resolution) and an individual task (backward masking) that purportedly tap different aspects of auditory processing (spectral and temporal, respectively) and yet share the procedural demands of a tone in masking noise paradigm. This suggests that performance across different psychoacoustic tasks may be more determined by procedural aspects of the test paradigm used than any purportedly specific auditory-processing ability.

The Holistic Assessment

It is widely thought that cognitive factors, including general intellectual ability, auditory memory, and attention, contribute strongly to the performance of even basic auditory tasks. In children, support for this comes from studies showing that young children rarely attain adultlike performance, even at "easy" stimulus levels (Allen & Wightman, 1994; Werner & Gray, 1998), although their peripheral auditory system appears to be well developed by the age of 2 years (Moore, 2002). Furthermore, general cognitive ability has been found to be correlated with, and even dependent on performance on a range of psychophysical tasks (Ahissar, Protopapas, Reid, & Merzenich, 2000; Deary, 1999). For example, better performance on both frequency selectivity and backward masking tasks has been associated with higher IQ scores (Hartley, Wright, Hogan, & Moore, 2000) and attention (Sutcliffe, 2003). An individual's auditory processing ability should be regarded within the context of the individual's other cognitive abilities. Otherwise, a nonspecific attention disorder or general cognitive impairment may be the primary cause of the auditory processing difficulties rather than an auditory modality-specific disorder (Cacace & McFarland, 2005).

The dangers of overinterpreting auditory processing data without controlling for attention have been shown in a study by Sutcliffe and Bishop (2002). They tested children aged 6 and 7 years on a variety of AP, language, reading, and attention tests. It was found that both reading and language measures were significantly correlated with auditory processing performance (using a frequency discrimination task). When the data were reanalyzed, but controlling for the effects of attention, these significant correlations disappeared. Therefore, assessment of APD needs to be comprehensive in scope and based on significant discrepancies between test scores rather than poor performance on tests of auditory processing alone.

From a clinical perspective, accounting for the individual's attention, memory, language, and general cognitive abilities is essential in being able to formulate why a listener may be experiencing certain difficulties. Unfortunately, the primacy given to auditory processing abilities has resulted at times in the neglect of other cognitive factors. In light of this, it is promising that there is a general agreement among researchers of the importance of the multidisciplinary assessment of individuals with suspected APD (Musiek, Bellis, & Chermak, 2005).

The importance of an integrated and comprehensive cognitive assessment of individuals with suspected APD has been embodied in the work of the MRC-IHR group with the development of the Children's Auditory Processing Evaluation (CAPE) battery (Cowan, 2007). This battery consists of measures of peripheral function (pure-tone audiometry, tympanometry and OAE) to determine the involvement of the peripheral auditory system, speech intelligibility tests to capture the nature of the presenting complaint, auditory processing tests to explore whether auditory processing impairments underpin any receptive language difficulties, and a range of cognitive measures to account for potential other factors impacting on the child's functioning, including general cognitive ability, attention, memory, phonological processing, language, and literacy.

This work has led to a greater awareness of the mismatch between the skills needed to conduct a holistic assessment of children with suspected APD and those available to the clinical audiologist working in isolation. The importance of a multidisciplinary assessment can be illustrated by the child who has been given a diagnosis of APD and who, if formally assessed by a multidisciplinary team including a speech and language therapist and clinical psychologist, could also be given a diagnosis of ADHD, SLI, or dyslexia. Reaching an understanding of the full clinical presentation of a child with any developmental cognitive disorder is beyond the pale of the audiologist working in isolation.

Psychometric Standards

The importance of establishing the psychometric robustness of measures used in characterising auditory processing is a frequent call from researchers (e.g., Katz et al., 2000), largely concerning the reliability and validity of the measure. Reliability is particularly relevant when assessing children because of their generally high variability on auditory processing tests (Allen & Wightman, 1994; Allen, Wightman, Kistler, & Dolan, 1989). An apparent deficit in performance on an auditory processing test may well "resolve" itself on repeated administration of the same test. In terms of the validity of measures used to assess for APD, the auditory repetition test, a measure used to test the "temporal processing hypothesis" has been shown to be assessing abilities other than simple temporal processing (Bishop, Carlyon, Deeks, & Bishop, 1999). A clear theoretical rationale, supported by empirical evidence of validity, is needed for the use of any test.

With this in mind, a body of developmental normative data has been collected for a range of auditory processing tasks administered concurrently (Cowan, 2007). Although these norms will be specific to the test paradigms, procedures, and population used, the creation of this corpus of normative developmental data on a range of auditory processing tasks will permit the characterization of children with suspected APD, especially as particular consideration was given to reporting the psychometric properties of the auditory processing measures.

The MRC-IHR study considered the reliability of the auditory processing measures, both within and between test sessions. Of considerable relevance to the use of auditory processing measures within the clinical setting was the finding that, despite the modest or better correlations within test session performance ($r = 0.51$ to 0.73), test-retest reliability deteriorated markedly between test sessions ($r = 0.16$ to 0.68) (Cowan, 2007). It is from this increased attention to the psychometric standards of tests that interesting features are beginning to emerge about the nature of performance

impairments on auditory processing tasks; namely, whether these deficits are persistent in nature or whether performance variability is the key index of reported auditory processing impairments (Heath, Bishop, Hogben, & Roach, 2006).

There is general agreement that test-retest reliability is fundamental to understanding performance on psychoacoustic tests. This is even more pertinent when dealing with clinical cases or evaluating the outcome of auditory training (Agnew, Dorn, & Eden, 2004; Moore, Rosenberg, & Coleman, 2005). Furthermore, the variability in performance typically found in children suggests that a variety of paradigms and procedures ultimately may be useful for more fully describing the impairments associated with APD, for example, the use of auditory event-related potentials (Liasis et al., 2003).

Research Methodologies for Improving Our Understanding of APD

The research methodologies that are likely to be fruitful in coming years include clinical studies, and epidemiologic and longitudinal research. The first two of these are currently being pursued by different research groups.

Maintaining a focus on clearly defined clinical populations is fundamental if the work into auditory processing is to maintain any sense of clinical utility. The importance of auditory processing is potentially undermined by recent evidence indicating that auditory processing impairments may not be a significant risk factor for subsequent speech and language development or later academic achievement (Roberts et al., 2004; Rosen, 2003). However, it remains the case that health care professionals are struggling to understand and manage a cluster of patients with similar clinical presenting features, driving the need to further our understanding of this group. Similar to studies of clinical populations with established disorders such as SLI or dyslexia, in which the role of auditory processing impairments is explored (Hulslander et al., 2004; McArthur & Bishop, 2004), the existence of these impairments needs to be explored in children who are given clinical diagnoses of APD. These investigations will better characterize the nature of the clinical condition, inform how clinical assessments are best conducted, and, importantly, the potential of specific remedial clinical interventions.

Epidemiologic research of auditory processing abilities in the general population (e.g., Watson & Kidd, 2002; Watson et al., 2003) can provide the basis of our understanding of the consequences and significance of auditory processing impairments. An example of such an approach is the large scale multicenter epidemiologic study of auditory processing abilities in over 1500 typically developing children, currently being undertaken by the MRC-IHR group. It is anticipated that this population-based approach, which incorporates audiometric, cognitive, and speech perception as well as auditory processing tests, will provide further evidence of the developmental trajectories of auditory processing abilities and their relationship to other cognitive abilities.

The measurement of auditory-processing abilities in longitudinal studies can shed light on their significance for development. To date, the significance of auditory processing impairments in development has been challenged by evidence from clinical populations with hearing loss (Briscoe, Bishop, & Norbury, 2001; Roberts et al., 2004), in children with language impairments (Bishop et al., 1999; Halliday & Bishop, 2006) and from large scale epidemiologic studies of children with normal hearing (Watson et al., 2003). This evidence supports the view that low-level auditory deficits are not the sole prerequisite for the development of dyslexia or SLI and may be, at most, an associated marker of neurodevelopmental impairment (Bishop et al., 1999; Mody, Studdert-Kennedy, & Brady, 1997; Rosen, 2003). However, the fact that auditory processing abilities are consistently found to be sensitive predictors of children at risk from maturational delay in their cognitive development (Bishop & McArthur, 2005) supports further investigations employing a longitudinal design. As mentioned previously, disparate patterns of impairments are likely to have differing developmental trajectories and it could be important to consider whether, for example, the infant showing markedly atypical performance on an auditory processing task becomes a child with a language impairment.

And Finally

The identification of a group of patients, presenting with a typical cluster of symptoms, as having APD is not a modern phenomenon, and has existed under various guises, including King-Kopetzky syndrome (King & Stephens, 1992) and obscure auditory dysfunction (Saunders & Haggard, 1992). What is a departure from the past is the recent surge of interest in, and efforts to understand, the phenomenon. It is anticipated that a clearer understanding of the relative contributions of perceptual and non-sensory, unimodal, and supramodal factors to performance on psychoacoustic tests may well be the key to unraveling the clinical presentation of these individuals.

References

Agnew, J. A., Dorn, C., & Eden, G. F. (2004). Effect of intensive training on auditory processing and reading skills. *Brain and Language, 88,* 21-25.

Ahissar, M., Protopapas, A., Reid, M., & Merzenich, M. M. (2000). Auditory processing parallels reading abilities in adults. *Proceedings of the National Academy of Sciences of the United States of America, 97,* 6832-6837.

Allen, P., & Wightman, F. (1994). Psychometric functions for children's detection of tones in noise. *Journal of Speech and Hearing Research, 37,* 205-215.

Allen, P., Wightman, F., Kistler, D., & Dolan, T. (1989). Frequency resolution in children. *Journal of Speech and Hearing Research, 32,* 317-322.

APA. (1995). *Diagnostic and statistical manual of mental disorders: DSM-IV* (4th ed., International version). Washington, DC: American Psychiatric Association.

ASHA. (2005). (Central) auditory processing disorders, American Speech-Language-Hearing Association (Vol. 2005): American Speech-Language-Hearing Association.

Bishop, D. V. M. (1997). Cognitive neuropsychology and developmental disorders: Uncomfortable bedfellows. *Quarterly Journal of Experimental Psychology: Human Experimental Psychology, 50A,* 899-923.

Bishop, D. V. M., Carlyon, R. P., Deeks, J. M., & Bishop, S. J. (1999). Auditory temporal processing impairment: Neither necessary nor sufficient for causing language impairment in children. *Journal of Speech, Language, and Hearing Research, 42,* 1295-1310.

Bishop, D. V. M., & McArthur, G. M. (2005). Individual differences in auditory processing in specific language impairment: A follow-up study using event-related potentials and behavioural thresholds. *Cortex, 41,* 327-341.

Briscoe, J., Bishop, D. V. M., & Norbury, C. F. (2001). Phonological processing, language, and literacy: A comparison of children with mild-to-moderate sensorineural hearing loss and those with specific language impairment. *Journal of Child Psychology and Psychiatry, 42,* 329-340.

BSA. (2005). Steering Group on Auditory Processing Disorder. Retrieved March 29, 2007, from http://www.thebsa.org.uk/apd/Home.htm#working%20def

Bushara, K. O., Weeks, R. A., Ishii, K., Catalan, M. J., Tian, B., Rauschecker, J. P., et al. (1999). Modality-specific frontal and parietal areas for auditory and visual spatial localization in humans. *Nature Neuroscience, 2,* 759-766.

Cacace, A. T., & McFarland, D. J. (2005). The importance of modality specificity in diagnosing central auditory processing disorder. *American Journal of Audiology, 14,* 112-123.

Cowan, J. A. (2007). *Auditory processing disorder in children*: Doctoral thesis, University of Nottingham.

Dallos, P. (1992). The active cochlea. *Journal of Neuroscience, 12,* 4575-4585.

Deary, I. J. (1999). Intelligence and visual and auditory information processing. In P. Ackerman, P. Kyllonen, & R. Roberts (Eds.), *Learning and individual differences: process, trait and content determinants.* Washington, DC: American Psychological Association.

De Santis, L., Clarke, S., & Murray, M. M. (2007). Automatic and intrinsic auditory "what" and "where" processing in humans revealed by electrical neuroimaging. *Cerebral Cortex, 17,* 9-17.

Domitz, D. M., & Schow, R. L. (2000). A new CAPD battery—multiple auditory processing assessment: factor analysis and comparisons with SCAN. *American Journal of Audiology, 9,* 101-111.

Fodor, J. A. (1983). *The modularity of mind: An essay on faculty psychology.* Cambridge, MA: MIT Press.

Gadian, D. G., Aicardi, J., Watkins, K. E., Porter, D. A., Mishkin, M., & Vargha-Khadem, F. (2000). Developmental amnesia associated with early hypoxic-ischaemic injury. *Brain, 123*(Pt. 3), 499-507.

Gatehouse, S., Naylor, G., & Elberling, C. (2003). Benefits from hearing aids in relation to the interaction between the user and the environment. *International Journal of Audiology*, *42*, S77–S85.

Grati, M., Scheider, M E., Lipkow, K., Stehler, E. E., Wenthold, R. J., & Kachar, B. (2006). Rapid turnover of stereocilia membrane proteins: evidence from the trafficking and mobility of plasma membrane Ca(2^{+})-ATPase2. *Journal of Neuroscience*, *26*, 6386–6395.

Griffiths, T. D., Kumar, S., Warren, J. D., Stewart, L., Stephan, K. E., & Friston, K. J. (2007). Approaches to the cortical analysis of auditory objects. *Hearing Research*, *229*, 46–53.

Griffiths, T. D., Warren, J. D., Scott, S. K., Nelken, I., & King, A. J. (2004). Cortical processing of complex sound: A way forward? *Trends in Neuroscience*, *27*, 181–185.

Halliday, L. F., & Bishop, D. V. (2006). Is poor frequency modulation detection linked to literacy problems? A comparison of specific reading disability and mild to moderate sensorineural hearing loss. *Brain and Language*, *97*, 200–213.

Hartley, D. E., Wright, B. A., Hogan, S. C., & Moore, D. R. (2000). Age-related improvements in auditory backward and simultaneous masking in 6- to 10-year-old children. *Journal of Speech, Language, and Hearing Research*, *43*, 1402–1415.

Heath, S. M., Bishop, D. V. M., Hogben, J. H., & Roach, N. W. (2006). Psychophysical indices of perceptual functioning in dyslexia: A psychometric analysis. *Cognitive Neuropsychology*, *23*, 905–929.

Hulslander, J., Talcott, J., Witton, C., DeFries, J., Pennington, B., Wadsworth, S., et al. (2004). Sensory processing, reading, IQ, and attention. *Journal of Experimental Child Psychology*, *88*, 274–295.

Karmiloff-Smith, A., Thomas, M., Annaz, D., Humphreys, K., Ewing, S., Brace, N., et al. (2004). Exploring the Williams syndrome face-processing debate: The importance of building developmental trajectories. *Journal of Child Psychology and Psychiatry*, *45*, 1258–1274.

Katz, J. K., Johnson, C. D., Tillery, K. L., Bradham, T., Brandner, S., Delagrange, T. N., et al. (2000). Clinical and research concerns regarding Jerger and Musiek (2000) APD recommendations. *Audiology Today*, *14*, 14–17.

Keith, R. W. (1995). Development and standardization of SCAN-A: Test of auditory processing disorders in adolescents and adults. *Journal of the American Academy of Audiology*, *6*, 286–292.

Keith, R. W., Rudy, J., Donahue, P. A., & Katbamna, B. (1989). Comparison of SCAN results with other auditory and language measures in a clinical population. *Ear and Hearing*, *10*, 382–386.

Kelley, M. W. (2006). Hair cell development: Commitment through differentiation. *Brain Research*, *1091*, 172–185.

King, K., & Stephens, D. (1992). Auditory and psychological factors in "auditory disability with normal hearing." *Scandinavian Audiology*, *21*, 109–114.

Liasis, A., Bamiou, D. E., Campbell, P., Sirimanna, T., Boyd, S., & Towell, A. (2003). Auditory event-related potentials in the assessment of auditory processing disorders: A pilot study. *Neuropediatrics*, *34*, 23–29.

Marriage, J., King, J., Briggs, J., & Lutman, M. E. (2001). The reliability of the SCAN test: Results from a primary school population in the UK. *British Journal of Audiology*, *35*, 199–208.

McArthur, G. M., & Bishop, D. V. M. (2004). Frequency discrimination deficits in people with specific language impairment: Reliability, validity, and linguistic correlates. *Journal of Speech, Language, and Hearing Research*, *47*, 527–541.

Mody, M., Studdert-Kennedy, M., & Brady, S. (1997). Speech perception deficits in poor readers: Auditory processing or phonological coding? *Journal of Experimental Child Psychology*, *64*, 199–231.

Moore, D. R. (2002). Auditory development and the role of experience. *British Medical Bulletin*, *63*, 171–181.

Moore, D. R., Rosenberg, J. F., & Coleman, J. S. (2005). Discrimination training of phonemic contrasts enhances phonological processing in mainstream school children. *Brain Lang*, *94*, 72–85.

Musiek, F. E., Bellis, T. J., & Chermak, G. D. (2005). Nonmodularity of the central auditory nervous system: implications for (central) auditory processing disorder. *American Journal of Audiology, 14,* 128–138; discussion 143–150.

Neijenhuis, K. A. (2003). *Auditory processing disorders: Development and evaluation of a test battery.* Nijmegem, The Netherlands: Catholic University of Nijmegen.

Oxenham, A. J., & Bacon, S. P. (2003). Cochlear compression: perceptual measures and implications for normal and impaired hearing. *Ear and Hearing, 24,* 352–366.

Polster, M. R., & Rose, S. B. (1998). Disorders of auditory processing: Evidence for modularity in audition. *Cortex, 34,* 47–65.

Poremba, A., Saunders, R. C., Crane, A. M., Cook, M., Sokoloff, L., & Mishkin, M. (2003). Functional mapping of the primate auditory system. *Science, 299,* 568–572.

Roberts, J., Hunter, L., Gravel, J., Rosenfeld, R., Berman, S., Haggard, M., et al. (2004). Otitis media, hearing loss, and language learning: controversies and current research. *Journal of Developmental and Behavioral Pediatrics, 25,* 110–122.

Rosen, S. M. (2003). Auditory processing in dyslexia and specific language impairment: Is there a deficit? What is its nature? Does it explain anything? *Journal of Phonetics, 31,* 509–527.

Saunders, G. H., & Haggard, M. P. (1992). The clinical assessment of "Obscure Auditory Dysfunction" (OAD) 2. Case control analysis of determining factors. *Ear and Hearing, 13,* 241–254.

Shallice, T. (1988). *From neuropsychology to mental structure.* Cambridge: Cambridge University Press.

Sutcliffe, P. A. (2003). *Auditory processing performance in young children: Attention is needed.* University of Oxford.

Sutcliffe, P. A., & Bishop, D. V. M. (2002). *Age-related changes in frequency discrimination: Tone duration and training can affect performance.* Paper presented at the ISCA Workshop on Speech Perception, Aix-en-Provence, France.

Temple, C. M. (1986). Developmental dysgraphias. *Quarterly Journal of Experimental Psychology: Human Experimental Psychology, 38,* 77–110.

Temple, C. M., & Marshall, J. C. (1983). A case study of developmental phonological dyslexia. *British Journal of Psychology, 74,* 517–533.

Temple, C. M., & Richardson, P. (2004). Developmental amnesia: A new pattern of dissociation with intact episodic memory. *Neuropsychologia, 42,* 764–781.

Vargha-Khadem, F., Gadian, D. G., Watkins, K. E., Connelly, A., Van Paesschen, W., & Mishkin, M. (1997). Differential effects of early hippocampal pathology on episodic and semantic memory. *Science, 277,* 376–380.

Watson, C. S., & Kidd, G. R. (2002). On the lack of association between basic auditory abilities, speech processing, and other cognitive abilities. *Seminars in Hearing, 23,* 83–93.

Watson, C. S., Kidd, G. R., Homer, D. G., Connell, P. J., Lowther, A., Eddins, D. A., et al. (2003). Sensory, cognitive, and linguistic factors in the early academic performance of elementary school children: The Benton-IU project. *Journal of Learning Disabilities, 36,* 165–197.

Werner, L. A., & Gray, L. (1998). Behavioral studies of hearing development. In E. W. Rubel, A. N. Popper, & R. R. Fay (Eds.), *Development of the auditory system. Springer handbook of auditory research* (Vol. 9, pp. 12–79). New York, London: Springer.

WHO. (1980). *International classification of impairments, disabilities and handicaps.* Geneva: World Health Organization.

Ziegler, J. C., Pech-Georgel, C., George, F., Alario, F. X., & Lorenzi, C. (2005). Deficits in speech perception predict language learning impairment. *Proceedings of the National Academy of Sciences of the United States of America, 102,* 14110–14115.

CHAPTER 12

Modality Specificity and Auditory Processing Disorders

DENNIS J. MCFARLAND AND ANTHONY T. CACACE

Introduction

There have been a number of definitions of central auditory processing disorder (CAPD; also known as auditory processing disorder, APD) offered over the years. Central auditory processing disorder has been defined anatomically in terms of the integrity of the auditory nervous system (Rintelmann, 1985). Katz (1992) described auditory processing as "what we do with what we hear." McFarland and Cacace (1995) define CAPD as a modality specific perceptual dysfunction (not due to peripheral hearing loss). A task force for the American Speech, Language, and Hearing Association (ASHA, 1996) defined auditory processing in terms of performances on a selected group of auditory tasks. In the ASHA Task Force definition, CAPD/APDs were considered to be any observed deficits in one or more of these so-called "behaviors." However, inclusive conceptualizations of CAPD/APD have been criticized based on the lack of diagnostic specificity (e.g., Cacace & McFarland, 1998; Rees, 1973). Therefore, modality specificity and its conceptual framework have been advocated as a way to improve the CAPD/APD diagnosis (Cacace & McFarland, 1998, 2005; McFarland & Cacace, 1995).

The concept of modality specificity can be traced to Teuber (1955) in the neuropsychology literature and Thompson, Johnson, and Hoopes (1963) in the neurophysiology literature. In fact, in the domain of neurophysiology, Mountcastle (1997) described modality specificity as a defining characteristic of sensory cortex. Humes, Christopherson, and Cokely (1992) were first to discuss modality specificity as it relates to evaluating CAPD/APD. Subsequently, McFarland and Cacace (1995) and Cacace and McFarland (1998, 2005), developed this argument in more detail. The basic idea behind modality specificity is that any test result is the product of multiple factors, such as perception, attention, motivation, language abilities, decision processes, motor skills, and so forth. To be a useful construct, CAPD/APD should be conceptualized as producing poor performance that is relatively specific to tasks involving auditory stimuli. If a relative deficit with auditory stimuli is obtained when test performance is also evaluated on matched tasks in other sensory modalities, like vision, then alternative nonsensory explanations can be ruled out, thus enhancing the diagnostic significance of this term.

Advocates of the inclusive approach to CAPD/APD talk about "auditory behaviors" (e.g., Musiek, Bellis, & Chermak, 2005). This orientation follows from the ASHA Task Force definition that associates auditory processing with performances on specific *unimodal* auditory tests. In contrast, it is our contention that auditory perception and auditory processing are theoretical constructs. They are not directly observable behaviors; therefore, in order to fully appreciate this distinction, it is necessary to consider what a theoretical construct is and how it functions in the development and application of testing paradigms.

Auditory Processing as a Theoretical Construct

Deciding what is and what is not a CAPD/APD is a matter of arriving at a useful definition. This process is not simply an empirical matter, as no amount of observation can generate a definition. To be a *useful* definition, there must be consensus within the scientific community; to be *effective*; the definition must also function within a practical theory. As discussed by Hood and Berlin (1992), auditory perception cannot be measured directly. They suggest as an alternative, the term "auditory processing." However, auditory processing cannot be measured directly either and this term still requires explication to be useful. We next consider whether auditory processing should be viewed as an observation or as a theoretical construct, which by its very nature requires some form of hypothesis testing to distinguish it from other concerns.

Conceptualizations of test validation have a long history within the field of individual differences. As noted by Smith (2005), the notion that tests are indexes of unobservable hypothetical constructs was quite foreign to thinking prior to Cronbach and Meehl (1955). At that time, the prevailing view held that it was pure speculation to claim that a test measures anything over and above the criterion on which it was validated. Cronbach and Meehl (1955) also assert that test validation is part of the process of theory construction. Thus, the validity of a test is related to the validity of the theory from which it is derived. To quote Smith (2005), "if I develop a measure of hypothetical construct *A*, I can only validate my measure if I have some theoretical argument that, for instance, *A* relates positively to *B*, but is unrelated to *C*. If I have such a theory, and if I have measures of constructs *B* and *C*, I can test whether my measure of *A* performs as predicted by my theory." In a related development, Campbell and Fisk (1959) have emphasized the importance of using different methods to measure hypothetical traits. This approach is refered to as "the multitrait-multimethod technique." In this framework, multiple tests measuring multiple traits are compared to evaluate whether a given test correlates with those measures with which it is theorized to be related to, but does not correlate with measures in which theory suggests it should not be correlated with. Multiple tests of each trait are deemed necessary, as no single test is considered to be a pure index of the construct being assessed. This method provides a means of developing converging evidence for both the theory and the specific tests of the hypothetical trait in question.

How then does the multitrait-multimethod framework apply to the development and validation of tests of CAPD/APDs? It is our position that we never actually observe a CAPD/APD. We must infer this from a consistent pattern of "test results" across different times and situations. We might suspect a CAPD/APD in a child who often misunderstands what is said; such a scenario could be apparent after a teacher in a classroom environment poses a question. However, it would be rash to reach any conclusion based solely on one specific event. An example of such an event might involve a child having difficulty understanding oral instructions for performing a mathematical calculation. Observation of this one behavior would not be sufficient for a diagnosis, as alternative possibilities could be postulated. He or she might have been fatigued due to lack of sleep, the child could be unmotivated to answer, or for that matter, the individual might have problems performing mathematical operations, rather than processing auditory-based materials per se. We would also want to verify whether there were problems with additional sorts of material that involved other domains of knowledge. This would serve to eliminate the possibility that problems with mathematics were at issue, rather than speech perception per se. Furthermore, we might also want to evaluate this child's ability to follow written instructions, so as to demonstrate specificity to the auditory modality. The point here is that a CAPD/APD is not a behavior, but rather, it is an abstract concept that describes a disposition (i.e., a tendency to have difficulty processing auditory stimuli). A second point is that individuals can be characterized by more than one disposition, such as one dealing with auditory abilities and another with mathematical abilities, and so forth. Thus, any specific observed behavior is a reflection of the combination of several hypothetical dispositions.

Whereas the recognition that human abilities are theoretical constructs rather than observable behaviors complicates the test construction process, it also increases substantially the generalizability of the findings. If auditory processing is narrowly defined in terms of the performance on a single specific test, then the results will *not* be of use outside the testing situation. Many tests currently used in the diagnosis of CAPD/APD are not typically encountered in everyday life and therefore are not of interest in and of themselves. Performance on tests of CAPD/APD is important to the extent that we can make inferences about behavior in other situations. In order to make an inference about performance in everyday situations, we must also consider the prognostic value of the construct the test measures, that is, its *ecological validity*. Proponents of the current generation of CAPD/APD tests appear to have an implicit theory that assumes that there is something common to CAPD/APD test performance and everyday tasks such as listening in a noisy classroom. If so, then consideration of this "implicit theory" reveals that the specific construct "auditory processing" is more than what is operationalized simply in terms of specific tests of CAPD/APD. The problem with an implicit theory, however, is that it is not stated explicitly, and as such, leads to confusion and difficulty in testing its assumptions.

The inclusive approach currently advocated by some (e.g., Musiek, Bellis, & Chermak,

2005), conceptualizes auditory behaviors as observables. According to the ASHA technical report (ASHA, 2005) "Screening for CAPD typically involves systematic observation of listening behavior and/or performance on tests of auditory function." Conceptualizing "listening behaviors" as observables leads to the view that difficulty with a test that uses auditory stimuli is direct evidence for a CAPD/APD. Alternatively, conceptualizing CAPD/APD as a hypothetical disposition leads to the use of multiple tests that serve the purpose of evaluating alternative hypotheses concerning the nature of observed behavioral deficits.

It could be argued that the various ASHA working groups (1996, 2005) have specified an implicit theory on which to base predictions. They list a series of "auditory behavioral phenomena" that includes constructs such as "temporal aspects of audition." These temporal aspects of audition are said to include temporal resolution, temporal masking, temporal integration, and temporal ordering. However, there are no citations of empirical research offered to support this taxonomy. Although this classification scheme may have face validity, a casual examination of the literature suggests that there are a number of outstanding questions that need to be resolved. Included within this framework is whether or not these types of tasks all measure the same underlying temporal factor and whether or not temporal processing is modality specific. We now consider these issues.

Temporal processing deficits are one of several popular explanations for language and reading-related problems in children, although there is by no means consensus on this issue (e.g., Bishop, Carlyon, Deeks, & Bishop, 1999; Wright, Lombardino, King, Purnanik, Leonard, & Merzenich, 1997; Zhang & Formby, 2007). Moreover, as noted by Farmer and Klein (1995), the modality-specific nature of these effects is uncertain. Walker, Hall, Klein, and Phillips (2006) examined eight temporal processing tasks and five language/reading tasks in a group of 120 children. They concluded, "the umbrella term 'temporal processing' encompasses fundamentally different sensory and cognitive processes that may contribute differentially to language and reading performance, which may have different developmental trajectories and be differentially susceptible to pathology." There may be considerable heterogeneity even within one specific temporal processing paradigm. For example, when evaluating five different temporal-order tasks which included frequency and level discriminations in the auditory modality and size, orientation, and color discriminations in the visual modality, McFarland, Cacace, and Setzen (1998) found both modality and submodality differences in thresholds for temporal-order discrimination. Fink, Ulbrich, Churan, and Wittmann (2006) extended these findings by examining the intercorrelations between scores on several temporal-order tasks. They found evidence for both feature-specific mechanisms and for a more general modality-independent timing mechanism. In the context of examining modality specificity of temporal-order discriminations in a clinical sample of remediation-resistant reading-impaired children, Cacace, McFarland, Ouimet, Schrieber, and Morrow (2000) showed reliable temporal processing deficits in dyslexic children, but found that these effects were neither modality specific nor temporal specific.

As a consideration of empirical data on temporal processing shows, it cannot be taken for granted that the different temporal processing tasks listed by the ASHA working groups all measure some unitary auditory temporal processing factor. What is required to establish an empirically derived evidence-based classification scheme is a systematic study of the intercorrelations between different measures and the way that they relate to the criteria of interest, whether it be speech perception, reading ability, language abilities, or some other skill. This should also be done in a manner that allows for alternative hypotheses concerning the nature of temporal processing abilities to be evaluated. Examining modality specificity allows for an evaluation of the hypothesis that there are specific auditory-based temporal processing skills. This can be contrasted to the alternative hypothesis that temporal processing skills are measures of an *amodal* factor such as processing speed, which in turn is theorized to be a component of general intelligence (e.g., Rammsayer & Brandler, 2007).

Bellis (1996) provides a more explicit example of theorizing in the CAPD/APD literature. She asserts that there are specific auditory processes that may be affected in CAPD/APD; one of which is "auditory closure." Auditory closure is said to refer to "the ability of listeners to utilize intrinsic and extrinsic redundancy to fill in missing or distorted portions of the auditory signal." She further asserts that individuals with an auditory closure deficit will perform poorly on low-pass filtered speech, time-compressed speech, and speech-in-noise tests. Examination of this construct indicates that auditory closure is an abstract hypothetical term that functions to account for performances on several specific tests. It is not defined solely in terms of these test results however, as it is said to affect understanding of everyday speech. Another interesting feature of the discussion of auditory closure championed by Bellis (1996) is that these assertions and the entire discussion about this issue are *not* accompanied by any citations to the literature. Consequently, if the concept of auditory closure as proposed by Bellis (1996)

is valid, then it should be possible to demonstrate meaningful correlations between tests of filtered speech, time-compressed speech, speech-in-noise, and measures of everyday speech. Without this information, the auditory closure construct lacks evidence for its convergent validity (Campbell & Fisk, 1959). In any case, auditory closure is an abstract concept involving the relationship between multiple measures. It is not an observable behavior.

In summary, auditory perception and auditory processing are abstract/theoretical terms; they are not specific observable behaviors. In contrast, auditory stimuli can be considered as observable/physical events in the sense that they can be heard from speakers or head phones and the physical dimensions of the stimuli (frequency, duration, or sound pressures levels) can be measured via laboratory instrumentation as two-dimensional time domain representations when their outputs from an artificial ear are viewed on an oscilloscope and measured by a sound level meter or transformed to the frequency domain and viewed as simple or complex spectra.

Modality Specificity as a Means to Determine the Domain of APD

As we have argued previously, the performance on any given test can be seen as the product of multiple factors (Cacace & McFarland, 2005; McFarland & Cacace, 1995). In addition, tests of CAPD/APD have been criticized for their potential sensitivity to factors such as attention (Cacace & McFarland, 2006; Gascon, Johnson, & Burd, 1986; Grundfast, Berkowitz, Conners, & Belman, 1991) and language abilities (Friel-Patti,

1999; Rees, 1973), particularly if verbal materials are used as stimuli in the assessment process. These views can be seen as alternative hypotheses for poor performance on tests of CAPD/APD. Moreover, these issues involve questions such as (1) what aspects of speech perception should be considered the domain of auditory processing, and (2) are there auditory specific attention deficits? One way to evaluate such alternative hypotheses is to examine performances on tests that depend on matched stimuli presented in other sensory modalities. For example, the amodal language hypothesis predicts that poor test performance will occur with both visual and auditory presentation of linguistic stimuli. The supramodal attention hypothesis makes similar predictions with the exception that linguistic features are not critical. In either case, hypothesis testing based on multimodal tests using matched stimuli can be directed at the question concerning whether a disorder is modality specific or supramodal. The answer to this query needs to be demonstrated; it cannot be assumed or taken for granted.

Ways of Demonstrating Modality Specificity

There are two basic ways to demonstrate modality specificity. One way employs the experimental approach. As an example, Cacace, McFarland, Emrich, and Haller (1992) showed that a patient with a posterior temporal lobe lesion performed poorly on a task using binary sequential auditory frequency patterns and normally on a task using binary sequential visual color patterns. In contrast, a second patient with a more anterior temporal lobe lesion performed poorly on a binary sequential visual color pattern task and normally on a binary sequential auditory frequency pattern task. In this instance, we demonstrate a "double-dissociation" between visual and auditory performances. Such findings show that modality-specific results can be obtained using tests that are psychometrically matched for other task-related features. The double dissociation paradigm is a powerful way to demonstrate both the sensitivity of the task (binary sequential patterns in the auditory and visual modalities) and the modality specificity of the deficit.

A second way to examine modality specificity is to examine the patterns of intercorrelations between tests in several modalities. An example of this approach is the recent study of Riccio, Cohen, Garrison, and Smith (2005) in which a battery of CAPD tasks (Staggered Spondaic Word Test and a Screening Test for Auditory Processing Disorders, SCAN test battery) were administered along with tests of memory and attention (Test of Variables of Attention, TOVA). The TOVA is a continuous performance test (CPT) that makes use of visual stimuli. In as much as TOVA scores were not significantly correlated with scores on either CAPD battery, these authors concluded that, "auditory processing may not necessarily be associated with ADHD or attention deficits." Unfortunately, there were methodological problems with this study that limit its generalizability. For example, the TOVA and CAPD tests were not "psychometrically matched" so that a third factor, not related to auditory processing or to the TOVA, could account for these results. More importantly however, the intertest correlations, based on the Pearson's r metric between TOVA commission errors and SCAN scores ranged from $r = -0.49$ to -0.59. These values are in the same absolute range reported between SCAN subtests ($r = 0.25$ to 0.53). Consequently, these correlations were probably not significant due to the small sample size available for the TOVA data ($n = 16$). Nevertheless, although the low power for these comparisons makes the conclusions derived from this study tenuous, it provides an example of how an analysis of intertest correlations can address the issue of modality specificity.

Demonstrating the modality specificity of poor test performance serves to characterize the domain of observed processing difficulties as being auditory in nature. To the extent that tests used to demonstrate modality specificity are matched for characteristics other than the sensory modality (psychometrically matched), alternative explanations of poor performance can be ruled out. Bellis (1996) has stated, "Simply identifying the presence of a disorder is not enough. Instead, the disorder must be qualified so that insightful intervention and educational planning can occur." We concur. This is precisely the reason that we advocate multimodal testing. This allows for the planners to predict whether deficits will be restricted to auditory materials or whether deficits should be expected across multiple modalities.

Bellis, Billiet, and Ross (2008) compared recall of dichotic digits and an analogous visual task in children with CAPD and controls. The dichotic digits task was a standard instrument frequently used in CAPD batteries (Musiek, 1983). The analogous visual task consisted of using an LCD monitor to present each member of the same digits pairs simultaneous on different sides of a fixation cross. Bellis et al. (2008) found that controls recalled significantly more digits than children with the CAPD diagnosis for both auditory and visual presentations. Fur-

thermore, they report several significant positive correlations between auditory and visual recall. These authors suggest that similar mechanisms might be recruited for both tasks and conclude that the results argue against the complete modality-specificity of CAPD.

The assertion of Bellis et al. (2008) that a failure to demonstrate modality specificity in children diagnosed with CAPD argues against the concept of modality specificity follows from the position that poor performance on auditory tasks is sufficient for the diagnosis. However, we would take these results as support for the necessity of doing multimodal testing. These findings show that the children diagnosed with CAPD may have problems with factors common to both auditory and visual tasks and question the logic of describing their problems as being auditory in nature.

Having a battery of tests in multiple sensory modalities allows for a description of the examinee's abilities in terms of relative strengths and weaknesses. Terms such as CAPD or APD suggest that performance on tests using auditory material should be affected more than those tests that do not use auditory material. If performance is uniformly poor across visual and auditory sensory modalities, then the description of the deficit should *not* be CAPD or APD; to the contrary, a more accurate representation would be "amodal processing disorder," "supramodal processing disorder," "pansensory processing disorder," and so on. Such a general disorder of sensory information processing implies that an individual would show uniformly poor performance on tests of these abilities. This is exactly what would be predicted in individuals with low intelligence (Johnson, Bouchard, Krueger, McGue, & Gottesman, 2004). Batteries that are designed to measure general intelligence include tests that use auditory stimuli, such as digit-span testing on the Wechsler Adult Intelligence Scale (WAIS). An inclusive view might lead to the conclusion that poor performance on an auditory digit-span task is sufficient evidence for the diagnosis of CAPD/APD. However, we contend that in order to have a construct distinct from general intelligence, it is necessary to show that the deficit on the auditory version of this task is relatively greater than that observed on digit-span testing using visual presentation of stimuli.

Attention deficit is another construct that might show potential overlap with CAPD/APD in terms of behavioral observations and test performances (e.g., Cacace & McFarland, 2006; Grundfast, Berkowitz, Conners, & Belman, 1991). Attention deficit hyperactivity disorder (ADHD) is currently viewed as an "executive" dysfunction that results in poor performance across sensory modalities (e.g., Seidman, 2006). For example, children diagnosed with ADHD show more errors on both visual and auditory versions of a CPT (Tinius, 2003). Again, the key to establishing CAPD/APD as a construct independent of ADHD, is in showing modality-specific effects.

In order to have a precise meaning, a specific disorder of information processing needs to be conceptualized in terms of the domain of tasks that show poor performance as well as the domain of tasks on which performance is relatively spared. For CAPD/APD, the domain of affected tasks includes those that use auditory stimuli and the domain of spared tasks includes those that do not. This is the purpose of including tests measuring multiple constructs in the multitrait-multimethod approach (Campbell & Fisk, 1959). Measures of alternative traits provide a means of demonstrating *discriminant validity*.

Modality Specificity and Auditory Neuroscience

A traditional view in neurophysiology is that areas of cortex can be subdivided into sensory, associative, and motor domains. Accordingly, sensory cortexes are those areas that are modality specific as indexed, for example, by their electrophysiologic response properties to specific sensory stimulation (Thompson, Johnson, & Hoopes, 1963). The importance of sensory interactions recently has been emphasized by some (e.g., Laurienti, Burdette, Wallace, Yen, Field, & Stein, 2002). The extreme position is that there are, in fact, few if any modality-specific brain regions (Ghazanfar & Schroeder, 2006). This later point of view has a counterpart in information processing models that assume an interaction between top-down cognitive and bottom-up perceptual processes. For example, McClellan, Mirman, and Holt (2006) assert that there are lexical influences on phonological processes that are generally considered to be prelexical in nature. Specifically, the identification of speech tokens is influenced by the context in which they occur. McClellan, Mirman, and Holt (2006) explain such effects in terms of top-down influences on early perceptual processing. This position is not universally accepted however. For example, McQueen, Norris, and Cutler (2006) contend that these effects can be accounted for solely in terms of perceptual mechanisms. They suggest that feedback adjusts the perceptual system, but not during on-line processing. Thus, both neurophysiologic and information processing models exist that minimize the role of modality specific processes. The problem is that the processes postulated by these models are not directly observed.

Sensory System Interactions: The Role of "Drivers" and "Modulators"

Accumulating data on the existence of extensive feedback connections between all levels of the nervous system serves as part of the argument against modularity in sensory systems. For example, the auditory cortex sends massive efferents to the thalamus, midbrain, and brainstem (Winer, 2005). This observation suggests the possibility of interactions between top-down and bottom-up processing. However, it is important to examine the nature of these interactions. Sherman and Guillery (1998) are proponents of the view which argues that a distinction should be made between "drivers" and "modulators." By this view, drivers transmit the receptive field properties of neurons, whereas modulators are seen as altering the probability of certain aspects of that transmission (i.e., the gain of the unit). As an example, consider the computation of interaural intensity differences; an important process involved in binaural hearing and localization of objects in space. For any given sound event, the specific intensity cue for location originates in the environment and is transmitted along the ascending auditory pathways. The descending efferent feedback pathway appears to maintain an appropriate balance in the overall sensitivity of the two cochleas (Darrow, Maison, & Liberman, 2006). This adjustment mechanism in gain allows the auditory system to function optimally, but this latter process does not provide specific information on the location of the auditory objects. In this example, descending efferent input to the cochleas serves as a modulator. In this context, efferent feedback serves to adjust the

sensitivity of the ascending auditory afferents, but they do not provide detailed information about specific sensory events.

There are also extensive reciprocal connections between sensory cortexes and supramodal association areas. We can again ask whether the feedback from association areas to primary sensory cortexes serve as drivers or modulators. This issue is more difficult to reconcile than the modulation induced by olivocochlear efferents, as the connections are more extensive and our knowledge of this type of information processing is in a much earlier stage of development (Romanski, 2007). Nonetheless, we will consider some possibilities. A number of studies have reported cross-modal interactions assessed by functional magnetic resonance imaging (*f*MRI), an indirect measure of neural activity based on the hemodynamic response of the brain induced by sensory, motor, or cognitive activations. For example, Laurienti, Burdette, Wallace, Yen, Field, and Stein (2002) found that presentation of visual stimuli resulted in *increased* blood oxygenated level-dependent (BOLD) response in visual cortex and a *reduced* BOLD response (deactivation) in auditory cortex. Presentation of auditory stimuli resulted in *increased* BOLD response in auditory cortex and *reduced* BOLD response in visual cortex. Thus, in this example, the cross-modal modulation of activity took the form of deactivations; an effect that is highly dependent on prestimulus baseline activity. Baier, Kleinschmidt, and Muller (2006) found that visual and auditory interactions depend on both the relevance of the sensory modality to the task under consideration and the statistical relationship between the sensory events. When visual-auditory pairings occurred by chance, activations occur in the relevant modality and deactivations occur in the irrelevant modality. When the information in the two modalities is reliably associated, activity is enhanced in both. These cross-modal interactions observed in *f*MRI experiments are commonly discussed in terms of attention-related modulations.

Cross-modal attention effects appear to be modulated by a system of amodal structures. For example, Dosenbach, Visscher, Palmer, Miezin, Wenger, Kang, et al. (2006) examined *f*MRI activations occurring across tasks varying in input (auditory vs. visual), processing requirements, and output modalities. They found that several areas including the anterior cingulate and the frontal operculum were active across all task conditions and appeared to represent a "core" task-set system.

However, simply describing cross-modal modulations as being related to attention does not clarify their relevance for discussions of modality specificity. It is necessary to consider the manner in which attention operates on different levels of sensory information processing. One could hypothesize that attention modulates the overall gain of a particular modality without selectively biasing the system toward one or another specific percept. An alternative hypothesis could argue that attention selectively enhances specific percepts. These two alternatives correspond roughly to the distinction between drivers and modulators discussed earlier (Sherman & Guillery, 1998). Fritz, Elhilali, and Shamma (2005) examined receptive fields in behaving ferrets making spectral and temporal discriminations. They found that task-specific receptive field changes occurred within minutes of task onset. Their results indicate that attention can bias neural units to respond to specific stimulus classes. However, these effects are still relatively tonic (occurring within minutes) and the phasic response of units is presumably driven by input from the external auditory environment. Consequently,

whereas attention may adjust the tuning of auditory cortical units, these units are still processing auditory information.

Musacchia, Sams, Nicol, and Kraus (2006) describe the results of an experiment that demonstrates audiovisual interactions occurring as early as 11 milliseconds (msec) postacoustic stimulation. They recorded evoked potentials while subjects were instructed to either count the number of /da/ tokens heard in a presentation of only auditory stimuli, or count the number of /du/ tokens presented in a sequence of visual stimuli that were occasionally discordant with an auditory sequence of only /da/ tokens. In the first case, successful counting required attending to the auditory modality and in the second case, successful counting required attending to the visual modality. They found shorter latency and larger amplitude evoked potentials occurring in the unimodal acoustic condition as compared to the bimodal condition. The authors rule out an explanation in terms of an interaction of modalities at the time of acoustic onset given the short latency of the response. Rather, they suggest that the effect must be due to the processing of visual information that precedes acoustic stimulation. One such mechanism they suggest is cortical gating of subcortical acoustic processing (i.e., attention).

The issue here is whether or not results such as those reported by Musacchia et al. (2006) argue against the modality specificity of early auditory pathways. It has been known for some time that supramodal attention can modulate the activity of brainstem auditory pathways. One of the earliest examples of this phenomenon was based on studies performed by Hernandez-Peon, Scherrer, and Jouvet (1956). Hernandez-Peon and colleagues showed that activity recorded from the cochlear nucleus of cats in response to click stimuli was reduced when they were shown a mouse in a jar. In the context of our general argument, should we view this effect as evidence that the cochlear nucleus is processing visual information or should we consider an alternative explanation? The authors suggest that the sensitivity of the cochlear nucleus is modulated by descending influences. Our knowledge of the anatomy and physiology of the auditory system should convince us that auditory sensory afferents represent the drivers for the neurons of the cochlear nucleus. In contrast, descending efferents modulate the sensitivity of these units in a relatively nonspecific manner and thus should be viewed as modulators.

Current research also demonstrates that the representation of stimulus events in primary sensory areas is modified by experience; that is, they are reactive, malleable, and therefore plastic. This representational plasticity appears to be driven by amodal neural systems. For example, Weinberger (2007) has reviewed studies demonstrating changes in the receptive fields of units in auditory cortex that are the result of classical and instrumental conditioning. These effects appear to depend on basal forebrain cholinergic inputs to the auditory cortex. Representational plasticity has been demonstrated in auditory, somatosensory, and visual sensory cortices (e.g., Blake, Byl, & Merzenich, 2002; Chen & Yan, 2007; Gu, 2003; Weinberger, Hopkins, & Diamond, 1984).

The basal forebrain cholinergic system receives inputs from many cortical and subcortical sites and projects to all areas of cortex (Saper, 1984). Thus, areas that are not modality specific drive plasticity of auditory receptive fields. However, although these amodal cholinergic afferents are involved in the poststimulus tuning of sensory receptive fields, they have not been reported to modulate the stimulus-induced real-time topography of unit activation in sensory cortex. That is, the cholinergic afferents are involved in the post-hoc tuning of the way auditory cortex units respond to auditory stimuli. They do not serve as an alternative source for receptive field properties.

In summary, there is ample evidence to suggest that structures traditionally considered to be components of the auditory nervous system receive inputs from areas that have not traditionally been considered to be modality specific. However, more likely than not, these inputs serve to modulate the response to acoustic stimulation via processes such as attention and perceptual learning. Thus, central auditory pathways may best be conceptualized as being specialized for processing acoustic information.

Some have taken demonstrations of cross-modal modulations to indicate that the concept of modality specific sensory areas should be abandoned (e.g., Stoffregen & Bardy, 2001). Although it is possible to show that cortex traditionally considered to be primary sensory projection areas are influenced by cross-modal effects, at present, it is not clear that this extreme view is warranted. In the first place, demonstrating a cross-modal effect does not mean that a given region of cortex is not specialized for processing sensory-specific information. Although it may be modulated by amodal areas, a given brain area may still be primarily involved in processing modality specific information. Studies that dissociate modality specific and cross-modal abilities provide evidence for the utility of the existence of modality specific brain systems.

Modality specific disorders of auditory processing such as pure word deafness (Stefanatos, Gershkoff, & Madigan, 2005), cortical deafness, auditory agnosia, and phonagnosia have been reported in the literature (e.g., Polster & Rose, 1998) and provide evidence for modularity in human auditory pathways. Likewise, it appears that the ability to integrate auditory and visual language cues can be disrupted by focal lesions, while leaving unimodal auditory abilities intact. Along these lines, Hamilton, Shenton, and Coslett (2006) describe a patient with an acquired audiovisual speech integration deficit. This patient showed no McGurk effect and was less accurate on speech tasks when the sight of lip movements was present. Such examples illustrate that modality specific and cross-modal abilities can be dissociated. We emphasize and reiterate here again, that what is important for understanding the neural substrates of human abilities is the relative specificity of information processing. This needs to be based on a quantitative assessment, rather than simply a demonstration of effects that may be minor in size and significance.

The issue of the cognitive penetrability of perception has been the subject of debate in the field of philosophy as well. In this context, Churchland (1979) has argued that our perception is influenced by cognition, which has been referred to as the "theory-ladenness of perception." This view has been considered a threat to realism and has resulted in considerable debate (e.g., Fodor, 1983). It is sufficient to say that this issue continues to be a point-of-contention within the domain of philosophy (Raftopoulos, 2001).

Issues such as the modular organization of the brain and whether perception is cognitively penetrable are currently the subject of debate in multiple areas including: philosophy (Raftopoulos, 2001), psychology (Pylyshyn, 1999), and neuroscience (Shimojo & Shams, 2001). A casual look at these citations will show that there is by no means a consensus on these issues. Consequently, it seems inappropriate for the ASHA working group to flatly assert that modality specificity is neurophysiologically untenable (ASHA, 2005); such a position is

premature, controversial, and uncalled for. The technical report states, "An extensive literature in neuroscience influenced the Working Group's conclusion that the requirement of "modality specificity" as a diagnostic criterion of CAPD/APD is not consistent with how processing actually occurs in the [central nervous system]. Basic cognitive neuroscience has shown that there are few, if any, entirely compartmentalized areas in the brain that are solely responsible for a single sensory modality (Poremba, Saunders, Sokoloff, Crane, Cook & Mishkin, 2003; Salvi, Lockwood, Frisina, Coad, Wack, Frisina, 2002, p. 2).

This statement concerning modality specificity is made without any substantial discussion of the philosophical and scientific literature. Furthermore, the interpretation of Poremba et al. (2003) used by Musiek and colleagues (2005) to discount modality specificity is *not* consistent with the actual data or conclusions of the authors. According to Poremba et al. (2003), "The present results suggest that an auditory region resembling and paralleling the unimodal, ventral visual pathway extends through the entire length of the supratemporal plane together with the exposed surface of the superior temporal gyrus; like the ventral visual pathway, *this auditory region appears to be modality specific*, suggesting that it is dedicated to analyzing acoustic stimulus quality for purposes of stimulus identification and recognition, just as the ventral visual pathway does for visual stimulus quality. In contrast, other large auditory sectors overlap extensively with visual areas" (p. 570). In an extension of this work, Poremba and Mishkin (2007) suggest that there are at least three different cortical processing streams in audition paralleling visual processing streams: "a modality specific ventral stream for processing acoustic stimulus quality or auditory 'objects,' analogous to the one in the visual system for processing visual objects; a modality-non-specific dorsal stream for processing the spatial source of acoustic stimuli, analogous to, and overlapping with, the one in vision for processing spatial location; and a second modality non-specific stream, this one coursing through the upper bank of the superior temporal sulcus and possibly processing auditory motion, by analogy to the visual stream in this same location that processes visual motion," (p. 18).

In his discussion of extra-auditory influences, Zatorre (2007) states that his purpose is not to abandon the classical definitions of auditory cortex. Rather, he suggests that it is necessary to " . . . consider more broadly how the auditory cortex works within a highly distributed system." The available data are consistent with many models of cortical functioning and there are good reasons for assuming that certain parts of cortex are specialized for processing modality specific information. Whether modality specific specialization rules out cognitive penetrability is a matter for further experimentation and theoretical debate.

The issue of modality specificity can be viewed in terms of a continuum. We can ask how far into the nervous system sensory inputs remain modality specific. At one extreme, it may be argued that only the inner and outer hair cells of the cochlea or the rods and cones of the retina are modality specific. At another extreme, it may be that a high degree of modality specificity is maintained as far as the parabelt regions of auditory and visual cortices (Kaas & Hackett, 2000), and perhaps even into modality-specific frontal areas (Romanski, 2004; 2007). From a scientific perspective, it is a complex issue concerning both theory and empirical observations that remains to be resolved. However, it is an issue that defines the domain of CAPD/APDs. For without

modality specificity, the concept of a CAPD/APD has little explanatory power; indeed, without modality specificity the concept of CAPD/APD does not make sense. Arguing against the application of modality specificity in neuroscience (e.g., Musiek et al, 2005) only restricts the domain of CAPD/APD; it does *not* negate the necessity of demonstrating modality specificity. If an area of the brain is involved in *amodal* information processing, then it makes *no* sense to describe it as being auditory. Moreover, if a test of human abilities is related to a general *amodal* factor, then it makes *no* sense to describe it as a test of auditory abilities. The modifier "auditory" clearly implies some sort of specificity. Otherwise, why use it?

Modality Specificity and Psychometrics

Neuroscience potentially provides the theory for CAPD/APD, but many issues are unsettled. As we have noted previously (McFarland & Cacace, 1995) and given such uncertainties, it may be more practical to define CAPD/APD in functional terms at present. This can involve specifying the patterns of intercorrelations that are to be expected between tests of CAPD/APD and other measures. As we have emphasized throughout this chapter, this process involves establishing the convergent and divergent validity of such tests (Campbell & Fisk, 1959).

Schow, Seikel, Chermak, and Berent (2000) administered a battery of auditory processing tests to a group of children and evaluated the pattern of intercorrelations with structural equation modeling. In theory, this procedure is appropriate as it provides a means of evaluating alternative hypotheses about the theoretical constructs that determine test performance. Unfortunately, these investigators included only auditory tests and evaluated only the ASHA (1996) model. McFarland and Cacace (2000) reanalyzed these data and showed that a model that included a single general factor could account for their results just as well as the ASHA model that included four factors. On the basis of parsimony, the simpler model is preferred. Thus, these results provide very little support for the four-factor model. As no tests involving nonauditory stimuli were included, it was not possible to evaluate the modality specificity of the tests in question.

This example illustrates an approach that can be taken to develop valid tests of auditory processing. Multiple tests can be given and the resulting matrix of correlations can be evaluated with structural equation modeling. In this way, alternative hypotheses about what these tests measure can be evaluated. However, the design should include more tests than those used by Schow et al. (2000). As we have noted, the lack of tests in more than one modality makes it impossible to interpret results in terms of modality-specific factors, and from a diagnostic standpoint, one could argue that the unimodal approach to testing results in an "indeterminate diagnosis." Therefore, the unimodal approach to testing is not a viable approach to apply in the clinic. Demonstrating modality specificity is necessary to establish *discriminant validity* (i.e., showing that a test does not correlate with factors that it theoretically shouldn't be related to). It is also necessary to include multiple measures of the same trait so as to establish *convergent validity* (i.e., showing that the test correlates with measures it is theoretically expected to correlate with).

As noted earlier, concern has been expressed about what tests of auditory processing measure. If verbal materials are used, then it is reasonable to suggest that these tests are confounded by language abilities (Reese, 1973; Cowan, Rosen, and Moore, Chapter 11, this volume) or attention (Gascon et al., 1986). This is the question of discriminative validity, and it is established by showing that tests of auditory processing do not correlate with factors that they are theoretically expected to be independent of. One way to rule out this type of effect is to include tests of these other abilities and show that the resulting matrix of inter-correlations is best accounted for by including modality specific factors in the model. However, existing tests of language abilities and attention may be less than ideal, so an even better approach is to include psychometrically matched tests in at least two modalities, such as vision and audition. In this way, the stimulus modality can be directly modeled and the hypothesis that modality matters, can be directly tested.

The other component of Campbell and Fisk's (1959) multitrait-multimethod procedure concerns convergent validity. This concept deals with whether or not a test correlates with what it is expected to correlate with. For example, as discussed earlier, the ASHA (2005) model implies that tests of "temporal aspects of audition" should all inter-correlate. In addition, they should also correlate with measures that temporal aspects of audition are theoretically supposed to predict. These could include practical measures of speech perception, reading abilities, or some other relevant practical skill. Convergent validity has been demonstrated for measures of general intelligence and this provides a good model for CAPD/APD test development. For example, Johnson, Krueger, McGue, and Gottesman (2006) showed that composite scores for three different intelligence batteries correlated highly with a single factor. Kuncel, Hezlett, and Ones (2004) showed that a test of general intelligence could predict a variety of educational and work-related outcomes. This is the sort of evidence that supports the convergent validity of a test that we strive to attain.

Summary and Conclusions

Tests currently available for evaluation of CAPD/APDs have been criticized based on their lack of specificity. This problem exists because none of these tests have been properly validated. This validation process should involve an ongoing process of evaluating hypotheses concerning what is measured by these tests.

Moreover, this validation process should start with a clear theoretical rational for the procedural basis of the test in question. Modality specificity needs to be part of the theoretical definition of an "auditory" processing disorder because as we mentioned previously and reiterate again here, without specificity, the concept of a CAPD/APD has little explanatory power, and more importantly, without specificity CAPD/APD makes little sense. Modality specificity provides a means of ruling out various amodal factors such as language abilities, supramodal attention, or polysensory deficits as factors accounting for poor test performance.

Some researchers have suggested that the concept of modality specificity is unrealistic (e.g., Katz & Tillery, 2005; Musiek et al., 2005). This argument is based in part on a Boolian logic, which views a single case as sufficient evidence to disprove a hypothesis. Thus, if a case of visual influences on auditory perception can be demonstrated (e.g., the McGurk effect), then the utility of viewing the auditory system as being modality specific is discounted. However,

the appropriate paradigm for reasoning in abilities testing is a quantitative statistical logic. For any given test, empirical research is needed to determine the amount of variance in performance that can be attributed to modality-specific factors, supramodal factors, and measurement error. Currently, this field lacks such logic, and remains in a holding pattern, waiting for more serious research to be performed.

References

American Speech-Language-Hearing Association. (1996) Central auditory processing: Current status of research and implications for clinical practice. *American Journal of Audiology, 5,* 41–54.

American Speech-Language-Hearing Association. (2005). (Central) auditory processing disorders—the role of the audiologist [Position statement]. Available at http://www.asha.org/members/deskref-journals/deskref/default

Baier, B., Kleinschmidt, A., & Muller, N. G. (2006). Cross-modal processing in early visual and auditory corticies depends on expected statistical relationship of multisensory information. *Journal of Neuroscience, 26,* 12260–12265.

Bellis, T. J. (1996). *Assessment and management of central auditory processing disorders in the educational setting: From science to practice.* San Diego, CA: Singular.

Bellis, T. J., Billiet, C., & Ross, J. (2008). Hemispheric lateralization of bilaterally presented homologous visual and auditory stimuli in normal adults, normal children, and children with central auditory dysfunction. *Brain and Cognition, 66,* 280–289.

Bishop, D. V., Carylon, R. P., Deeks, J. M., & Bishop, S. J. (1999). Auditory temporal processing impairment: neither necessary nor sufficient for causing language impairment in children. *Journal of Speech, Language and Hearing Research, 42,* 1295–1310.

Blake, D. T., Byl, N. N., & Merzenich, M. M. (2002). Representation of the hand in the cerebral cortex. *Behavioral and Brain Research*, *135*, 179–184.

Cacace, A. T., & McFarland, D. J. (1998). Central auditory processing disorder in school-aged children: A critical review. *Journal of Speech, Language and Hearing Research, 51*, 355–373.

Cacace, A. T., & McFarland, D. J. (2005). The importance of modality specificity in diagnosing central auditory processing disorder. *American Journal of Audiology*, *14*, 112–123.

Cacace, A. T., & McFarland, D. J. (2006). Delineating auditory processing disorder (APD) and attention deficit hyperactivity disorder (ADHD): A conceptual, theoretical, and practical framework. In T. K. Parthasarathy (Ed.), *An introduction to auditory processing disorders in children*, (pp. 39–61). Mahwah, NJ: Lawrence Erlbaum.

Cacace, A. T., McFarland, D. J., Emrich, J. F., & Haller, J. S. (1992). Assessing short-term recognition memory with forced-choice psychophysical methods. *Journal of Neuroscience Methods*, *44*, 145–155.

Cacace, A. T., McFarland, D. J., Ouimet, J. R., Schrieber, E. J., & Marro, P. (2000). Temporal processing deficits in remediation-resistant reading-impaired children. *Audiology and Neuro-Otology*, *5*, 83–97.

Campbell, D. T., & Fisk, D. W. (1959). Convergent and discriminant validation by the multitrait-multimethod matrix. *Psychological Bulletin*, *56*, 81–105.

Chen, G., & Yan, J. (2007). Cholinergic modulation incorporated with a tone presentation induces frequency-specific threshold decreases in the auditory cortex of the mouse. *European Journal of Neuroscience, 25*, 1793–1803.

Churchland, P. M. (1979). *Scientific realism and the plasticity of mind*. Cambridge University Press.

Chronbach, L. J., & Meehl, P. E. (1955). Construct validity in psychological tests. *Psychological Bulletin*, *52*, 281–302.

Cowan, J., Rosen, S., & Moore, D. R. (in press). Putting the auditory processing back into auditory processing disorders in children. In

A. T. Cacace & D. J. McFarland, *Current controversies in CAPD*. San Diego, CA: Plural Publishing.

Darrow, K. N., Maison, S. F., & Liberman, M. C. (2006). Cochlear efferent feedback balances interaural sensitivity. *Nature Neuroscience*, *9*, 1474–1476.

Dosenbach, N., Visscher, K., Palmer, E., Miezin, F., Wenger, K., Kang, H., Burgund, E., Grimes, A., Schlaggar, B., & Petersen, S. (2006). A core system for the implementation of task sets. *Neuron*, *50*, 799–812.

Fink, M., Ulbrich, P., Churan, J., & Wittmann, M. (2006). Stimulus-dependent processing of temporal order. *Behavioral Processes*, *71*, 344–352.

Fodor, J. A. (1983). *The modularity of mind*. Cambridge, MA: MIT Press.

Friel-Patti, S. (1999). Clinical decision-making in the assessment and intervention of central auditory processing disorders. *Language, Speech, and Hearing Services in the Schools*, *30*, 345–352.

Fritz, J., Elhilali, M., & Shamma, S. (2005). Active listening: Task-dependent plasticity of spectrotemporal receptive fields in primary auditory cortex. *Hearing Research*, *206*, 159–176.

Gascon, G. G., Johnson, R., & Burd, L. (1986). Central auditory processing and attention deficit disorders. *Journal of Child Neurology*, *1*, 27–33.

Ghazanfar, A. A., & Schroeder, C. E. (2006). Is neocortex essentially multisensory? *Trends in Cognitive Sciences*, *10*, 278–285.

Grundfast, K. M., Berkowitz, R. G., Conners, C. K., & Belman, P. (1991). Complete evaluation of the child identified as a poor listener. *International Journal of Pediatric Otorhinolaryngology*, *21*, 65–78.

Gu, O. (2003). Contribution of acetylcholine to visual cortex plasticity. *Neurobiology of Learning and Memory*, *80*, 291–201.

Hamilton, R. H., Shenton, J. T., & Coslett, H. B. (2006). An acquired deficit of audiovisual speech processing. *Brain and Language*, *98*, 66–73.

Hernandez-Peon, R., Scherrer, H., & Jouvet, M. (1956) Modification of electrical activity in cochlear nucleus during "attention" in unanesthetized cats. *Science, 123,* 331–332.

Hood, L. J., & Berlin, C. I. (1992). Central auditory function and disorders. In S. J. Segalowitz & I. Rapin (Eds.), *Handbook of neuropsychology, Vol. 7: Child neuropsychology* (pp. 459–486). Baltimore: Elsevier.

Humes, L., Christopherson, L., & Cokey, C. (1992). Central auditory processing disorders in the elderly: Fact or fiction? In J. Katz, N. Stecker, & D. Henderson (Eds.), *Central auditory processing: A transdisciplinary view* (pp. 141–149). St. Louis, MO: Mosby.

Johnson, W., Bouchard, T. J., Krueger, R. F., McGue, M., & Gottesman, I. I. (2004). Just one g: Consistent results from three test batteries. *Intelligence, 32,* 95–107.

Kass, J. H., & Hackett, T. A. (2000). Subdivisions of auditory cortex and processing streams in primates, *Proceedings of the National Academy of Sciences, 97,* 11793–11799.

Katz, J. (1992). Classification of auditory processing disorders. In J. Katz, N. Stecker, & D. Henderson (Eds.), *Central auditory processing: A transdisciplinary view*. St. Louis, MO: Mosby.

Kuncel, N. R., Hezlett, S. A., & Ones, D. S. (2004). Academic performance, career potential, creativity, and job performance: Can one construct predict them all? *Journal of Personality and Social Psychology, 86,* 148–161.

Laurienti, P. J., Burdette, J. H., Wallace, M. T., Yen, Y., Field, A. S., & Stein, B. E. (2002). Deactivation of sensory-specific cortex by cross-modal stimuli. *Journal of Cognitive Neuroscience, 14,* 420–429.

McClelland, J. L., Mirman, D., & Holt, L. L. (2006). Are there interactive processes in speech perception? *Trends in Cognitive Sciences, 10,* 363–369.

McFarland, D. J., & Cacace, A. T. (1995). Modality specificity as a criterion for diagnosing central auditory processing disorders. *American Journal of Audiology, 4,* 36–48.

McFarland, D. J., & Cacace, A. T. (2000). Factor analysis in CAPD and the "unimodal" test battery: Do we have a model that will satisfy? *American Journal of Audiology, 11,* 9–12.

McFarland, D. J., Cacace, A. T., & Setzen, G. (1998). Temporal-order discrimination for selected auditory and visual stimulus dimensions. *Journal of Speech and Hearing Research, 41,* 300–314.

McQueen, J. M., Norris, D., & Cutler, A. (2006). Are there really interactive processes in speech perception? *Trends in Cognitive Sciences, 10,* 533.

Mountcastle, V. B. (1997). The columnar organization of nerocortex. *Brain, 120,* 701–722.

Musacchia, G., Sams, M., Nicol, T., & Kraus, N. (2006). Seeing speech affects acoustic information processing in the human brainstem. *Experimental Brain Research, 168,* 1–10.

Musiek, F. E., Bellis, T. J., & Chermak, G. D. (2005). Nonmodularity of the central auditory nervous system: Implications for (central) auditory processing disorder. *American Journal of Audiology, 14,* 128–138.

Polster, M. R., & Rose, S. B. (1998). Disorders of auditory processing: Evidence for modularity in auditory. *Cortex, 34,* 47–65.

Poremba, A., & Mishkin, M. (2007). Exploring the extent and function of higher-order auditory cortex in rhesus monkeys. *Hearing Research 229,* 14–23.

Poremba, A, Saunders, R. C., Sokoloff, L., Crane, A., Cook, M., & Miskin, M. (2003). Functional mapping of the primate auditory system. *Science, 299,* 568–572.

Pylyshyn, Z. (1999). Is vision continuous with cognition? *Behavioral and Brain Sciences, 22,* 341–365.

Raftopoulos, A. (2001). Is perception informationally encapsulated? The issue of the theory-ladenness of perception. *Cognitive Science,* 423–451.

Rammsayer, T. H., & Brandler, S. (2007). Performance on temporal information processing as an index of general intelligence. *Intelligence, 35,* 123–139.

Rees, N. (1973). Auditory processing factors in language disorders: The view from Procrustes' bed. *Journal of Speech and Hearing Disorders, 38,* 304–315.

Riccio, C. A., Cohen, M. J., Garrison, T., & Smith, B. (2005). Auditory processing measures: Correlation with neuropsychological measures of attention, memory, and behavior. *Child Neuropsychology, 11,* 363-372.

Rintelmann, W. F. (1985). Monaural speech tests in the detection of central auditory disorders. In M. L. Pinheiro & F. E. Musiek (Eds.), *Assessment of central auditory dysfunction: Foundations and clinical correlates* (pp. 173-200). Baltimore: Williams & Wilkins.

Romanski, L. M. (2004). Domain specificity in the primate prefrontal cortex. *Cognitive, Affective, and Behavioral Neuroscience, 4,* 421-429.

Romanski, L. M. (2007). Representation and integration of auditory and visual stimuli in the primate vertral lateral prefrontal cortex. *Cerebral Cortex,* e-pub ahead of print.

Salvi, R. J., Lockwood, A. H., Frisina, R. D., Coad, M. L., Wack, D. S., & Frisina, D. R. (2002). PET imaging of the normal human auditory system: Responses to speech in quiet and in background noise. *Hearing Research, 170,* 96-106.

Saper, C. B. (1984). Organization of cerebral cortical afferent systems in the rat. II. Magnocellular basal nucleus. *Journal of Comparative Neurology, 20,* 313-342.

Schow, R. L., Seikel, J. A., Chermak, G. D., & Berent, M. (2000). Central auditory processing and test measures: ASHA 1996 revisited. *American Journal of Audiology, 9,* 63-68.

Seidman, L. J. (2006). Neuropsychological functioning in people with ADHD across the lifespan. Clinical *Psychology Review, 26,* 466-485.

Sherman, S. M., & Guillery, R. W. (1998). On the actions that one nerve cell can have on another: Distinguishing "drivers" from "modulators." *Proceedings of the National Academy of Sciences, 95,* 7121-7126.

Shimojo, S., & Shams, L. (2001). Sensory modalities are not separate modalities: Plasticity and interactions. *Current Opinions in Neurobiology, 11,* 505-509.

Smith, G. T. (2005). On construct validity: Issues of method and measurement. *Psychological Assessment, 17,* 396-408.

Stefanatos, G. A., Gershkoff, A., & Madigan, S. (2005). On pure word deafness, temporal processing, and the left hemisphere. *Journal of the International Neuropsychology Society, 11,* 456-470.

Stoffregen, T. A., & Bardy, B. G. (2001). On specification and the senses. *Behavioral and Brain Sciences, 24,* 195-213.

Teuber, H. K. (1955). Physiological psychology. *Annual Review of Psychology, 9,* 267-296.

Thompson, R. F., Johnson, R. H., & Hoopes, J. J. (1963). Organization of auditory, somatic sensory, and visual projection to associative fields of the cerebral cortex in the cat. *Journal of Neurophysiology, 26,* 343-364.

Tinius, T. P. (2003). The intermediate visual and auditory continuous performance test as a neuropsychological measure. *Archives of Clinical Neuropsychology, 18,* 199-214.

Walker, K. M. M., Hall, S. E., Klein, R. M., & Phillips, D. P. (2006). Development of perceptual correlates of reading performance. *Brain Research, 1124,* 126-141.

Weinberger, N. M. (2007). Auditory associative memory and representational plasticity in the primary auditory cortex. *Hearing Research, 229,* 54-68.

Weinberger, N. M., Hopkins, W., & Diamond, D. M. (1984). Physiological plasticity of single neurons in auditory cortex of the cat during acquisition of the papillary conditioned response: I primary field (AI). *Behavioral Neuroscience, 98,* 171-188.

Winer, J. A. (2005) Decoding the auditory corticofugal systems. *Hearing Research, 207,* 1-9.

Wright, B. A., Lombardino, L. J., King, W. M., Puranik, C. S., Leonard, C. M., & Merzenich, M. M. (1997). Deficits in auditory temporal and spectral resolution in language-impaired children. *Nature, 387,* 176-178.

Zatorre, R. J. (2007). There's more to auditory cortex than meets the ear. *Hearing Research, 229,* 24-30.

Zhang, T., & Formby, C. (2007). Effects of cueing in auditory temporal masking. *Journal of Speech, Language, and Hearing Research, 50,* 564-575.

CHAPTER 13

Associations Between Auditory Abilities, Reading, and Other Language Skills, in Children and Adults

CHARLES S. WATSON AND GARY R. KIDD

Introduction and Summary

The Benton-IU Project was an epidemiologic study of variables associated with children's success in learning to read (Watson, Kidd, Horner, et al., 2003). This project was epidemiologic in the sense that it included 96% of the children entering the four elementary schools of Benton County, Indiana, over a three-year period and its goal was to determine the incidence of severe reading deficits and other academic problems and the associations between those deficits and other variables. Unlike most other research discussed in this volume, the purpose of this study was not to investigate central auditory

processing disorder (CAPD), although measures commonly used to categorize children as CAPD were administered to all children, together with a wide range of other sensory and perceptual (auditory and visual), linguistic, intellectual, and cognitive variables. The goal of predicting the acquisition of reading skills in grades 1 through 4 was achieved, based on a principal components analysis of all of these variables. Measures of auditory processing were found to have almost no association with the development of reading or language skills in this population. Whether this result has any relevance to understanding CAPD has been questioned (see discussion by Cacace & McFarland, 2005) but that issue is not addressed here. This chapter simply describes the Benton-IU study and its findings in terms of the balance of several influences that are significantly related to success in learning to read and in other academic achievements. The somewhat surprising (to some investigators) finding that, in this population, individual differences in auditory spectral-temporal acuity have little or nothing to do with the development of language skills or with reading achievement is interpreted in terms of associations among these and other related variables in adult populations. Research is reviewed that demonstrates that in adults with normal auditory sensitivity, speech recognition abilities under difficult listening conditions do not covary with measures of spectral or temporal resolution. A theoretical interpretation of these results explains the apparent disagreement between the results of the Benton study and earlier studies of clinical samples tested on one or a few measures of auditory processing.

An ongoing controversy in the CAPD literature concerns the possible roles of certain auditory abilities in a variety of behavioral or social difficulties experienced by children. Difficulty in unraveling this problem begins with the lack of a definitive diagnostic test or battery of tests. That, in turn, reflects the vague understanding of the nature and number of distinct auditory abilities that humans possess. An ideal research study designed to address this problem would include several critical elements. First, it would not compare a clinical sample of children considered to be afflicted with CAPD, or with a language disorder, to a sample considered to be "normal." That design, unfortunately, confounds the criteria used to select the clinical sample with the study's outcome variables. Instead, the ideal study would include an unselected sample, representative of the general popu-

lation of children, large enough to be virtually certain to include some who would be identified as instance of CAPD (assuming the prevalence estimates of 1–5% or more to be correct). Second, a broad range of predictor and outcome variables should be measured on every child. Third, to establish both reliability and their value as predictors, the measurements should be obtained at least twice, at points in time sufficiently separated to provide a longitudinal view. The "broad range" of predictor variables should be based on current theoretical understanding, meaning the sensory, perceptual, linguistic, and cognitive measures implicated by previous research as possible causes of developmental, behavioral, or academic difficulties. A large order indeed. This is the sort of design that is often rejected as a "fishing trip" by reviewers of grant proposals. Fortunately, as in the landmark Isle of Wight Study (Rutter, 1989), such projects are occasionally accomplished, with major impact on both theory and practice. The work described in this chapter was in part motivated by Rutter's excellent example; it is hoped that it can offer a fraction of its benefits. Although our project was not specifically aimed at CAPD, that construct was among the theoretical predictors considered in assembling a battery of tests for use in a longitudinal, epidemiologic study.

Overview of the Benton-IU Project

This project was conducted in response to a request from the Benton County School Corporation for assistance in identifying children who might need special help in learning to read. This request was routed to the Indiana University School of Optometry, however the clinicians and scientists there advised that, although vision might indeed be part of the problem, it was a complex issue and several other disciplines should be included in the discussion. The result was the formation of a group of university investigators representing optometry, audiology, clinical psychology, cognitive science, experimental psychology, developmental linguistics, speech-language pathology, and special education. A review by this group of the relevant literature confirmed their preliminary conclusions that (1) there is some evidence supporting at least six or seven alternative explanations of difficulty in learning to read, and (2) no single study yet conducted has provided a comprehensive assessment of the relative contributions of the full range of hypothesized causes of reading failure.

The Benton school system therefore was advised that it could make a significant contribution to the understanding of reading problems by allowing the conduct of a large-scale study within its grade schools. In order to achieve sufficient statistical power to differentiate among the effects of several alternative postulated causes of reading problems, it was recommended that all first-grade children in Benton County should be tested for three consecutive years, which would yield a sample of approximately 500 children. Then, the entire testing program should be repeated when the children reached the fourth grade. Such a project, requiring eight hours of individual testing per child, clearly would be disruptive of regular school activities. Thus, the immediate acceptance of this proposal by the school system came as somewhat of a surprise. Not only did they provide space for the testing and help to coordinate the movement of children in and out of classes, they also provided transportation for the children's 100-mile trip to Indianapolis where the optometric and audiologic assessments were made. Parents served as chaperones on these many trips. Language skills, perception, and other cognitive tests were administered in the schools by teams of graduate students from optometry, audiology, and speech-language pathology, under the supervision of certified clinicians or special-education specialists. Possibly as a result of the favorable terms in which teachers and school administrators presented the project to the parents, participation included 96% of the children entering first grade.[1] The children in the Benton project were followed from first through fourth grades. Because three annual cohorts were included in the study, the year after the third cohort completed first grade, the first cohort had reached fourth grade and was retested on all of the same measures. Testing of all cohorts was thus completed over a period of six years.

---

[1]For others who may attempt similar projects, some common responses to funding requests for this project deserve comment. Studies not clearly motivated by a single theoretical perspective and which include a large array of measures are likely to provoke the criticism that, "It is merely a fishing trip." Another common criticism of such projects is that, "It has all been done before." Both criticisms occurred in this case, and both were wrong. Several discrete hypotheses were tested. No prior study had included the needed array of measures, sufficient numbers of unselected children, or a longitudinal design, to provide comparisons among the hypothesized causes of reading disorders. The Benton Project was, however, supported by funds obtained from Indiana University, sufficient for travel costs for the testing teams. Because the investigators had previously had considerable success in obtaining support for within-discipline projects, the largely negative responses of federal agencies to this multidisciplinary effort was unexpected. Agencies that publically support cross-disciplinary work seem remarkably unreceptive when actually confronted with multidisciplinary proposals.

Measures

We will not devote space to a justification of each of the individual measures used in this project. They are summarized in Table 13-1 and are discussed in detail in Watson et al. (2003). This list of variables may be best understood as the result of committee discussions, in which the investigators had a range of viewpoints nearly as broad as that represented in the literature on the subject of read-

TABLE 13–1. Summary of Tests Used in Grades 1 and 4 in the Benton-IU Project

Benton-IU Tests	Grade 1	Grade 4
Clinical Hearing Assessment	✓	✓
Clinical Vision Assessment	✓	✓
Developmental Test of Visual Perception (DTVP)	✓	✓
Flicker Fusion Test	✓	
SCAN test battery	✓	✓
Indiana Test of Auditory Memory and Processing Rate (ITAMPR)	✓	✓
Backward Masking		✓
Backward Digit Recall		✓
Test of Language Development (TOLD)	✓	✓*
Syntax Test	✓	✓
Morphology Test	✓	✓
Comprehensive Test of Reading Related Phonological Processes (CTRRPP)	✓	✓
Woodcock Reading Mastery Test	✓	✓*
Conner's Rating Scales	✓	✓
School-administered tests		
Comprehensive Test of Basic Skills (CTBS)	✓	
Primary Test of Cognitive Skills (PTCS)	✓	
Terra Nova (Basic Skills)		✓
Test of Cognitive Skills (TCS/2)		✓
Other measures		
ISTEP (Grade 3 only)		
SES (free lunch program)	✓	
Teacher-assigned grades (1–4)	✓	✓

*New version for Grade 4.

ing disorders. In all but a few instances, tests were selected because they were in common use in the United States by clinicians and researchers from the eight disciplines mentioned earlier. One exception was the temporal-order task developed by Tallal and Piercy (1974), for which permission could not be obtained for use in this project. A new task was therefore developed, using similar stimuli (sequences of /ba/ and /da/), and designed to independently measure temporal processing ability and memory capacity, tests of which are often confounded (Watson, Eddins, & Kidd, 1999). In general, the tests were selected to assess the contributions to reading achievement of: (1) auditory and visual sensitivity and resolving power, (2) auditory and visual perceptual processing abilities, including speech recognition under difficult listening conditions, (3) linguistic abilities, including phonological awareness and grammar, and (4) general intellectual abilities, both verbal and nonverbal.

In addition to the tests administered by the project, the schools also made available several other measures of these children's abilities and academic achievement, including tests of basic academic skills (Comprehensive Tests of Basic Skills in grade 1 and TerraNova CTBS in grade 4) and cognitive skills (Primary Test of Cognitive Skills in grade 1 and Test of Cognitive Skills in grade 4) from CTB/McGraw-Hill, as well as teacher-assigned grades for the first four years of elementary school.

The means and variances of the specific tests administered to both the first- and fourth-grade children are shown in Table 13-2. Performance of the population on these measures clearly demonstrated it to be representative of national averages for all measures, and thus likely to provide evidence that might be generalized to most other school populations in the United States.

Analyses

As noted earlier, this project was designed to determine the relative influence of various basic cognitive/intellectual, sensory-perceptual, and linguistic skills on reading achievement in the early grades. The investigators decided against preassignment of individual measures to hypothesized categories of causes, such as linguistic development, peripheral sensory resolving power, auditory or visual processing, or general intellectual ability. The reasoning was that such arbitrary assignments are generally based on untested (and sometimes unwarranted) assumptions, for example, that a given measure reflects sensory rather than intellectual or linguistic ability. Instead, the test scores were examined, through a principal components analysis, to determine how many functionally independent abilities, or factors, were required to account for the patterns of covariation among the scores.

The results of the principal components analyses (after varimax rotation) are shown in Figures 13–1A (for the data obtained in the first grade) and 13–1B (for the data obtained in the fourth grade). In Figure 13–1, the individual tests are each assigned to the factor on which they have the highest loading, with the tests ordered within each factor according to the relative strength of their loadings. Also shown for each test are the cross-loadings on each of the other three factors.

For those less familiar with factor-analytic methods presented in this format, a brief explanation may be helpful. Principal components analysis is a procedure that is commonly used to determine the number of underlying variables necessary to account for the variance in a larger set of measures.

TABLE 13–2. Stability of Measures, as Indexed by the Correlation Between Scores in First and Fourth Grades

Test	Grade	Mean	Std. Dv.	f(X,Y)
Reading Composite (CTBS, TerraNova)	1	508.76	57.17	
	4	631.80	34.75	0.63
General Visual Perception	1	98.83	12.21	
	4	101.81	11.39	0.59
Cognitive Skills Index (PTCS, TCS/2)	1	96.63	14.08	
	4	100.87	13.38	0.56
Motor-Reduced Perception	1	94.30	13.79	
	4	99.25	15.78	0.56
Rapid Digit Naming	1	34.22	10.06	
	4	17.80	4.63	0.54
Reading Comprehension	1	498.94	72.38	
	4	633.23	39.10	0.52
SCAN: Competing Words	1	9.60	2.73	
	4	9.80	3.03	0.52
Morphology	1	13.96	5.53	
	4	32.02	5.60	0.51
Reading Vocabulary (CTBS, TerraNova)	1	60.72	26.08	
	4	56.08	25.50	0.50
Math Concepts and Applications (CTBS, TerraNova)	1	525.05	68.51	
	4	626.90	36.50	0.50
Word Identification (Woodcock)	1	110.20	11.33	
	4	99.82	11.58	0.49
Math Grades (Teacher Assigned)	1	3.17	0.67	
	4	2.94	0.69	0.49
SCAN: Composite score	1	99.72	13.21	
	4	102.14	15.71	0.48
Picture Vocabulary (TOLD)	1	9.39	2.39	
	4	9.71	2.61	0.47
Word Attack (Woodcock)	1	104.22	12.04	
	4	101.35	12.98	0.47
Visual-Motor Integration (DTVP)	1	103.99	13.14	
	4	103.55	11.27	0.47
Phoneme Blending	1	14.50	5.08	
	4	21.83	3.52	0.46
ITAMPR: Rats	1	1.79	0.39	
	4	2.02	0.48	0.44
Reading Grades (Teacher Assigned)	1	2.88	1.01	
	4	2.72	0.86	0.44

TABLE 13–2. *continued*

Test	Grade	Mean	Std. Dv.	f(X,Y)
Attentiveness (Conner's Factor)	1	−0.06	0.96	
	4	0.00	1.01	0.44
Defiance (Conner's Factor)	1	−0.03	0.94	
	4	−0.06	0.93	0.45
Spatial/Nonverbal skills (PTCS, TCS/2)	1	335.03	62.68	
	4	458.54	54.41	0.45
Verbal Reasoning (CTBS, TerraNova)	1	321.89	58.49	
	4	426.81	49.59	0.41
Concepts/Nonverbal skills (PTCS, TCS/2)	1	307.71	67.87	
	4	458.54	54.41	0.41
Elision	1	9.27	4.45	
	4	19.72	4.40	0.40
Visual Memory	1	0.79	0.38	
	4	0.95	0.36	0.34
Sensitive (Conner's Factor)	1	0.01	0.99	
	4	0.01	1.00	0.32
SRT—right ear	1	8.75	7.09	
	4	7.98	7.16	0.32
SRT—left ear	1	8.14	7.33	
	4	7.54	6.96	0.31
ITAMPR: Number	1	4.84	0.97	
	4	4.02	0.86	0.30
Grammatic Completion (TOLD)	1	8.03	2.55	
	4	9.93	2.87	0.28
Syntax Test	1	39.76	5.77	
	4	45.81	3.33	0.28
SCAN—Figure-Ground	1	10.46	2.84	
	4	9.92	2.65	0.25
Memory (PTCS, TCS/2)	1	305.12	63.43	
	4	422.94	45.96	0.22
SCAN—Filtered Sounds	1	11.07	2.84	
	4	11.63	2.77	0.19
Word Recognition— right ear	1	95.44	4.69	
	4	96.57	8.92	0.10
Word Recognition— left ear	1	93.37	7.18	
	4	94.15	7.83	0.07

Measures are sorted in order of decreasing stability.

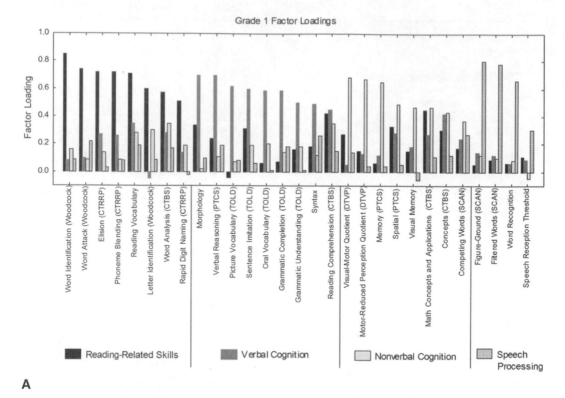

A

Figure 13–1. Factor loadings for measures obtained in the Benton-IU Project. **A.** Measures obtained in the first grade. **B.** Measures obtained in the fourth grade. The measures are grouped according to the factor on which they have the highest loading, and within each factor they are arranged from highest to lowest loading on that factor. *continues*

After measuring a group of subjects with a large number of tests, a principal components model is fitted to the data, and the proportion of the total variance accounted for is computed as the number of components (independent factors) postulated in the model is increased. A factor solution is found by identifying the number of components/factors, above which the incremental proportion of variance accounted for becomes relatively small, and the interpretation of additional factors becomes difficult. Once a solution is found, the variables can be grouped according to the factor loadings, which are the correlations between the measured variables and the derived factors. Thus, the factors can be thought of as representing independent underlying abilities, and the factor loadings indicate the degree to which performance on each test is influenced by each of the underlying abilities. The common practice is to assign names to the factors on the basis of the tests that are loaded most strongly on each of them, under the assumption that the test with the highest loading is the closest to being a pure measure of that factor.

It must be understood that, because the tests are arbitrarily selected in advance, the set of tests actually used may or may not

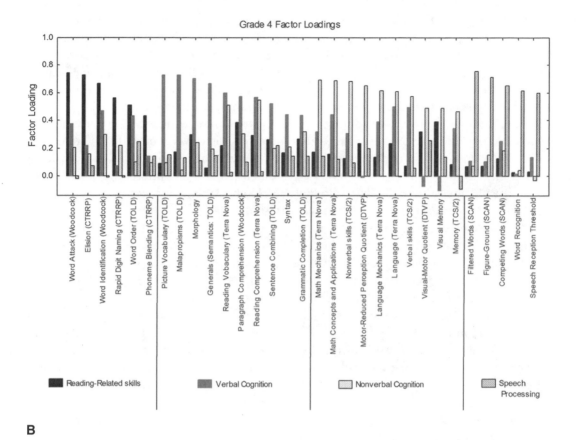

B

Figure 13–1. *continued*

happen to include measures that are highly sensitive to the strength of a specific ability. For this reason, the underlying structure of abilities is most likely to be revealed not by a single factor-analytic study, but rather by comparison among numbers of such studies, each of which utilizes different but overlapping sets of measures.

The value of principal-components interpretations of test battery data can be appreciated if one considers the volume of evidence that can be summarized by such a model. The analysis is addressed to information that can also be displayed in a correlation matrix. Thus, with 39 independent measures on each child in the current project, the resulting correlation matrix includes 741 independent correlations. One might search among these for hypothesized patterns of covariation, but a principled process for conducting this search, a formal factor analysis, is less sensitive to subjective biases and the limits of human apprehension span. The weakness of the approach is that it can yield valid estimates of the number and nature of human abilities *only if tests of each ability are included in the battery*. This limitation, however, also characterizes a great deal of research that has bypassed the test battery approach. Most studies begin with the apparent assumption that the investigators already know enough about the structure of human abilities to choose tests of them without any prior evidence of their existence. Thus, for example, it may be posited that there is a discrete auditory temporal processing ability, and that some particular test is a good measure of it. Then it might be hypothesized that this ability, of which the test is assumed to be a valid measure, is likely to predict speech recognition accuracy, which in turn might predict language development or reading achievement. This sort of theorizing would be advanced by evidence that specific abilities in fact exist, prior to conducting research on the relation between those hypothesized abilities and aspects of human development.

In the history of the study of intellectual abilities, the factor analytic techniques, originally developed by the statistical pioneer, L. L. Thurstone (1938, 1947), have been applied in hundreds of investigations. These studies mainly have been aimed at the identification of the number and nature of "primary mental abilities." This body of research was elegantly summarized by Carroll in 1993, in a text in which he reanalyzed data from a number of studies conducted over a half century of research on individual differences in cognitive abilities. For the present purpose, the most important observation included in Carroll's summary is that there appear to be independent auditory abilities for speech recognition (or "social sounds" as he termed them) and for auditory spectral-temporal acuity. That individual differences in the resolution of nonspeech sounds might *not* be closely related to the ability to understand speech seemed a surprising result, in light of the subtle spectral and temporal differences that signify different phonemes, or syllabic constituents. This conclusion is also at odds with the com-

monly accepted view that hearing-impaired persons have difficulty understanding amplified speech because they have poorer spectral or temporal acuity than normal-hearing listeners. Finally, it is also contrary to the view, among some recent theorists, that the negative consequences of CAPD for language and reading development often stem from temporal processing deficits that adversely affect speech perception (e.g., Tallal, Miller, & Fitch, 1993). A recent ASHA Working Group (2005) has concluded, for example, that (C)AP includes the auditory mechanisms that underlie (among other aspects of auditory processing) "temporal aspects of audition, including temporal integration, temporal discrimination (e.g., temporal gap detection), temporal ordering, and temporal masking." We return to this issue later, after a discussion of the factor analyses of the data collected in the Benton-IU Project.

As may be seen from the results shown in Figure 13–1A, first-grade students appear to differ in at least the following independent abilities: Factor 1. Reading-related skills (primarily, word identification and phonological awareness); Factor 2. Verbal cognition (primarily linguistic abilities); Factor 3. Nonverbal cognition (visual-spatial, visual-motor, and nonverbal conceptual abilities); Factor 4. Speech processing under difficult conditions. Comparison of the factor structure for the first-grade data (see Figure 13–1A) and that for the fourth-grade data (see Figure 13–1B) shows some slight variation, but the overall pattern of independent abilities appears remarkably similar at these two points in the children's development. The main differences are higher loadings for reading measures on the verbal cognition factor in the fourth grade and a greater prevalence of relatively large cross-loadings on the verbal and nonverbal factors for other measures in the fourth grade. The prevalence of cross-loadings on these two factors suggests that reading and other conceptually demanding tasks at the fourth-grade level place stronger demands on general intellectual abilities than at earlier ages.

Prediction of Reading Achievement

When factor models are fitted to sets of data, as illustrated by the factors illustrated in Figures 13–1A (first grade) and 13–1B (fourth grade), one consequence of that modeling is that a set of factor scores may then be computed for each individual student. These scores express each student's relative strengths on each of the factors (or factor-implied abilities). A multiple regression coefficient can be computed using factor scores for each student as predictors of that student's reading achievement. For the purposes of predicting reading achievement, the composite reading scores from the CTBS/4 (grade 1) and TerraNova CTBS (grade 4) were used as the measures of reading, and two new principal components analyses were performed with the

CTBS reading measures excluded. The new analysis produced the same four factors, and correlations between loadings for corresponding factors in the two solutions at each grade level were greater than 0.99. Multiple regression predictions of reading achievement based on first-grade factor scores and fourth-grade factor scores are shown in Table 13–3. The multiple R values for predictions of reading in grade 1 and grade 4 on the basis of measures obtained in the first grade show only a slight decrease over time, accounting for over half of the variance at both points in time. The prediction of fourth grade reading from test data collected in that same grade is somewhat better than within-year predictions of first grade reading and, as expected, substantially better than the prediction from first-grade data, accounting for roughly 74% of the variance.

An important difference between the multiple-R predictions of reading achievement in grades 1 and 4 is that they involve quite different weightings of the four factorial predictors, as shown in Table 13–3. Early reading skills measured in the first

TABLE 13–3. Correlations and Multiple-Regression Coefficients for Factor Scores from Grade 1, Predicting Reading Achievement in the First Two Grades and in Fourth Grade

| Factor | Predictions from Grade 1 Measures | | Predictions from Grade 4 Measures |
	Grade 1	Grade 4	Grade 4
Reading Related Skills	0.56	0.37	0.31
Verbal Cognition	0.43	0.48	0.60
Nonverbal Cognition	0.36	0.34	0.54
Speech Processing	0.19	0.13	0.05
Multiple R	0.81	0.73	0.86

grade were most strongly predicted by the reading-skills factor (primarily due to phonological awareness measures). The second strongest predictor was the verbal cognition factor, and the third was the nonverbal cognition factor. Ability to understand speech under difficult listening conditions (the factor including SCAN tests and other measures of speech perception), as reflected in Factor 4, was close to being a nonpredictor.

In the case of fourth-grade reading, the strongest predictor is no longer the reading skills factor (or phonological awareness), but instead it is the verbal-cognition factor. This shift is even more apparent when predicting from abilities measured in the fourth grade. The contribution of reading-related skills is somewhat lower than in predictions from first-grade data, and the contributions of both verbal and nonverbal abilities are considerably greater. This shift from lower level coding skills explaining the largest portion of the variance in early reading achievement, to higher-level cognitive functions as the dominant predictor of later reading has had many precedents in the literature. This same conclusion has been supported by longitudinal studies by Storch and Whitehurst (2002) and by Wagner, Torgeson, Rashote, Hecht, Barker, Burgess, et al. (1997). Of course, this finding does not suggest that the abilities summarized in the reading skills factor are no longer a major determinant of reading success, but rather that nearly all children have achieved them by fourth grade and therefore individual differences in some other abilities begin to account for differential reading achievement. Those other abilities appear to be verbal and nonverbal cognitive skills. This should be expected, as reading tests from fourth grade forward stress higher level abilities, for example, sentence and paragraph comprehension rather than word recognition.

Another approach to evaluating the role of various abilities in the development of reading skills is to simply examine the correlations between the individual tests and reading achievement. Table 13–4 lists all of the tests administered in the first grade, in order of their correlations with several measures of reading achievement. In this table are some measures that were not included in the principal components analyses discussed above. (These measures were excluded because they were not available for a substantial portion of the children or because they were composite measures based on other measures in the analysis.) In addition to the large drop in the apparent influence of phonological awareness measures and the increasing importance of language measures, the consistently low correlations with auditory measures also can be seen. In particular, the three measures of the ability to identify the sequence of

TABLE 13–4. Correlations Between Individual Measures Obtained in Grade 1 and Measures of Reading Achievement (CTBS Reading Composite scores) in the First and Fourth Grades. Tests Are Ordered by the Magnitude of the Correlation with Reading Achievement in Grade 1

Grade 1 Measure	Grade 1 Reading	Grade 4 Reading
Math Concepts and Analysis (CTBS)	0.64	0.50
Cognitive Skills Index (PTCS)	0.63	0.61

TABLE 13–4. *continued*

Grade 1 Measure	Grade 1 Reading	Grade 4 Reading
Word Analysis (CTBS)	0.62	0.54
Word Identification (Woodcock)	0.60	0.47
Verbal Reasoning (PTCS)	0.60	0.53
Elision (CTRRP)	0.59	0.43
Phoneme Blending (CTRRP)	0.56	0.39
Concepts (PTCS)	0.55	0.49
Morphology	0.53	0.50
TOLD (overall mean)	0.52	0.54
Word Attach (Woodcock)	0.51	0.40
Spatial (PTCS)	0.51	0.43
Letter Identification (Woodcock)	0.47	0.34
Visual-Motor Quotient (DTVP)	0.46	0.37
Sentence Imitation (TOLD)	0.45	0.49
General Vision Perception Quotient (DTVP)	0.44	0.38
Rapid Naming (CTRRPP)	0.40	0.41
Syntax	0.40	0.36
Conner Factor 3 (Attentiveness)	0.40	0.38
SCAN Composite Score	0.40	0.41
Grammatic Understanding (TOLD)	0.39	0.36
Competing Words (SCAN)	0.37	0.38
Memory (PTCS)	0.37	0.35
Oral Vocabulary (TOLD)	0.35	0.34
Picture Vocabulary (TOLD)	0.31	0.30
Grammatic Completion (TOLD)	0.31	0.35
Motor-Reduced Perception Quotient (DTVP)	0.30	0.33
Filtered Words (SCAN)	0.28	0.28
Figure-Ground (SCAN)	0.28	0.20
Visual Memory	0.27	0.31
Word Recognition (Auditory)	0.23	0.12
Speech Reception Threshold	0.21	0.16
Conner Factor 2 (Sensitivity)	−0.21	−0.13
Number-Rate (ITAMPR)	0.19	0.23
Number (ITAMPR)	0.18	0.14
Rate (ITAMPR)	0.16	0.22
Conner Factor 1 (Defiance)	−0.04	−0.05

/ba/ and /da/ syllables, derived from a test designated the ITAMPR (Indiana Test of Auditory Memory and Processing Rate), had low correlations not only with reading, but with all other variables. It is interesting that these measures do not correlate strongly with the speech measures, as some authors have assumed that poor performance in repeating heard sequences of /ba/ and /da/ syllables should be strongly related to word recognition and, indirectly, to the acquisition of vocabulary and the development of language skills (Tallal et al., 1993).

Cluster Analyses

Although conclusions based on averages are helpful, understanding why specific children have academic problems in reading or other disciplines can also be advanced by considering the special characteristics of the children who fail. One approach to determining why certain children fail is illustrated in Figure 13–2. Each child in the Benton-IU Project was characterized by a "profile" represented his or her four factors scores (reading-related skills, visual-cognitive skills, verbal-cognitive skills, and speech processing) derived from the tests administered in the first grade. The profiles were then subjected to a *k*-means cluster analysis, to identify subsets of students with similar profiles. The determination of the number of clusters is somewhat arbitrary in that the investigator selects the number of clusters into which the subjects are to be partitioned. The most useful number of clusters is just large enough to capture meaningful differences between groups of children, while preserving reasonable homogeneity within clusters. After the number of clusters has been chosen, the clustering algorithm partitions the data into that number of clusters

in such a way that the ratio of between- to within-cluster variance is maximized.

In this case, nine clusters were found to partition the children into subgroups that could be described in meaningful terms, as shown in Figure 13–2. At the extremes were clusters (Clusters 1 and 9) that included children who had uniformly high or low scores on all of the factors (abilities). The other clusters contained children with various other patterns, including high scores on one or more abilities and low on others. The children within these clusters were then identified as either successful or failing readers in grades 1 and 2, as indicated by reading grades (the composite of three reading grades assigned by two teachers, later validated by correlations with performance on standardized tests). In the clusters, failing readers are represented by solid lines and successful ones by dotted lines. The percentage of failing readers (PRF) within each cluster is indicated in the upper left corner of each panel. The percentage of math failures (PMF) among those same children is indicated in the upper right. Mean reading grades (MRG) and mean math grades (MMG) are also given, expressed in normalized (Z-score) units. Examination of these clusters reinforces the conclusions based on the multiple-regression modeling described earlier. The one constant that is associated with a high likelihood of reading failure is poor reading-related skills, and this can occur in combination with either very high or very low scores on the speech factor (which is largely determined by performance on the SCAN battery), as shown by Clusters 7 and 8. In Cluster 4, the children had below-average scores on the speech processing factor, but average abilities on all other factors. It may be informative that Cluster 4 was tied with two others for the lowest number of reading failures (2).

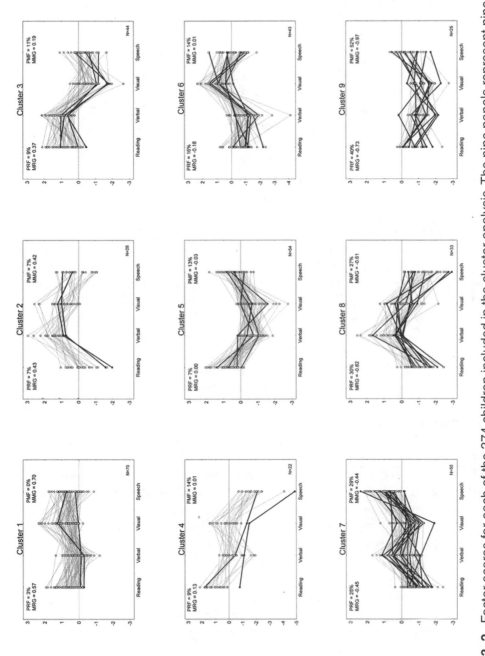

Figure 13–2. Factor scores for each of the 374 children included in the cluster analysis. The nine panels represent nine clusters of children with similar factor-score profiles. Children with unsatisfactory reading achievement (defined as more than 1 SD below the mean reading grade) are represented by solid lines and the others are represented by dotted lines. The percentage of reading failures (*PRF*), percentage of math failures (*PMF*), mean reading grade (*MRG*, in Z-score units), and mean math grade (*MMG*) are provided for each cluster. The total number (*n*) of children in each cluster is also provided in the lower right of each cluster plot.

Understanding the Weak Relations Between Spectral-Temporal Acuity and Language Skills

Some authors have predicted strong relations between individual differences in spectral-temporal acuity and speech recognition and, in turn, between speech recognition and language development. A similar case has sometimes been made for a strong relation between all of these variables and reading achievement (Bellis, 2003; Tallal et al., 1993). But the data presented in the previous section fail to support such causal connections between auditory or speech-recognition skills and these other variables. One possible explanation for this failure is that there are many reasons that children perform poorly on psychophysical tasks, only some of which are related to speech, language, and reading. Children are less able to stay on task than adults, as demanded by many sensory and perceptual tests. Thus, it is possible that strong relations between auditory acuity measures and reading or language may be obtained in adults, whereas they might have been obscured by behavioral "noise" in children (see arguments supporting this interpretation of sensory measures in young children by Viemeister and Schlauch (1992) and by Wightman and Allen (1992). Several studies of individual differences in auditory processing abilities in adults, however, have found a *dissociation* between individual differences in auditory spectral-temporal acuity and speech recognition that might also exist among the Benton children. In a study of college students, in which subjects with average or better reading skills were compared to those with reading disabilities, Watson and Miller (1993) found that auditory temporal processing ability was not a predictor of reading level. They did, however, note that poor performance on difficult psychophysical tasks might be a "marker" variable that indicates some cognitive deficits.

Studies of individual differences in auditory abilities in adult listeners with normal auditory sensitivity have been conducted by several investigators over the past 75 years. As mentioned above, the earlier studies are described in a review and reanalysis of most of the factor-analytic studies of cognitive abilities (intellectual abilities, visual and auditory processing, musicianship, and many others) by Carroll (1993). One of the few early studies of auditory abilities was by Karlin (1942), who reported that there seemed to be only very weak associations between listeners' abilities to recognize speech and their basic auditory abilities measured with nonspeech sounds. This result was replicated almost 50 years later by Surprenant and Watson (2001), who found that tests conducted with speech and nonspeech sounds loaded on different factors. However, that study used only a small number of speech tasks and did not include measures of several abilities that have been hypothesized to be critical for speech processing. The most widely discussed of these were measures of temporal resolution, especially that required for the detection of silent gaps and for gap discrimination (e.g., Glasberg & Moore, 1989; Snell, Mapes, Hickman, & Frisina, 2002; Tyler, Summerfield, Wood, & Fernandes, 1982).

In order to extend the study by Surprenant and Watson (2001), Kidd, Watson, and Gygi (2007) administered a battery of 19 auditory tests to 338 normal-hearing college students. The tests are listed in Table 13–5, together with the performance expressed in threshold units (Hz, milliseconds, or dB, as appropriate to each test) for each decile of the sample. Examination of these data

TABLE 13–5. Threshold (70% correct) Estimates for Each Decile for All 19 Subtests of the TBAC-E

Subtest	1	2	3	4	5	6	7	8	9	10
1. Pitch (ΔF, Hz)	36.27	15.45	13.99	12.55	10.96	8.78	7.88	6.59	4.95	3.08
2. Intensity (ΔI, dB)	2.37	1.16	0.84	0.70	0.65	0.55	0.48	0.45	0.34	0.29
3. Duration (ΔT, ms)	67.20	41.34	30.58	27.47	24.71	22.54	19.67	18.04	14.11	9.68
4. Pulse train (ΔT, ms)	22.83	14.92	11.53	10.38	9.69	7.94	7.26	6.21	4.93	3.22
5. Embeded tone (T, ms)	55.95	42.64	35.89	33.54	28.16	25.15	21.73	19.49	15.75	10.63
6. Temporal order tones (T, ms)	119.97	77.73	64.74	56.97	51.22	45.99	41.65	35.73	28.13	21.96
7. Temporal order syllables (T, ms)	256.11	159.45	135.64	114.15	105.42	100.10	86.94	87.59	80.89	73.70
8. Syllable ID: VC [P(c)]	0.61	0.69	0.71	0.73	0.74	0.75	0.77	0.78	0.80	0.84
9. SAM 8 Hz (mod. depth, dB)	−16.34	−20.52	−22.60	−23.48	−25.02	−25.90	−26.48	−27.31	−28.25	−29.73
10. SAM 20 Hz (dB)	−14.05	−16.52	−20.84	−22.60	−23.94	−24.53	−26.08	−26.81	−27.61	−30.87
11. SAM 60 Hz (dB)	−12.95	−17.70	−19.82	−20.60	−21.38	−22.38	−22.94	−23.55	−24.37	−25.88
12. SAM 200 Hz (dB)	−7.08	−14.30	−16.32	−16.97	−17.34	−17.94	−18.52	−19.13	−20.12	−22.04
13. Ripple noise (dB)	0.64	−1.75	−3.58	−4.70	−5.06	−5.90	−7.43	−8.08	−8.65	−11.00
14. Gap detection (T, ms)	5.10	3.06	2.59	2.34	2.00	1.83	1.54	1.40	1.09	0.71
15. Gap discrimination (ΔT, ms)	67.68	48.91	46.56	41.73	37.04	31.39	30.93	28.24	24.36	14.61
16. Syllable ID (CVC) (S/N)	−4.49	−5.77	−6.53	−7.08	−7.62	−8.03	−8.45	−8.82	−9.41	−9.35
17, Word ID (S/N)	−7.37	−9.23	−9.56	−9.96	−10.46	−10.73	−11.04	−11.54	−11.99	−13.39
18. Sentence ID (S/N)	−7.07	−7.70	−7.88	−8.05	−8.25	−8.34	−8.39	−8.57	−8.84	−9.22
19. Environmental sounds ID (S/N)	−10.73	−11.98	−12.42	−12.91	−12.94	−13.15	−13.53	−13.72	−14.17	−14.92

revealed a considerable range of performance among these "normal-hearing" (in terms of pure-tone sensitivity) subjects. The results were subjected to a principal components analysis similar to that used in the Benton study. Figure 13–3 shows the resulting four-factor solution. Factor 1 is most strongly related to energy integration, as measured either by intensity discrimination for constant-duration tones or by duration discrimination for constant-amplitude tones. Factor 2 included three tests of the depth of modulation required to discriminate between a nonmodulated noise burst and one that is temporally modulated with a sinusoid, at rates of 8, 20, or 60 cycles per second. Measurement of the detection of sinusoidal amplitude modulation of noise bursts (termed SAM noises) is considered one of the most

fundamental means of characterizing a listener's temporal resolving power (e.g., Viemeister, 1979). These measures may be used to derive temporal modulation transfer functions (TMTFs), which could represent a form of personal temporal-detail filter through which each listener must listen. This factor also included gap detection, which requires detection of a different type of amplitude modulation. One of the SAM noise tests, that for the 200-Hz modulation rate, loaded more strongly on Factor 1. This may reflect a difference in neural coding for events as rapid as 200 times per second versus those with the lower rates. Factor 3 included several tests of speech recognition, for sentences, words, and nonsense syllables, making it quite similar to the speech recognition factor identified in the Benton

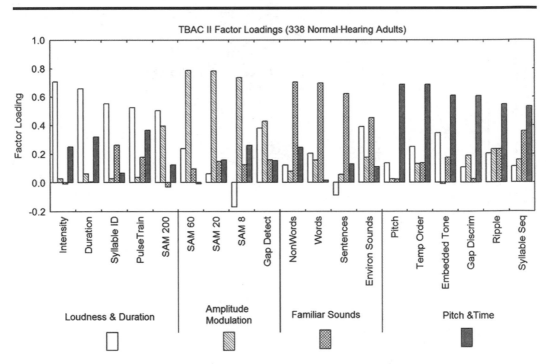

Figure 13–3. Factor loadings for each of the 19 TBAC-E subtests. Subtests are grouped according to the factor on which they have the highest loading and ordered within each factor according to the magnitude of the primary loading on that factor.

study. However, Factor 3 also included recognition accuracy for familiar environmental sounds, including dogs barking, doors closing, cars starting, electric saws, and so forth. This intercorrelation of tests for speech and nonspeech sounds leads us to characterize this ability as *familiar sound recognition* (FSR), rather than speech processing. Factor 4 included several measures of discrimination for simple and complex *unfamiliar sounds*, including word-length multitone patterns.

In addition to the auditory tests administered to the 338 listeners in the study just described, measures of their intellectual abilities were also available, in the form of their performance on the Scholastic Aptitude Tests (SATs). With the listeners' permissions, verbal and quantitative SAT scores were obtained for the subset of 235 students for whom the university had those scores on file (many had not taken those tests, or their scores were unavailable for unexplained reasons). Figure 13–4 shows the correlations between the various auditory tests and SAT scores. It can be seen that, although there were significant correlations with either verbal or quantitative SAT scores for several of the 19 subtests, all correlations were less than 0.3, indicating very weak associations between auditory abilities and intellectual abilities, as measured by these tests. Recent

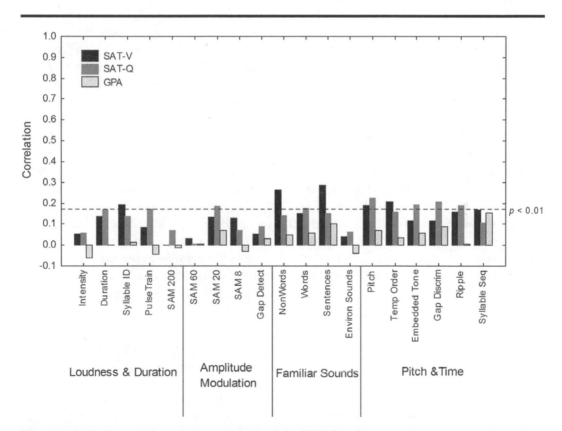

Figure 13–4. Correlations between each of the TBAC subtests and measures of intellectual abilities. The three intellectual measures shown are Verbal (*SAT-V*) and Quantitative (*SAT-Q*) Scholastic Achievement Test scores and college grade point average (*GPA*).

evidence has shown a close correspondence between SAT measures and other measures of general intelligence (IQ) (Beaujean, Firimin, Knoop, Michonskim Betty, & Lowrie, 2006; Frey & Detterman, 2004).

Space has been devoted to describing this study of auditory abilities for adult listeners with normal hearing because its results clearly support a specific interpretation of the data obtained with children in the Benton-IU Project. Speech recognition under difficult conditions, in both adults and children, appears to have little association with individual differences in either auditory acuity or general intellectual competence. But how, many will ask, can this be rationalized in light of the wealth of research showing the need to resolve the subtle spectral-temporal details that distinguish among meaningful elements of the speech code? The answer, now supported by a growing literature, is that speech is such an excellent, highly redundant code that virtually all normal-hearing listeners have sufficiently precise resolving power that they can recognize its sounds nearly perfectly, despite the considerable range of spectral-temporal acuity in this population. This conclusion, however, is restricted to relatively quiet listening conditions. When confronted with a good deal of background noise, either speech or nonspeech masking sounds, there is a considerable range of speech-to-noise ratios (S/N) required for individual listeners to recognize words or sentences at some criterion level of performance. Surpranant and Watson (2001) found this range to be roughly 7 to 8 dB, for 50% words correctly recognized, in a background of Gaussian noise. Kidd, Watson, and Gygi (in press) found ranges of 5, 6, and 2 dB S/N for words, nonsense syllables, and sentences, respectively (for 70% correct, based on the difference between the best and worst 10% of the subjects). But, in these

adult studies, it was found that speech recognition performance, even with masking noise, did not correlate with measures of spectral or temporal acuity, as discussed earlier. Watson, Qui, Chamberlin, and Li (1996) reported stronger correlations between speech recognition by eye (lip reading, with no auditory input) and pure auditory speech recognition, than between any of these recognition measures and spectral-temporal acuity. This apparently means that there is a higher level (cognitive) skill by which perceived fragments of familiar stimuli can be used to identify the stimulus of which the fragments are a part. Some listeners (or viewers) require more or better defined fragments than others to solve the problem of the identity of the stimulus. This ability was termed FSR in the earlier discussion, and it is possible that the children who score poorly on the SCAN, or have low scores on the speech processing factor in the Benton-IU Project, in fact, have poor FSR abilities. But they probably do not have problems with spectral or temporal acuity, as far as can be told from the studies reviewed here. This would be consistent with the existence of some children who have greater difficulty understanding their teacher in a noisy class room. But the Benton project data show no evidence that such a deficit in speech recognition is associated with below-average reading, language development, or other academic achievement (especially mathematics).

What Is CAPD?

This chapter began with a disclaimer, indicating that the studies described in it were not designed as investigations of CAPD. Some of the results obtained with children and with adult listeners may have some relevance to that topic, but only if questions of the association of that disorder with reading or language development are of interest. There is, however, one way that the data from the Benton project might provide direct evidence about the nature of CAPD. The study of human intellect has had definitional difficulties somewhat similar to those encountered by working groups attempting to delineate the nature of CAPD. Although there are many nuanced definitions of IQ, a pragmatic approach has been to assert that *IQ is whatever IQ tests measure*. Without intending to demean the thoughtful efforts of working groups who have attempted definitions of CAPD, it might be suggested that, as the SCAN battery is the most common single instrument used to identify persons with that disorder, one might, as a working definition, consider the possibility that *CAPD is whatever the SCAN measures*. Trivial as this suggestion may appear, it is surely true that much of the use of CAPD as a diagnostic category has been consistent with such a definition. It might therefore be of some interest to take a close look at what the SCAN appears to measure or what abilities appear to influence performance on that set of tasks. Because it was used in first and fourth grades with the Benton children, there are a large number of correlations available between the SCAN and various other measures.

Table 13–6 presents correlations between the SCAN and a selection of the primary measures of reading, language, and cognitive abilities. Correlations with the other auditory measures (the ITAMPR, Word Recognition, and Speech Reception Thresholds) are also included. (The ITAMPR includes a Number subtest, which varies the number of CVs to be recalled, and a Rate subtest, which varies the rate of presentation.) Correlations are shown in two sections in Table 6, for first- and fourth-grade mea-

sures. Examination of these correlational data should be done with an understanding of the rather low reliability of the SCAN measures (Amos & Humes, 1998), which will limit the correlations with any other variables. On the other hand, it is true that, although low reliability limits clinical usefulness, it does not render meaningless the correlations between a test and other measures. With those caveats, there does not appear to be any pattern of strong associations between the SCAN measures and any other tests administered in the Benton study. The highest correlations (those greater than 0.3, shown in bold) are those with reading, language, and cognitive skills. These correlations indicate that, although the SCAN test is a poor predictor of reading and language development, it does appear to provide some measure (albeit unreliable) of general intellectual abilities.

Correlations between the SCAN tests and other speech recognition tests are also among the highest. This, combined with the grouping of these measures in the factor analysis, suggests that the SCAN test may also be an index of the general ability to recognize speech on the basis of perceived fragments, the "FSR ability" discussed earlier. However, correlations with the ITAMPR are generally low, as are correlations between the ITAMPR and all other measures. Thus, individual differences in auditory memory and processing rate do not appear to be related to differences in the FSR ability or in any other ability measured by this large collection of tests.

The correlations in Table 13–6, along with the factor analyses of the Benton data, provide some addition information concerning the relations among the SCAN subtests and between the individual subtests and other measures. The competing words subtest has a higher correlation with the composite score and higher loadings on

TABLE 13–6. Correlations Between Auditory Processing Tests (SCAN and ITAMPR) and the School-Administered Achievement and Aptitude Tests in Grade 1 and Grade 4

Grade 1

Selected Measures	SCAN				ITAMPR	
	Filtered Words	Figure-Ground	Competing Words	Composite	Number	Rate
Vocabulary	0.29	0.28	0.31	0.35	0.16	0.13
Comprehension	0.23	0.24	0.35	0.36	0.17	0.15
Reading Composite	0.28	0.28	0.37	0.40	0.18	0.16
Math Concepts and Applications	0.15	0.18	0.29	0.29	0.19	0.16
Word Analysis	0.27	0.27	0.34	0.37	0.14	0.16
Cognitive Skills Index	0.22	0.25	0.36	0.38	0.19	0.29
Spatial	0.16	0.17	0.20	0.22	0.17	0.21
Memory	0.06	0.10	0.20	0.19	0.12	0.17
Concepts	0.19	0.21	0.29	0.31	0.13	0.24
Verbal Reasoning	0.25	0.29	0.22	0.28	0.17	0.24
TOLD (overall mean)	0.25	0.25	0.37	0.40	0.19	0.28
Word Recognition	0.36	0.39	0.08	0.23	0.04	0.10
Speech Reception Threshold	−0.16	−0.23	−0.22	−0.25	−0.07	0.02
SCAN: Filtered Words	1.00	0.52	0.24	0.52	0.09	0.12
SCAN: Figure-Ground	0.52	1.00	0.26	0.52	0.14	0.15
SCAN: Competing Words	0.24	0.26	1.00	0.91	0.14	0.17
SCAN: Composite Score	0.52	0.52	0.91	1.00	0.16	0.20
ITAMPR: Number	0.09	0.14	0.14	0.16	1.00	0.45
ITAMPR: Rate	−0.12	−0.15	−0.17	−0.20	−0.45	1.00

Grade 4

Selected Measures	SCAN				ITAMPR	
	Filtered Words	Figure-Ground	Competing Words	Composite	Number	Rate
Reading	0.20	0.21	0.32	0.30	0.14	0.18
Vocabulary	0.14	0.19	0.30	0.28	0.19	0.19
Reading Composite	0.19	0.22	0.34	0.32	0.18	0.20
Language	0.17	0.17	0.30	0.27	0.18	0.17
Language Mechanics	0.14	0.15	0.24	0.22	0.17	0.18
Language Composite	0.17	0.18	0.30	0.27	0.20	0.19
Math	0.18	0.20	0.33	0.30	0.23	0.13
Math Computation	0.23	0.22	0.28	0.29	0.20	0.14
Math Composite	0.23	0.23	0.33	0.33	0.24	0.15
Cognitive Skills Index	0.20	0.23	0.36	0.34	0.22	0.19
Nonverbal	0.15	0.17	0.28	0.26	0.20	0.15
Memory	0.07	0.13	0.16	0.16	0.11	0.09
TOLD (overall mean)	0.28	0.26	0.43	0.42	0.22	0.24
Word Recognition	0.29	0.35	0.23	0.32	0.10	0.03
Speech Reception Threshold	−0.42−	−0.28−	−0.29−	−0.36−	−0.13−	0.05
SCAN: Filtered Words	1.00	0.48	0.47	0.67	0.16	0.12
SCAN: Figure-Ground	0.48	1.00	0.47	0.69	0.13	0.13
SCAN: Competing Words	0.47	0.47	1.00	0.91	0.22	0.23
SCAN: Composite Score	0.67	0.69	0.91	1.00	0.23	0.22
Vearbal Reasoning	0.15	0.15	0.28	0.26	0.17	0.15
ITAMPR: Number	0.16	0.13	0.22	0.23	1.00	0.46
ITAMPR: Rate	−0.12−	−0.13−	−0.23−	−0.22−	−0.46−	1.00

verbal and nonverbal cognition factors than do the figure-ground and filtered-words subtests. In the first grade, this discrepancy is greater than in the fourth grade, and the competing words subtest loads highest on the verbal cognition factor (with a relatively strong cross-loading on the speech-processing factor, which includes the other two SCAN subtests). This pattern is likely due, at least in part, to the relatively low reliability of the figure-ground and filtered-word subtests (Amos & Humes, 1998), which may be lower for the first-grade children than for the fourth-grade children. However, the data also indicate that the competing words subtest differs from the other two subtests, not because it represents a separate auditory ability (as suggested by Schow, Seikel, Chermak, & Berent, 2000), but because it is more strongly (or more reliably) associated with verbal and nonverbal cognition than the other subtests.

Overall, the magnitude and pattern of these correlations provide no hints regarding the use of this battery for clinical purposes. As a further consequence, if CAPD were in fact what the SCAN appears to measure, the use of CAPD as a diagnostic category would not be supported.

General Conclusions

1. Auditory processing abilities are not significantly related to reading achievement or to the development of language skills in grades 1 through 4, in a sample of children that is closely representative of national norms in intelligence and socioeconomic status.
2. Reading achievement can be predicted with considerable accuracy on the basis of tests administered in the first grade.
3. The primary predictors of reading achievement in grades 1 and 2 are measures of phonological awareness.
4. The primary predictors of reading achievement in grade 4 are verbal and nonverbal cognitive abilities.
5. One of the main dimensions, or abilities, on which both children and adults show significant individual differences is their recognition of speech under difficult listening conditions. Adult data show this to be an ability associated with familiar sounds in general, not simply with speech, and it is therefore termed a Familiar Sound Recognition (FSR) ability.
6. The FSR ability is remarkably independent of both intellectual abilities and academic achievement.
7. If CAPD were defined as *that which the SCAN tests measure*, no meaningful clinical application could be found for it in the data from the Benton-IU Project.

References

American Speech-Language-Hearing Association. (2005). *(Central) auditory processing disorders. Report of CAPD Working Group.* Available at http://www.asha.org/members/deskref-journals/deskref/default

Amos, N. E., & Humes, L. E. (1998). SCAN test-retest reliability for first- and third-grade children. *Journal of Speech, Language, and Hearing Research, 41,* 834–845.

Beaujean, A. A., Firmin, M. W., Knoop, A. J., Michonski, J. D., Betty, T. P., & Lowrie, R. E. (2006). Validation of the Frey and Detterman (2004) IQ prediction equations using the Reynolds Intellectual Assessment Scales. *Personality and Individual Differences, 41,* 353–357.

Bellis, T. J. (2003). *Assessment and management of central auditory processing disorders in the educational setting: From science to practice.* Clifton Park, NY: Thomson.

Cacace, A. T., & McFarland, D. J. (2005). Response to Katz and Tillery (2005), Musiek, Bellis, and Chermak (2005), and Rosen (2005). *American Journal of Audiology, 14,* 143–150.

Carroll, J. B. (1993). *Human cognitive abilities: A survey of factor-analytic literature.* Cambridge, UK: Cambridge University Press.

Frey, M. C., & Detterman, D. K. (2004). Scholastic assessment or g? The relationship between the scholastic assessment test and general cognitive ability. *Psychological Science, 15,* 373–378.

Glasberg, B. R., & Moore, B. C. J. (1989). Psychoacoustic abilities of subjects with unilateral and bilateral cochlear hearing impairments and their relationship to the ability to understand speech. *Scandinavian Audiology, Supplement, 32,* 1–25.

Karlin, J. E. (1942). A factorial study of auditory function. *Psychometrika, 7,* 251–279.

Kidd, G. R., Watson, C. S., & Gygi, B. (2007). Individual differences in auditory abilities. *Journal of the Acoustical Society of America, 122,* 418–435.

Rutter, M. (1989). Isle of Wight revisited: Twenty-five years of child psychiatric epidemiology. *Journal of the American Academy of Child and Adolescent Psychiatry, 28,* 633–653.

Schow, R. L., Seikel, J. A., Chermak, G. D., & Berent, M. (2000). Central auditory processes and test measures: ASHA 1996 revisited. *American Journal of Audiology, 9,* 63–68.

Snell, K. B., Mapes, F. M., Hickman, E. D., & Frisina, D. R. (2002). Word recognition in competing babble and the effects of age, temporal processing, and absolute sensitivity. *Journal of the Acoustical Society of America, 112,* 720–727.

Storch, S.A., & Whitehurst, G. J. (2002). Oral language and code-related precursors to reading: Evidence from a longitudinal structural model. *Develomental Psycholology, 38,* 934–947.

Surprenant, A. M., & Watson, C. S. (2001). Individual differences in the processing of speech and nonspeech sounds by normal-hearing listeners. *Journal of the Acoustical Society of America, 110,* 2085–2095.

Tallal, P., Miller, S., & Fitch, H. A. (1993). Neurobiological basis of speech: A case for the preeminence of temporal processing. In P. Tallal, A. M. Galaburda, R. R. Llinas, & C. v. Euler (Eds.), *Temporal information processing in the nervous system: Special reference to dyslexia and dysphasia, Annals of the New York Academy of Sciences* (Vol. 682, pp. 27–47). New York: NYAS.

Tallal, P., & Piercy, M. (1974). Developmental aphasia: Rate of auditory processing and selective impairment of consonant perception. *Neuropsychologia, 12,* 83–93

Thurstone, L. L. (1938). *Primary mental abilities.* Chicago: University of Chicago Press.

Thurstone, L. L. (1947). *Multiple-factor analysis.* Chicago: University of Chicago Press.

Tyler, R. S., Summerfield, Q., Wood, E. J., & Fernandes, M. A. (1982). Psychoacoustic and phonetic temporal processing in normal and hearing impaired listeners. *Journal of the Acoustical Society of America, 72,* 740–752.

Wagner, R. K., Torgesen, J. K., Rashotte, C. A., Hecht, S. A., Barker, T. A., Burgess, et al. (1997). Changing relations between phonological processing abilities and word-level reading as children develop from beginning to skilled readers: A 5-year longitudinal study. *Developmental Psychology, 33,* 468–479.

Watson, B. U., & Miller, T. K. (1993). Auditory perception, phonological processing, and reading ability/disability. *Journal of Speech and Hearing Research, 36,* 850–863.

Watson, C. S., Eddins, D. A., & Kidd, G. R. (1999). The Indiana Test of Auditory Memory and Processing Rate (ITAMPR). *Journal of the Acoustical Society of America, 105,* 1236.

Watson, C. S., Kidd, G. R. , Horner, D. G., Connell, P. J., Lowther, A., Eddins, D. A., et al. (2003). Sensory, cognitive, and linguistic factors in the early academic performance of elementary school children: The Benton-IU Project. *Journal of Learning Disabilities, 36,* 165–197

Watson, C. S., Qiu, W. W., Chamberlain, M., & Li, X. (1996). Auditory and visual speech perception: Confirmation of a modality-independent source of individual differences in speech recognition. *Journal of the Acoustical Society of America, 100*, 1153–1162.

Wightman, F., & Allen, P. (1992). Individual differences in auditory capability among preschool children. In L. A. Werner & E. W. Rubel (Eds.), *Developmental psychoacoustics* (pp. 113–134). Washington, DC: American Psychological Association.

Viemeister, N. F. (1979). Temporal modulation transfer functions based on modulation thresholds. *Journal of the Acoustical Society of America, 66*, 1364–1380.

Viemeister, N., & Schlauch, R. S. (1992). Issues in infant psychoacoustics. In L. A. Werner & E. W. Rubel (Eds.), *Developmental psychoacoustics* (pp. 191–210). Washington, DC: American Psychological Association.

CHAPTER 14

Music Perception and Recognition Disorders

SIMONE DALLA BELLA

Introduction

Music is one of the highest human achievements, which transcends places and cultures. This form of art has its roots very deep in our evolutionary past. It is likely that music was not discovered by a few individuals who spread it to others. More likely, music emerged spontaneously around 40,000 years ago, as indicated by the discovery of bone flutes (Mithen, 2006; Wallin, Merker, & Brown, 2000). Even today, music appreciation and music making are not the privilege of the few. Musicians and nonmusicians alike can perceive, appreciate, and, to a certain extent, perform music (e.g., singing). Core music abilities do not require extended musical training or long-lasting exposure to music. The most elementary processes which represent the building blocks of adult music perception (e.g., the analysis of music contour or of dissonance) appear as soon as during infancy (see Trehub, 2003). In sum, there is increasing evidence that music may not be a mere cultural product

(i.e., a sort of spandrel, which appeared as a side effect of a true adaptation without a genuine adaptive function). Instead, music, at least in a very primitive form, may have played a relevant role during evolution (Huron, 2001; Mithen, 2006; Peretz, 2006; Wallin, Merker, & Brown, 2000).

The study of the neuronal underpinnings of musical processes is key to address the question of the biological roots of music. If music served a specific evolutionary purpose (e.g., to favor group cohesion; see Huron, 2001) then we expect that it should be supported by dedicated brain mechanisms which would not be recruited by other functions, such as language (herein the *specificity issue*). The interest in the neuronal underpinnings of music is not new. Neuroscientists have been fascinated by the relationship between music and the brain for more than a century (Critchley & Henson, 1977). Still, it is only during the last two decades that this topic reached momentum, as witnessed by a growing number of studies devoted to the neuronal bases of music. This increased interest has been favored by the application of neuroimaging techniques such as positron emission tomography (PET-scan) and functional magnetic resonance imaging (fMRI) to the study of the functional and neuronal organization of the musical brain. These advances recently culminated in the publication of three volumes devoted to the biological foundations of music (Avanzini et al., 2003; Peretz & Zatorre, 2003; Zatorre & Peretz, 2001) and of significant reviews of the literature (Peretz & Zatorre, 2005; Stewart et al., 2006).

A great deal of neuropsychological studies focussed on single-case studies where the effect of brain damage on musical processing was examined in individual patients. This chapter focuses on the disorders of music perception and music recognition that emerged as a consequence of brain damage (i.e., acquired amusia; Peretz, 2001). It also reviews studies on impaired music perception and recognition resulting from developmental music disorders, in absence of evident brain lesions (i.e., congenital amusia; Ayotte et al., 2002; Peretz et al., 2002; Peretz & Hyde, 2003). The behavior of patients suffering from acquired or congenital amusia is examined from the perspective of cognitive neuropsychology (Coltheart, 2001; Shallice, 1988). This approach postulates that the human mind can be modeled as an ensemble of components (i.e., modules) within a particular functional architecture (Fodor, 1983). Each module has a well-defined function (e.g., extracting melodic contour), and enjoys a certain degree of domain-specificity (e.g., Coltheart, 2001). The structure of this functional architecture is revealed by the behavior of patients following brain injury or with developmental disorders. In this framework, the performance of patients with acquired or congenital amusia is the basis for a model of the cognitive architecture underlying normal music perception and recognition.

This chapter first describes the processes underlying music perception and recognition in neurologically intact individuals, based on recent advances in music cognition. The next step is to describe various disturbances of the recognition of auditory stimuli (i.e., auditory agnosias) with particular attention to music recognition disorders. Furthermore, neuropsychological findings leading to a neuropsychological model of music recognition proposed by Peretz (1993a, 2001; Peretz & Coltheart, 2003) are reviewed. Finally, current issues in the field with regard to the functional and neuronal underpinnings of music perception and recognition are discussed.

Normal Music Recognition

Recognizing a well-known tune (e.g., "Happy Birthday") is a straightforward and effortless task for the majority of us. However, this apparent simplicity may be misleading. Music recognition is a complex function involving several cognitive operations. To recognize a well-known tune, perceptual features of the tune to be recognized, such as pitch and note durations, must be properly extracted from the auditory signal. This information is essential to construct a structural representation of the presented melody. When this percept matches with a representation stored in memory we start to feel that we know the tune. However, this is not sufficient to provide the title of the melody. The phonological representation of the title must be activated to articulate the correct title of the melody. The most important steps in music recognition and their underlying neuronal structures in healthy individuals are examined below.

Pitch Dimension

Pitch extraction and the computation of relative pitch distances in a melody is key to music recognition. Elementary pitch extraction is instantiated soon after the sound waves reach the eardrum at the level of cochlea (see Moore, 1997). From the cochlea to the primary auditory cortex through the brainstem and midbrain nuclei neuronal information is organized as a function of wave frequency (i.e., tonotopically). The right temporal cortex seems to play a priviledged role in pitch processing. For example, there is neuroimaging evidence that fine-grained pitch manipulations lead to greater activation in right auditory regions than in left regions (Zatorre, 2001; Zatorre & Belin, 2001; Zatorre, Belin, & Penhune, 2002). Both anterior and posterior secondary auditory cortex is likely involved in pitch processing (Griffiths et al., 1998; Hall et al., 2002; Hart et al., 2003). Still, it has been suggested that these regions are functionally separable (Warren et al., 2003). The posterior region would be mostly involved in processing *pitch height* (i.e., single pitch dimension, from low to high, where pitch is the logarithmic function of frequency) whereas the anterior region would be mostly involved in processing *pitch chroma* (i.e., the position of the notes relative to the musical octave, as indicated by note names).

Elementary pitch extraction is followed by further stages of melodic analysis consisting in processing *pitch contour* (i.e., the overall shape of the melody's ups and downs) and *pitch intervals* (i.e., frequency ratios between consecutive notes, indicating pitch distances) (for a review, see Dowling & Harwood, 1986). Contour is a global melodic property which is treated at the very beginning of the recognition process. The relevance of contour in recognition has been disclosed in tasks in which participants compared melodies that differed or not in terms of contour. For instance, with this paradigm, it was found that different atonal melodies were harder to discriminate when they shared the same contour than when they possessed a different contour (Dowling & Fujitani, 1971; Francès, 1958). In addition, contour is relevant in immediate recognition of novel melodies (Dowling, 1978) as well as in the recognition of familiar melodies. Distorted melodies (i.e., with changed intervals) in which the contour is spared are much easier to recognize than melodies in which the contour is destroyed (Dowling & Fujitani, 1971; White, 1960). The analysis of melodic intervals requires a more precise estimate of the pitch distance between subsequent notes (i.e., interval size). People are quite accurate in noticing distortions of intervals in familiar tunes (e.g., Bartlett & Dowling, 1980). Indeed, intervals are much more relevant to the recognition of familiar tunes stored in long-term memory than to immediate recognition of novel melodies (Dowling & Bartlett, 1981; see Dowling & Harwood, 1986, for a review). These functional differences between contour and interval processing have been mirrored by neuropsychological findings, revealing left-right brain asymmetries in the processing of these two components. The analysis of contour for melody discrimination engages right temporal structures. However, when discrimination is based on intervals, left or more bilateral involvement is observed (Peretz & Babaï, 1992; Peretz & Morais, 1988; Vignolo, 2003). A similar asymmetry was observed in infants (Balaban, Anderson, & Wisniewski, 1998).

Pitch processing cannot be limited to the analysis of contour and intervals, though. Notes and intervals exist within a given musical *scale* (e.g., C major), indicating a specific subset of pitch intervals or scale degrees (usually between five and seven). In western music the tones of the scale vary in terms of stability and are organized around a central tone, called the tonic (e.g., "C" in C major). Tones are related to each other according to a hierarchical structure (i.e., the tonal hierarchy) specifying their degree of importance (see Krumhansl, 1990, for a review). There is substantial evidence that listeners are sensitive to scale structure while perceiving and memorizing melodies (Krumhansl, 1990; Tillmann, Bharucha, & Bigand, 2000). Still, evidence is relatively scant regarding the localization of brain regions underlying the processing of the scale structure. The mesiofrontal cortex is engaged in scale processing and in treating sequences of keys activated throughout a piece (Janata et al., 2002). In other studies, simultaneously presented tones (i.e., chords) were used to evoke a tonality instead of sequential tones. The principles governing chord sequences in western music (i.e., harmonic rules) are similar to the rules governing the tonal hierarchy. For example, chords, as well as tones, are characterized by a hierarchy of stability, with the tonic chord indicating maximum stability. Neuroimaging studies showed that detecting deviations from harmonic expectancies in chord sequences engages the inferior frontal regions (the frontal operculum, corresponding to Broca's areas on the left side) bilaterally (Koelsch et al., 2002; Maess et al., 2001; Tillmann et al., 2003).

Temporal Dimension

The temporal dimension (i.e., perceived rhythm) can be divided into two main time relations. *Grouping* refers to the segmentation of an ongoing sequence into temporal groups of events (i.e., tones) based on their durational values. *Meter* indicates the extraction of the underlying temporal regularity or musical beat. Beat extraction is likely the result of attentional and/or perceptual entrainment to the temporal regularities (e.g., accent structure) of musical stimuli (Jones, 1976; Large & Jones, 1999; see London, 2004, for a review). Grouping and meter have been treated by some scholars as integrated in a hierarchical fashion, thus representing two facets of the same psychological process (Cooper & Meyer, 1960; Povel & Essens, 1985). In this case, the same pattern of accents would define both meter and the grouping structure. In contrast, others have argued that grouping and meter represent rather distinct processes (e.g., Drake, 1998; Lerdahl & Jackendoff, 1983).

Unfortunately, evidence is scant regarding the neuronal underpinnings of grouping and meter in healthy individuals. Yet, the hypothesis that grouping and meter are separate processes received some support. For example, it was shown that participants have fewer difficulties to tap a rhythmic pattern with their right hand and to tap the beat with the left hand than the reverse (Ibbotson & Morton, 1981). This suggests that grouping events based on their duration may be mostly under the control of the left hemisphere whereas beat extraction would rely mostly on the right hemisphere. In addition, there is evidence from neuroimaging that comparing metrical rhythms (i.e., sequences with time intervals characterized by integer ratios) and nonmetrical rhythms (i.e., with noninteger ratios) without reproduction may engage different neural circuitries at the level of frontal and cerebellar structures (Sakai et al., 1999). It is intriguing that areas related to motor processing (e.g., the cerebellum) are activated when perceiving and comparing rhythmic sequences (e.g., Xu et al., 2006). These findings point to a strong link between rhythm perception and motor processing. This is consistent with recent behavioral findings showing an effect of body movement (i.e., bouncing) on the way infants code meter in an auditory sequence (Phillips-Silver & Trainor, 2005).

Memory

In order for recognition to be achieved a structural representation of the tune to be recognized has to be matched to a representation stored in long-term memory. Recognition is successful when there is correspondence between the percept and stored representations. The study of the musical features involved in this matching process has received particular attention (see Snyder, 2000, for a review). For example, changes in melodic contour (Dowling & Fujitani, 1971; Dowling & Hollombe, 1977; Idson & Massaro, 1978; Kallman & Massaro, 1979) and in pitch chroma (Idson & Massaro, 1978; Kallman & Massaro, 1979; for a different view, see Deutsch, 1972) are both detrimental to recognition. In addition, the temporal dimension is less important for recognition than the pitch dimension (Hébert & Peretz, 1997; White, 1960). For instance, recognizing well-known melodies based on pitch variations is easier than when relying on melodies' rhythmic pattern (Hébert & Peretz, 1997). Still, little is known about the nature and the organization of representations in musical long-term memory. Behavioral studies in which participants were asked to sing well-known songs from memory (Levitin, 1994; Levitin & Cook, 1996) or to perform mental rehearsal (Halpern, 1988, 1989) indicate that memory representations maintain aspects of the

musical surface such as tempo and absolute pitch. However, more abstract melodic features (e.g., tonality) are also likely to be represented, as participants can recognize melodies when they are transposed to a different key (e.g., Dowling & Fujitani, 1971) and when tempo is changed (e.g., Warren et al., 1991). In addition, memory activation of the correct melody representation over time is thought to require the access and selection of potential candidates retrieved from long-term memory (Dalla Bella, Peretz, & Aronoff, 2003).

The neuronal underpinnings of musical memory are little investigated. The few neuroimaging studies devoted to this topic revealed either bilateral or preferentially left-hemisphere activations in the anterior portion of the superior temporal gyrus with additional involvement of inferior frontal and parahippocampal areas in familiarity tasks (Platel et al., 1997; Satoh et al., 2005). Another way to explore the characteristics of musical memory is to examine the brain circuitries involved in music imagery in healthy individuals. Music imagery refers to the experience of imagining music or specific musical properties in absence of actual sound stimulation. This activity requires the retrieval of musical features from long-term memory, thus uncovering their characteristics. Neuroimaging studies indicate that retrieving information from long-term memory, for example when producing a well-known tune, engages inferior frontal regions (Halpern & Zatorre, 1999; Zatorre et al., 1996). This is in keeping with the hypothesis that these regions play a relevant role in general for memory retrieval (Nyberg & Tulving, 1996). Yet, the present evidence is insufficient to draw firm conclusions about the neuronal circuitry involved in musical memory, a topic which awaits further research.

Auditory Recognition Disorders

Auditory Agnosias

It is well known that brain damage can disrupt the recognition of external stimuli (e.g., visual or auditory). The term "agnosia" indicates a loss of the ability to recognize objects, persons, sounds, shapes, or smells not resulting from elementary sensory dysfunctions. The recognition deficit can touch selectively one modality of stimuli, such as vision (e.g., Farah, 2004) or audition. In general, any impairment in the recognition of auditory events (such as speech, music, and environmental sounds) consequent to brain damage is referred to as "auditory agnosia" (Lichtheim, 1885; see Dalla Bella & Peretz, 1999; Peretz, 1993a, 2001, and Polster & Rose, 1998, for reviews). This disorder is limited to the auditory modality (recognition is possible by sight or touch) and cannot be explained by deafness or by difficulties in verbal expression.

Auditory agnosia usually occurs as a global impairment. The typical patient complains of being unable to recognize several categories of sounds (e.g., music or speech) and to hear different sounds as unintelligible noise. However, the patient can typically speak, read, and write. Yet, this impairment is not due to a deficient peripheral auditory system. Interestingly, the auditory deficit can be quite selective. A well-established distinction concerns verbal and nonverbal agnosias. The first refers to a selective loss of recognition abilities for speech sounds and the latter to a selective loss of recognition for nonverbal sounds, involving both music

and other familiar environmental sounds (e.g., animal cries, traffic noises, etc.). The existence of two kinds of auditory agnosias depending on the verbal nature of the auditory material is consistent with the hypothesis that there are two modes of auditory perception (Liberman et al., 1967; Mann & Liberman, 1983). One mode—the speech or phonetic mode—is responsible for speech processing; the other—the auditory mode— is a general-purpose system processing all the other kinds of sounds (i.e., music, environmental sounds, and voices). There is compelling neuropsychological evidence in support of this hypothesis. Several cases of agnosia for speech in absence of recognition deficits for music and/or environmental sounds were documented. Conversely, the recognition of music and/or environmental sounds can be impaired after brain injury, while speech recognition is spared. This double dissociation is illustrated in Table 14-1.[1] In cognitive neuropsychology, a "double dissociation" consists in finding at least two brain-damaged patients, one whose performance is impaired selectively in one of two tasks and a second patient with selective impairment in the other task. A double dissociation represents strong evidence in favor of functional independence between two mental faculties or processes (Coltheart, 2001; Shallice, 1988).

The distinction between verbal and nonverbal agnosias does not exhaust all possibilities, though. Music recognition abilities also fragment. Cases of selective sparing and of selective losses have been documented (see Table 14-1). The evidence is less clear for the category of environmental sounds. Although there are cases of selective sparing (Eustache et al., 1990; Tanaka, Yamadori, &

---

[1]Table 14-1 refers to data from auditory recognition tests both from patients with brain damage (i.e., with acquired amusia) and patients with developmental musical disorders in absence of brain lesions (i.e., with congenital amusia or tone deafness). The distinction between these two categories of musical disorders is discussed later.

TABLE 14–1. Case Reports of Selective Impairment in the Recognition of Speech Sounds, Music, and Environmental Sounds

Reports	Domain		
	Speech	*Music*	*Environmental Sounds*
Metz-Lutz & Dahl (1984)	−	+	+
Yaqub et al. (1988)	−	+	+
Takahashi et al. (1992)	−	+	+
Spreen et al. (1965)	+	−	−
Habib et al. (1995)	+	−	−
Laignel-Lavastine & Alajouanine (1921)	−	+	−
Godefroy et al. (1995)*	−	+	−
Mendez (2001), N.S.	−	+	−
Peretz et al. (1994), C.N. and G.L.	+	−	+
Peretz et al. (1997), I.R.	+	−	+
Griffith et al. (1997), H.V.	+	−	+
Piccirilli et al. (2000)	+	−	+
Steinke et al. (2001), K.B.	+	−	+
Ayotte et al. (2002), 11 cases of cong. amusia	+	−	+
Tanaka et al. (1987)	−	−	+
Mendez & Geehan (1988)*, case II	−	−	+
Eustache et al. (1990), case I	−	−	+
Motomura et al. (1986)*	+	+	−

+ = normal recognition; − = impaired recognition.
*during recovery.

Mori, 1987; Mendez & Geehan, 1988, during recovery), selective losses have never been observed at onset but only during recovery (Motomura, et al., 1986).

In sum, recognition processes for different auditory events are not subserved by a shared general-purpose system. More likely, recognition relies on multiple mechanisms enjoying domain-specificity. Multiple dissociations point toward two separable systems for auditory recognition, one devoted to speech and the other devoted to music. Recognition of environmental sounds may be subserved by a specialized system, as well. However, this latter category is ill-defined and requires further neuropsychological scrutiny. For the time being, the taxonomy of auditory agnosias involves verbal agnosia (or verbal deafness) and music agnosia. In addition, there are cases of patients with impaired recognition of the human voices (i.e., phonoagnosia; Van Lancker & Canter, 1982; Van Lancker & Kreiman, 1987). Phono-agnosia has been observed in absence of concurrent disorders in auditory speech comprehension (see Van Lancker & Kreiman, 1987). Still, to date, cases of impaired speech recognition with spared voice recognition have not been yet documented. However, brain areas dedicated to voice processing were uncovered in the superior temporal gyri, as revealed by neuroimaging studies (Belin et al., 2000). These findings suggest that recognizing voices may be supported by a specific neuronal mechanism. The following section focuses on music recognition disorders.

Music Agnosia

Music agnosia has been defined as a specific impairment in music recognition in absence of elementary perceptual deficits and general intellectual disorders (Peretz, 1993a, 2001). To illustrate the nature of these recognition deficits and their specificity for musical auditory material two examples of patients are described in some detail below. The first patient, IR (Peretz, Belleville, & Fontaine, 1997; Peretz, Gagnon, & Bouchard, 1998), is a right-handed woman with 10 years of formal education who was 40 years old at the time of testing. IR received little musical education. However, music represented an important part of her life. Raised in a musically inclined family (e.g., her only brother is a professional musician), IR was used to listen to music and to sing as an amateur before her brain accident. She was a restaurant manager when at 28 years of age she underwent successive brain surgeries for the repair of cerebral aneurysms on the right and left sides of the brain. After surgery, IR showed bilateral lesions invading the auditory cortex and extending to the frontal regions on the right side (e.g., Patel et al., 1998). When tested about 10 years following the cerebral accident, IR's cognitive abilities were relatively intact. IR had no trouble to carry a conversation, and her intellectual and memory abilities were normal for somebody with her level of education and age. The only salient deficits were a mild articulation difficulty and a left hemiplegic arm. Still, IR complained that she was not capable of perceiving and recognizing music as before the accident, and that she was no more able to carry a tune. IR is a pure case of *amusia without aphasia*, a neuropsychological condition which has been described for more than century (see Marin & Perry, 1999, for a review).

A thorough exam of IR's musical abilities confirmed that IR was incapable of providing the titles of well-known tunes, such as "Happy Birthday." Recognition improved when a IR had to choose the correct title in a forced-choice task. Still, IR's performance was definitely below the norm provided by a group of matched control participants. IR was unable to relearn melodies which she was no long able to recognize, as if novel melodies did not leave any trace in her memory. In contrast, IR's ability to recognize words, environmental sounds, and voices was spared, thus indicating that IR is a pure case of music agnosia. IR deficits were not limited to music recognition, though. Her performance was deficient when she was asked to discriminate melodies varying on the pitch or on the temporal dimension, revealing that her perception of relevant musical features was dramatically impaired. It is likely that impaired pitch and temporal perception hindered IR's ability to access the memory representations of well-known tunes. Curiously, however, despite her major perceptual deficits, IR claimed that she was still able to appreciate music. A further systematic assessment revealed that IR can still distinguish happy from sad music, and is sensitive to the manipulation of musical parameters, such as tempo and mode, which are relevant for emotional judgments (Peretz, Gagnon, & Bouchard, 1998). This intriguing finding points to a separation between the mechanisms responsible for music recognition and those involved in the recognition of emotions conveyed by music. Cases of music agnosias similar to IR were documented in the literature (e.g., Griffiths et al., 1997; Peretz et al., 1994; Peretz, 1996; see Peretz, 2001, for a review). Disorders of music recognition are in general associated with bilateral (Peretz et al., 1994; Peretz, 1996) or unilateral damage (Griffiths et al., 1997) of the superior temporal regions, in particular involving the right insula (see Ayotte et al., 2000).

IR is a pure case of music agnosia consequent to brain damage. However, a brain insult is not the only condition leading to impaired music recognition. Congenital brain anomalies can bring to a halt the development of processes needed for normal music perception and memorization. This condition, referred to in the literature as tone deafness, dysmusia, or dysmelodia has been thought to exist for more than a century (e.g., Geshwind, 1984; Grant-Allen, 1878; see Peretz & Hyde, 2003, for a review). Tone deafness has been recently named "congenital amusia" by Peretz and collaborators (Peretz et al., 2002; Peretz & Hyde, 2003), referring to the "observation of musical failures that cannot be explained by obvious sensory or brain anomalies, low intelligence nor lack of environmental stimulation to music" (Peretz & Hyde, 2003, p. 363). Congenital amusia is observed in about 4% of the population, as reported in a study conducted by Kalmus and Fry (1980) who asked a large group of participants to detect erroneous pitches inserted in well-known melodies. However, the drawback of this estimate is that it is based on a single task focussing on pitch processing abilities. The

incidence of congenital amusia may vary as a function of the task used to assess musical abilities.

Although congenital amusia has been "in the air" for a long time, this condition has been subjected to systematic scrutiny only during the last decade (e.g., Ayotte et al., 2002; Peretz et al., 2002; Peretz & Hyde, 2003). A prototypical case of congenital amusia named Monica was recently described by Peretz and collaborators (Peretz et al., 2002). Monica is a French-speaking woman in her early forties at the time of testing. She worked as a nurse before deciding to start a Masters degree in Mental Health (for a thorough description, see Peretz et al., 2002). Monica did not present signs of intellectual or neurologic disorders. In addition, she had no psychiatric and neurological history, and she presented normal hearing. Magnetic resonance imaging did not reveal any evidence of brain anomaly.

Monica responded to a newspaper advertisement addressed to people with musical difficulties (i.e., without musical ear, tone-deaf). She overtly complained of being "musically impaired." Interestingly, not all self-declared tone-deaf individuals are really impaired in formal tests (see Sloboda, Wise, & Peretz, 2005). However, Monica is a genuine congenital amusic. Like IR, she presented the typical profile of musical agnosia. Monica suffers from a lifelong disability to perceive and recognize music, sing, and synchronize with music (e.g., in dance). Unlike IR, however, Monica complained of being unable to appreciate music which sounded to her like noise. This impairment is unlikely the result of lack of exposure to music or of a musically deprived environment. During her childhood and adolescence, Monica took part in musical activities, such as a church choir and a high school band, which are normal at that age. Still, she did so mostly under social pressure, being aware of her difficulties with music.

Monica was submitted to a systematic exam of her intellectual, musical, and nonmusical abilities. Her performance was excellent in tests of general intellectual abilities, with an IQ of 111 (i.e., above average) and good memory for both verbal and nonverbal information. She was equally successful in tasks requiring the recognition of nonmusical auditory stimuli, such as spoken words and environmental sounds. Thus, Monica's recognition deficit is limited to the music domain. Monica's music perception and memory for music was dramatically impaired, as revealed by the Montreal Battery of Evaluation of Amusia (MBEA; Peretz, 1990; Peretz, Champod, & Hyde, 2003). MBEA is a battery which serves to test music perception and incidental memory for music usually in patients with brain damage (e.g., Peretz, 1990). The battery includes discrimination tests in which two novel short melodies are presented and participants have to say whether they are same or different. When different, melodies vary along either the pitch dimension (three tasks target different pitch aspects) or the time dimension (i.e., notes' duration). The battery includes an additional metrical task (i.e., novel musical sequences written in binary or ternary metrum must be classified as "marches" or "waltzes") and an incidental memory task. Monica performed most of these discrimination tasks involving pitch and temporal variations below chance. These tasks are typically performed with little effort by individuals without musical training of Monica's age. Interestingly, however, Monica performed above chance in the metrical task, thus indicating that she was still able to process durations in order to extract a metrical pattern from musical sequences.

These findings suggest that Monica's recognition deficits may be rooted mostly in her deficient pitch perception. This hypothesis has been examined by asking her to detect a pitch change (with various pitch distances) in a sequence of five tones (Peretz et al., 2002). In this test, Monica exhibited a striking deficit in the perception of pitch intervals, as she was unable to perceive a descending pitch interval of 11 semitones. With ascending intervals her performance improved, but she was still unable to perceive the smallest interval in western music (i.e., a semitone). Hence, it is likely that Monica's music agnosia stems mostly from her pitch discrimination deficit, which hinders the activation of the proper representation in musical memory.

Cases like Monica are not very rare in the general population. A few patients suffering from congenital amusia have been uncovered during the last years (e.g., Ayotte et al., 2002). These otherwise normal individuals have been characterized as congenital amusics based on the results obtained in the MBEA. Participants with a general MBEA score below two standard deviations from the mean of a group of nonmusicians were treated as congenital amusics (Peretz, Champod, & Hyde, 2003). This impairment was recently related to anatomic anomalies (i.e., a reduction in white matter concentration) in the right inferior frontal gyrus, as revealed by voxel-based morphometry (Hyde et al., 2006). Like Monica, other congenital amusics were always impaired in the pitch domain, whereas their time perception, as revealed by the MBEA, quite often was spared. This finding was confirmed in a further study contrasting pitch discrimination to time discrimination (Hyde & Peretz, 2004). However, further tests requiring beat and meter extraction (e.g., sensorimotor synchronization tasks) revealed that most congenital amusics are also impaired in temporal processing (Dalla Bella & Peretz, 2003). It is worth noting that the MBEA is biased toward the pitch dimension, because it includes three tasks tapping pitch processing abilities and two tasks requiring the processing of durations. In addition, it is possible that self-declared congenital amusics pay more attention to the fact of being out of tune than out of time (e.g., performing a wrong note when singing; see Sloboda, Wise, & Peretz, 2005). Thus, the prevalence of pitch discrimination disorders may be partly related to amusics' selection criteria and to the pitch-oriented definition of tone deafness in the general population. Finally, congenital amusia is diagnosed based on perceptual criteria through the MBEA. Still, deficits in music performance, such as poor singing, are often associated to tone deafness (Ayotte et al., 2002; Sloboda, Wise, & Peretz, 2005) and sometimes occur in a pure form in absence of perceptual impairments (Dalla Bella, Giguère, & Peretz, 2007). Thus, additional tasks including measures of music performance (e.g., synchronization in tapping tasks and singing) should complement the perceptual and memory tests of the MBEA.

To sum up, music perception and recognition disorders can emerge following brain damage or developmental music disorders. As the cases of IR and Monica illustrate, however, different causes can bring about recognition deficits (e.g., impaired pitch discrimination). The following section describes a neuropsychological model proposed by Peretz (1993a, 2001; Peretz & Coltheart, 2003) specifying the functional mechanisms underlying music recognition.

Fractionation of Musical Abilities

It is a regular observation in neuropsychology that brain injury can produce highly selective deficits by affecting one function

(e.g., speech recognition), while leaving other functions intact (e.g., music recognition). This observation is tied to the concept of specificity, indicating that the brain is structured in such a way that different cognitive functions are carried out by separate processes which are supported by dedicated neuronal circuitries. According to this idea, cognitive functions, or at least some of them, are likely to be functionally and anatomically independent in the brain, thus dissociable as a consequence of brain damage or developmental disorders. In neuropsychological terms, specificity can generally be assimilated to selectivity (Shallice, 1988).

Several double dissociations have been observed in patients with music agnosia (see Peretz, 2001, for a review), indicating that the music recognition system fractionates as a result of brain injury. Neuropsychological data have proven useful to build a viable model of the functional architecture of the normal music recognition system. A model has been put forward about 15 years ago by Peretz (1993a) and revised since based on new neuropsychological evidence (Peretz, 2001; Peretz & Coltheart, 2003; see also Carrol-Phelan & Hampson, 1996). The model specifies the perceptual and cognitive processes required to recognize a single musical excerpt formed by a single voice (i.e., without harmony), as compared to single word recognition. A simplified version of the original model proposed by Peretz and Coltheart (2003) is illustrated in Figure 14–1.[2] In the full version of the model, other modules related to emotional processing and to music performance (e.g., singing and tapping) were included. For simplicity, these processes have been omitted from Figure 14–1 as they do not pertain *strictu sensu* to music recognition.

---

[2]This model was built on the basis of neuropsychological evidence from patients with brain damage. Still, as it is a model of normal recognition, it can be used to identify the mechanisms whose development was brought to a halt in congenital amusia.

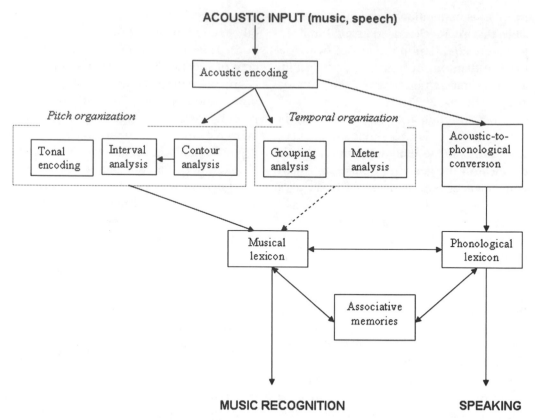

Figure 14–1. Cognitive model of music perception and recognition. Simplified version of Peretz and Coltheart's model (2003).

The model postulates that the auditory input (e.g., music or speech) undergoes elementary auditory analysis leading to the extraction of basic acoustical features. These processes, which are not specified in detail in the model, are common to the analysis of speech and music material. Deficits of the extraction of elementary acoustical traits would hinder the recognition of all categories of sounds. Following acoustical analyses, depending on the nature of the stimulus (e.g., linguistic or musical), the information is sent to one of two separate routes devoted to speech or music recognition. Each of these two routes can be independently disrupted, thus modelling purely musical and speech recognition disorders (see above). Note that the model suggests complete independence of the musical and speech recognition route. However, the extent to which different modules enjoy domain-specificity is a more complicated issue, which is discussed in the following section.

Melodic Processing Versus Time Processing

The music recognition system includes two main routes leading to a structural representation of the presented melody which will activate a representation in musical memory (i.e., the musical lexicon). The *melodic route* deals with the analysis of tunes' pitch organization (e.g., needed to provide the names of the notes contained in a melody). The *temporal route* is responsible for processing melodies' temporal organization (i.e., musical rhythm), and is important to determine when a given note occurs in time. According to the model, the analysis of the melodic and temporal information occurs independently and in parallel. This is not trivial. In music theory, the melodic and temporal dimensions have been often treated independently (e.g., Dowling & Harwood, 1986). Still, there is evidence in music cognition that melody and temporal information are processed in an integrated fashion both in perception and in memory (e.g., Bigand, 1997; Boltz & Jones, 1986; Jones, 1987). Neuropsychological data, however, point toward a separation of the two dimensions. Several double dissociations between melodic and temporal processing were reported in both music perception and performance. Isolated deficits of pitch processing with spared temporal processing following brain damage were documented in singing (see Dorgueille, 1966), music perception (Ayotte et al., 2002; Fries & Swihart, 1990; Liégeois-Chauvel, et al., 1998; Peretz, 1990; Peretz et al., 1994; Piccirilli et al., 2000; Satoh et al., 2005), and music reading (Brust, 1980, case 1; Fasanaro, et al., 1990; Judd, Gardner, & Geshwind, 1983; Horikoshi et al., 1997; see Hébert & Cuddy, 2006, for a review). In the perceptual domain, most of these patients were able to discriminate melodies based on their temporal structure; still, they were deficient in distinguishing two melodies when pitch was locally manipulated. A similar dissociation was observed in patients suffering from congenital amusia (Ayotte et al., 2002; Hyde & Peretz, 2004). The reverse dissociation (i.e., impaired rhythmic processing with spared melody) was described in patients with brain damage in perception (Brust, 1980, case 2; Mavlov, 1980) and reading

(Assal, 1973; Dorgueille, 1966; Midorikawa & Kamamura, 2000, 2003).

Although melodic and temporal processing nicely dissociate at a functional level, it is unclear whether these processes engage separate brain regions. Various lesions bring about disturbances of pitch or temporal processing (for a thorough review, see Stewart et al., 2006). Deficits of pitch processing were observed in particular following damage of the right temporal cortex (e.g., Zatorre, 1988). In general, this finding is consistent with the results obtained in neuroimaging studies. However, left temporal damage was found to disrupt melody discrimination based on specific pitch properties (i.e., interval information; Ayotte et al., 2000; Liégeios-Chauvel et al., 1990; Peretz, 1990), thus showing that both hemispheres are engaged in pitch processing. Deficits of temporal processing occurred after lesions of the right temporal auditory cortex (e.g., Fries & Swihart, 1990; Wilson, Pressing, & Wales, 2002), causing difficulties in generating a steady pulse and in tapping the beat. However, rhythmic deficits also resulted from left-hemisphere lesions (e.g., Mavlov, 1980). It is noteworthy that temporal processing has also been associated with subcortical structures, such as the basal ganglia and the cerebellum, which play a major role in motor and perceptual timing (e.g., Harrington, Haaland, & Hermanowicz, 1998; Ivry & Keele, 1989; see Ivry & Spencer, 2004, for a review). Still, in these studies timing was studied with stimuli which were not embedded in a musical context. Hence, it is difficult to draw firm conclusions on the brain localization of timing mechanisms in music.

Fractionation of Melodic Processes

The melodic route includes three modules devoted to the analysis of melodic contour (i.e., the overall shape of the melody's ups and downs), intervals (i.e., frequency ratios between consecutive notes, indicating pitch distances), and scale (i.e., specific subset of pitch intervals or scale degrees). Dissociations between these processes were found following brain injury. Patients with brain damage involving the left hemisphere exhibited difficulties to discriminate melodies based on interval information. Right-hemisphere lesions, in contrast, affected melody discrimination based on both contour and intervals (Ayotte et al., 2000; Liégeois-Chauvel et al., 1998; Peretz, 1990). A plausible interpretation of this finding is that global pitch features (i.e., melodic contour) are analyzed first, an activity which is likely to be supported by the right-hemisphere. Subsequently, melodic contour would pose the bases (i.e., provide anchorage points) needed for the extraction of finer pitch information (i.e., intervals). This activity would be supported by left-hemisphere structures (see Peretz, 2001). The dependence of the interval processing mechanisms on contour analysis is represented in the model by an arrow joining the two modules. The dissociation between contour and intervals is consistent with the results obtained in lateralization studies (e.g., Bever & Chiarello, 1974; Peretz & Babaï, 1992; see Peretz & Morais, 1988, for a review), showing that contour processing is tied to the right hemisphere whereas interval processing is linked to the left hemisphere.

The third component of the melodic route deals with scale processing (i.e., tonal encoding of pitch). Evidence is scant regarding tonal encoding in brain-damaged individuals. Hence, despite the fact that tonal encoding is mediated by several cognitive components, in the model the processes underlying tonal encoding have been summarized by a single module. Impaired tonal encoding was found in aphasic patients who did not exhibit the usual superiority

effect for tonal sequences over nontonal ones when comparing pairs of melodies (Francès, Lhermitte, & Verdy, 1973). A similar impairment was found in another patient (Peretz, 1993b) using the probe-tone paradigm (Krumhansl & Kessler, 1982; see Krumhansl, 1990, for a review). In this paradigm a context melody or chord is presented followed by a tone (i.e., the probe tone), selected among the degrees of the scale; participants have to rate to what extent the probe tone fits with the context. The obtained tonal profile reflects participants' sensitivity to the tonal structure of music. The patient reported by Peretz (1993b), GL, was not sensitive to the tonal structure of music, as assessed by the probe-tone task. Pitch was not coded in terms of its position within the musical scale. Still, GL was able to perceive pitch in terms of contour and intervals. The opposite dissociation was encountered in a patient who was able to encode pitch according to the scale, still exhibiting impaired pitch discrimination abilities (Tramo, Bharucha, & Musiek, 1990). Yet, these dissociations await empirical confirmation, as different methods and tasks were adopted in these case studies.

Fractionation of Temporal Processes

The temporal route includes only two separate components, one devoted to grouping processing (i.e., segmentation of an ongoing sequence into temporal groups of events based on their durational values), the other to meter (i.e., to the extraction of underlying temporal regularity or musical beat). Neuropsychological evidence in support of the distinction between grouping and meter comes from studies with the tapping paradigm, in which patients were asked to tap the beat or generate a steady pulse.

Patients with right temporal lesions were no longer able to extract the beat (i.e., they could not tap along with it) but were still able to discriminate and reproduce irregular temporal sequences (Fries & Swihart, 1990; Wilson, Pressing, & Wales, 2002). Additional evidence of a dissociation between meter and grouping was provided with perceptual tasks. Patients with right anterior lesions of the superior temporal gyrus had difficulties in categorizing the appropriate meter; yet, their ability to discriminate rhythmical patters was spared (Liégeois-Chauvel et al., 1998). The opposite dissociation (i.e., impared grouping with spared meter) was also observed in patients with a left-hemisphere lesion (Di Pietro et al., 2004).

Lesion localization in single cases leading to grouping or meter deficits is consistent with data from normal finger tapping, showing that meter processing involves right hemisphere structures whereas grouping engages the left hemisphere. To my knowledge, disturbances of the perception of grouping and meter in music after lesions of subcortical structures, such as the cerebellum and the basal ganglia, which are known to be involved in temporal processing, are little explored. In a recent study, however, it was found that dysfunctions of the basal ganglia-cortical circuitry, as observed in Parkinson's disease, affect sensorimotor synchronization with musical and nonmusical stimuli, but sparing time perception (Laskowska et al., 2006; but see Harrington, Haaland, & Hermanowicz, 1998).

Musical Long-Term Memory: The Musical Lexicon

According to the model, pitch and temporal information is sent to musical memory. This long-term memory system, referred to as "musical lexicon," "is a representational system that contains all the representations of the specific musical phrases to which one has been exposed during one's lifetime" (Peretz & Coltheart, 2003, p. 690). One strong assumption of the model concerns the nature of the representations contained in musical long-term memory. The musical lexicon is treated as "a perceptual representation system that mediates music recognition . . . representing information about the form and structure of events, and not the meaning or other associative properties" (Peretz, 2001, p. 533). It is noteworthy that pitch information has a privileged access to the musical lexicon, as compared to temporal information. This is underscored in the model by the full and dotted arrows indicating the flow of pitch and temporal information reaching the musical lexicon. That the temporal dimension is less important for recognition than the pitch dimension is known from the study of normal recognition (Hébert & Peretz, 1997; White, 1960). This is confirmed by neuropsychological evidence of patients with music agnosia exhibiting impaired pitch perception in absence of impairment in discriminating and retaining temporal patterns (Peretz et al., 1994). Even though these patients could theoretically use the spared temporal route to access the repertoire, thus leading to recognition, they still exhibited impaired performance at recognizing well-known tunes.

Lesion studies showed that, in most of the cases, disturbances of musical memory co-occur with deficient pitch processing (e.g., Ayotte et al., 2000; Peretz, 1994; Piccirilli et al., 2000). Still, there are cases where impaired recognition is observed in absence of major deficits in the perception of musical patterns (Eustache et al., 1990; Peretz, 1996). In these cases, recognition deficits are likely to result from impaired musical memory or impaired access to the repertoire. In addition, the impairment in recognizing well-known musical tunes can be very specific, in absence of concomitant deficits in recognizing songs' lyrics and environmental sounds (Peretz, 1996; see also Samson & Zatorre, 1992, with novel melodies). In sum, these findings point to recognition mechanisms for music in which perception and memory are separated. This is not unusual in neuropsychology and goes back to the distinction between apperceptive and associative agnosias put forward by Lissauer more than a century ago (1890). In apperceptive agnosias the recognition deficit is due to deficient perception which prevent from building an appropriate structural representation of the presented stimulus, thus hindering the activation of the matching memory representation. Associative agnosias are characterized by normal perception, but impaired association of the percept with the representation in memory. Similar distinctions between perception and memory characterize neuropsychological models of face, object, and word recognition (e.g., Ellis & Young, 1988; Rapp, 2001).

Right-temporal lesions have been found to affect retention of novel melodies more than left-hemisphere damage (Samson & Zatorre, 1992). However, right hemisphere dominance is less evident with recognition of well-known tunes. Impaired recognition of familiar melodies was observed following both left-hemisphere and right-hemisphere lesions (Ayotte et al., 2000; Peretz, 1996; Peretz et al, 1994). However, more evidence is needed to draw firm conclusions about the localization of long-term musical memory and of coding and retrieval mechanisms in the musical lexicon.

The model postulates separate memory representations for music and speech information (i.e., musical lexicon vs. phonological lexicon). This is particularly relevant in the case of songs, where music and language are strictly related. Whether music and text are represented separately in memory or rather in an integrated fashion is a long-lasting debate. This question has been addressed in normals by asking participants to recognize the music, the text, or both of novel songs previously heard. Neurologically intact listeners revealed better recognition when text was matched with music, as previously presented (i.e., match songs) than when the melody of one song and the lyrics of another song were matched (i.e., mismatch songs) (Crowder, Serafine, & Repp, 1990; Serafine, Crowder, & Repp, 1988; Serafine et al., 1986). Similar results were obtained in epileptic patients following unilateral temporal lobe resections (Samson & Zatorre, 1991). These findings were treated as evidence that melody and lyrics are integrated in memory. However, as mentioned above, brain injury can selectively impair musical memory for well-known songs while sparing the recognition of the lyrics (Peretz et al., 1994). This dissociation is supported by psychophysiological evidence, showing that incongruities in speech and music elicit distinctive brain potentials (Besson et al., 1998). In sum, the debate on the representation of text and music in songs is not closed, yet. There is a need for more neuropsychological studies assessing recognition for speech and lyrics using both familiar and unfamiliar materials, and more differentiated tasks.

After the Repertoire

The activation of the correct representation of the presented tune in the repertoire, typically accompanied by a feeling of knowing the melody, is followed by the production of the title. This signals the end of the recognition process. Title production requires the access to verbal memory for titles, to phonological representations, and eventually involves word articulation. All these mechanisms are not illustrated in the model, but summarized by the label "Recognition." A further link exists between the musical lexicon and associative memories, that is episodic memory traces tied to a given musical piece (e.g., the circumstances in which we listened to that musical piece for the first time). The activation of these memory traces can cue the appropriate representation in the musical lexicon, thus favoring recognition. Associative memories can be activated both from the musical code and from the linguistic code.

Current Issues

During the last two decades an increasing number of neuropsychological studies has led to a better understanding of the functional and neuronal processes underlying music perception and recognition. Nonetheless, there are a few issues which await further research, some of which are briefly mentioned here.

On major issue concerns the degree of specificity of the modules involved in music recognition (i.e., the specificity issue). Within the melodic route it is likely that the mechanisms engaged in processing melodic contour serve in general to treat pitch direction, regardless of the domain. Processing pitch direction in music and speech (i.e., intonation) may require the same brain circuitry. This possibility is supported by neuropsychological evidence. Bilateral temporal lesions were found to affect the processing of both melodic contour and speech prosody (Patel et al., 1998; see Patel & Peretz, 1997, for a review). To date, there is no report of dissociations between the perception of music contour and speech intonation following brain damage. In contrast, the processing of musical intervals and tonal encoding appear as more specific to the music domain than contour processing. Continuous pitch variations typical of speech intonation have little in common with discrete pitch units (i.e., notes), with stable intervals and ruled by a hierarchy of importance (i.e., the tonal hierarchy) as observed in music. Still, neuroimaging data suggest that the mechanism underlying expectancies engendered by music's tonal structure (i.e., musical grammar) and expectancies resulting from linguistic grammar may be mediated partly by similar brain regions (e.g., Koelsch et al., 2002; Maess et al., 2001; but see Bigand, Tillmann, & Poulin-Charronnat, 2006, for a critical view). Within the temporal route, it is likely that both grouping and meter processing are supported by general-purpose mechanisms rather than by domain-specific processes (Peretz & Coltheart, 2003). This is consistent with the general idea that durational patterns, regardless of the context in which they occur (e.g., musical or linguistic) and of the modality (e.g., visual or auditory), engage the same cognitive modules (see Buhusi & Meck, 2005, for a review). For example, the possibility of nonauditory supramodal mechanisms devoted to temporal pattern analysis and recognition which can be impaired following brain damage has been raised in the past (Mavlov, 1980). Yet, it is noteworthy that studies comparing different domains and different modalities with the same timing tasks (e.g., tapping) are rare (e.g., Dalla Bella & Peretz, 2003; Laskowska et al., 2006; Repp & Penel, 2002, 2004). Thus, the question of domain- and modality-specificity for grouping and meter processing needs further scrutiny.

In the full version of the model, the same modules which served for melody recognition are supposed to be engaged in other production tasks such as singing from memory or tapping along with the beat of music (see Peretz & Coltheart, 2003). The mechanisms underlying these production tasks are underspecified in the model (i.e., they are just labeled at the output side of the model), which is truly focused on perceptual and memory processes. Still, there are cases of patients with brain damage (Schön et al., 2004) or with developmental disorders (Dalla Bella, Giguère, & Peretz, 2007) revealing impaired vocal performance with spared perception. This indicates that the original neuropsychological model of music perception and recognition should be extended to account for deficits of music performance which are not the mere outcome of deficient perception (for an example, see Schön et al., 2004).

The last issue regards the explanatory power of the presented model. As several models in cognitive neuropsychology (see Rapp, 2001), Peretz and Coltheart's model provide a quite static description of cognitive processes, thus neglecting the time dimension. For example, the model does not account for the time course of the recognition process (e.g., when the feeling of knowing the melody emerges, when the listener is certain of the identity of the tune, and so forth). In this respect, it has been demonstrated that a cohort model of music recognition is quite appropriate to account for the time-course of melody recognition and for differences due to musical expertise and familiarity (Dalla Bella, Peretz, & Aronoff, 2003). Peretz and Coltheart's model would benefit from the introduction of more dynamic aspects (e.g., the progressive selection of candidates in the musical lexicon), which would increase the model's explanatory power.

Conclusions

This chapter thoroughly examined the main disorders of music perception and recognition, subsequent to brain damage (i.e., acquired amusias) or resulting from developmental music dysfunctions (i.e., congenital amusia). Acquired amusias have been related to the malfunctioning of various functional modules after brain damage, such as those responsible for treating melodic contour or grouping events into temporally meaningful units. The extent to which these processes are specific to music or rather general-purpose mechanisms (e.g., supra-modal processes) still remains a matter of discussion. Congenital amusia mostly has been treated as the outcome of a more elementary auditory deficit, involving deficient pitch discrimination. Interestingly, regardless of the different causes underlying acquired and congenital amusias, their outcome can be very similar. Patients are unable to recognize well-known music, to perceive music properly, and sometimes cannot appreciate music like others do. When music deficits emerge early during development, such as in the case of congenital amusia, these disturbances may significantly impact individuals' normal functioning. Music accompanies several social activities which are common during the school years (e.g., taking part in a church choir). In these contexts, the inability to react to music like others represents a source of stress, and sometimes can lead to group exclusion.

Neuropsychological findings, together with data from cognitive psychology and neuroimaging, provide converging evidence that, at least to some extent, music perception and recognition are subserved by separate mechanisms which are likely to enjoy domain-specificity. The functional architecture of the main mechanisms underlying music perception and recognition was summarized in Peretz and Coltheart's model (2003). This model, albeit in some respects still underspecified (e.g., with regard to tonal encoding or music performance), provides the bases for further systematic research on the functional and neuronal underpinnings of music perception and recognition.

Acknowledgments. This chapter was written while the author was supported by a Marie-Curie International Reintegration Grant (n. 14847) from the European Commission.

References

Assal, G. (1993). Aphasie de Wernicke chez un pianiste. *Revue Neurologique, 29*, 251–255.

Avanzini, G., Faienza, C., Minciacchi, D., Lopez, L., & Majno, M. (2003). The neurosciences and music. *Annals of the New York Academy of Sciences, 999*.

Ayotte, J., Peretz, I., & Hyde, K. (2002). Congenital amusia: A group study of adults afflicted with a music-specific disorder. *Brain, 125*(2), 238–251.

Ayotte, J., Peretz, I., Rousseau, I., Bard, C., & Bojanowski, M. (2000). Patterns of music agnosia associated with middle cerebral artery infarcts. *Brain, 123*, 1926–1938.

Balaban, M.T., Anderson L.M., & Wisniewski, A.B. (1998). Lateral asymmetries in infant melody perception. *Developmental Psychology, 34*, 39–48.

Bartlett, J. C., & Dowling, W. J. (1980). Recognition of transposed melodies: A key-distance effect in developmental perspective. *Journal of Experimental Psychology: Human Perception and Performance, 6*, 501–515.

Belin, P., Zatorre, R., Lafaille, P., Ahad, P., & Pike, B. (2000). Voice-selective areas in human auditory cortex. *Nature, 403*, 309–312.

Besson, M., Faïta, F., Peretz, I., Bonnel, A.-M., & Requin, J. (1998). Singing in the brain: Independence of lyrics and tunes. *Psychological Science, 9*(6), 494–498.

Bever, T., & Chiarello, R. (1974). Cerebral dominance in musicians and nonmusicians. *Science, 185*, 537–539.

Bigand, E. (1997). Perceiving musical stability: The effects of tonal structure, rhythm, and musical expertise. *Journal of Experimental Psychology: Human Perception and Performance, 23*, 808–822.

Bigand, E., Tillmann, B., & Poulin-Charronat, B. (2006). A module for syntactic processing in music? *Trends in Cognitive Sciences, 10*(5), 195–196.

Boltz, M., & Jones, M. R. (1986). Does rule recursion make melodies easier to reproduce? If not, what does? *Cognitive Psychology, 18*, 389–431.

Brust, J. (1980). Music and language: Musical alexia and agraphia. *Brain, 103*, 367–392.

Buhusi, C. V., & Meck, W.H. (2005). What makes us tick? *Nature Review Neuroscience, 6*(10), 755–765.

Carrol-Phelan, B., & Hampson, P. J. (1996). Multiple components of the perception of musical sequences: A cognitive neuroscience analysis and some implications for auditory imagery. *Music Perception, 13*, 517–561.

Coltheart, M. (2001). Assumptions and methods in cognitive neuropsychology. In B. Rapp (Ed.), *The handbook of cognitive neuropsychology* (pp. 3–21). Philadelphia: Psychology Press.

Cooper, G., & Meyer, L. (1960). *The rhythmic structure of music.* Chicago: Chicago University Press.

Critchley, M., & Henson, R.A. (1977). *Music and the brain: Studies in the neurology of music.* London: Heinemann.

Crowder, R., Serafine, M.L., & Repp, B. (1990). Physical interaction and association by contiguity in memory for the words and melodies of songs. *Memory and Cognition, 18*, 469–476.

Dalla Bella, S., & Peretz, I. (1999). Music agnosias: Selective impairments of music recognition after brain damage. *Journal of New Music Research, 28*, 209–216.

Dalla Bella, S., Giguère, J-F., & Peretz, I. (2007). Singing proficiency in the general population.

Journal of the Acoustical Society of America, 121, 1182-1189.

Dalla Bella, S., & Peretz, I. (2003). Congenital amusia interferes with the ability to synchronize with music. *Annals of the New York Academy of Sciences, 999*, 166-169.

Dalla Bella, S., Peretz, I., & Aronoff, N. (2003). Time course of melody recognition: A gating paradigm study. *Perception and Psychophysics, 65*, 1019-1028.

Deutsch, D. (1972). Octave generalization and tune recognition. *Perception and Psychophysics, 11*, 411-412.

Di Pietro, M., Laganaro, M., Leeman, B., & Schnider, A. (2004). Receptive amusia: Temporal auditory deficit in a professional musician following a left temporo-parietal lesion. *Neuropsychologia, 42*, 868-977.

Dorgeuille, C. (1966). *Introduction à l'étude des amusies.* Unpublished doctoral dissertation, Université de la Sorbonne, Paris.

Dowling, W. J. (1978). Scale and contour: Two components of a theory of memory for melodies. *Psychological Review, 85*, 341-354.

Dowling, W. J., & Bartlett, J. C. (1981). The importance of interval information in long-term memory for melodies. *Psychomusicology, 1*, 30-49.

Dowling, W. J., & Fujitani, D. S. (1971). Contour, interval, and pitch recognition in memory for melodies. *Journal of the Acoustical Society of America, 49*, 524-531.

Dowling, W. J., & Harwood, D. L. (1986). *Music cognition.* Orlando, FL: Academic Press.

Dowling, W. J., & Hollombe, A. W. (1977). The perception of melodies distorted by splitting into several octaves: Effects of increasing proximity and melodic contour. *Perception and Psychophysics, 21*, 60-64.

Drake, C. (1998). Psychological processes involved in the temporal organization of complex auditory sequences: Universal and acquired processes. *Music Perception, 16*, 11-26.

Ellis, A., & Young, A. (1988). *Human cognitive neuropsychology.* London: L. Erlbaum Assoc.

Eustache, F., Lechevalier, B., Viader, F., & Lambert, J. (1990). Identification and discrimination disorders in auditory perception: A report on two cases. *Neuropsychologia, 28*, 257-270.

Farah, M. J. (2004). *Visual agnosia* (2nd ed.). Cambridge, NA: MIT Press.

Fasanaro, A.M., Spitaleri, D.L.A., Valiani, R., & Grossi, D. (1990). Dissociation in musical reading: A musician affected by alexia without agraphia. *Music Perception, 7*, 259-272.

Fodor, J. (1983). *The modularity of mind.* Cambridge, MA.: MIT Press.

Francès, R. (1958). *La perception de la musique* [The perception of music]. Paris: J. Vrin.

Francès, R., Lhermitte, F., & Verdy, M. (1973). Le déficit musical des aphasiques. *Revue Internationale de Psychologie Appliquée, 22*, 117-135.

Fries, W., & Swihart, A. (1990). Disturbance of rhythm sense following right hemisphere damage. *Neuropsychologia, 28*, 1317-1323.

Geshwind, N. (1984). The brain of a learning-disabled individual. *Annals of Dyslexia, 34*, 319-327.

Godefroy, O., Leys, D., Furby, A., De Reuck, J., Daems, C., Rondepierre, P., et al. (1995). Psychoacoustical deficits related to bilateral subcortical hemorrhages: A case with apperceptive auditory agnosia. *Cortex, 31*, 149-159.

Grant-Allen. (1878). Note-deafness. *Mind, 10*, 157-167.

Griffiths, T., Buchel, C., Frackowiak, R. S. J., & Patterson, R. D. (1998). Analysis of temporal structure in sound by the human brain. *Nature Neuroscience, 1*, 422-427.

Griffiths, T., Rees, A., Witton, C., Cross, P., Shakir, R., & Green, G. (1997). Spatial and temporal auditory processing deficits following right hemisphere infarction: A psychophysical study. *Brain, 120*, 785-794.

Habib, M., Daquin, G., Milandre, L., Royere, M. L., Rey, M., Lanteri, A., Salamon, G., & Khalil, R. (1995). Mutism and auditory agnosia due to bilateral insular damage—role of the insula in human communication. *Neuropsychologia, 33*(3), 327-339.

Hall, D. A., Johnsrude, I., Haggard, M. P., Palmer, A.R., Akeroyd, M. A., & Summerfield, A. Q. (2002). Spectral and temporal processing in human auditory cortex. *Cerebral Cortex, 12*, 140-149.

Halpern, A. R. (1988). Mental scanning in auditory imagery for songs. *Journal of Experimental*

Psychology: Learning, Memory and Cognition, 14, 434–443.

Halpern, A. R. (1989). Memory for the absolute pitch of familiar songs. *Memory and Cognition, 17*(5), 572–581.

Halpern, A. R., & Zatorre, R. (1999). When that tune runs through your head: A PET investigation of auditory imagery for familiar melodies. *Cerebral Cortex, 9*, 697–704.

Harrington. D. L., Haaland, K., & Hermanowicz, N. (1998). Temporal processing in the basal ganglia. *Neuropsychology, 12*, 3–12.

Hart, H. C., Palmer, A. R., Hall, D. A. (2003). Amplitude and frequency-modulated stimuli activate common regions of human auditory cortex. *Cerebral Cortex, 13*, 773–781.

Hébert, S., & Cuddy, L. L. (2006). Music-reading deficiencies in the brain. *Advances in Cognitive Psychology, 2*(2–3), 199–206.

Hébert, S., & Peretz, I. (1997). Recognition of music in long-term memory: Are melodic and temporal patterns equal partners? *Memory and Cognition, 25*, 518–533.

Horikoshi, T., Asari, Y., Watanabe, A., Nagaseki, Y., Nukui, H., Sasaki, H., et al. (1997). Music alexia in a patient with mild pure alexia: Disturbed visual perception of nonverbal meaningful figures. *Cortex, 33*, 187–194.

Huron, D. (2001). Is music an evolutionary adaptation? *Annals of the New York Academy of Sciences, 930*, 43–61.

Hyde, K., & Peretz, I. (2004). Brains that are out of tune but in time. *Psychological Science, 15*(5), 356–360.

Hyde, K., Zatorre, R., Griffiths, T. D., Lerch, J. P., & Peretz, I. (2006). Morphometry of the amusic brain: A two-site study. *Brain, 129*, 2562–2570.

Ibbotson, N. R., & Morton, J. (1981). Rhythm and dominance. *Cognition, 9*, 125–138.

Idson, W. L., & Massaro, D. W. (1978). A bidimensional model of pitch in the recognition of melodies. *Perception and Psychophysics, 24*, 551–565.

Ivry, R. B., & Keele, S. (1989). Timing functions of the cerebellum. *Journal of Cognitive Neuroscience, 1*, 136–152.

Ivry, R. B., & Spencer, R. (2004). The neural representation of time. *Current Opinion in Neurobiology, 14*, 225–232.

Janata, P., Birk, J., Van Horn, J., Leman, M., Tillmann, B., & Bharucha, J. (2002). The cortical topography of tonal structures underlying western music. *Science, 298*, 2167–2170.

Jones, M. R. (1976). Time, our lost dimension: Toward a new theory of perception, attention, and memory. *Psychological Review, 83*, 323–355.

Jones, M. R. (1987). Dynamic pattern structure in music: Recent theory and research. *Perception and Psychophysics, 41*, 621–634.

Judd, T., Gardner, H., & Geshwind, N. (1983). Alexia without agraphia in a composer. *Brain, 106*, 435–457.

Kallman, H. J., & Massaro, D. W. (1979). Tone chroma is functional in melody recognition. *Perception and Psychophysics, 26*, 32–36.

Kalmus, H., & Fry, D. B. (1980). On tune deafness (dysmelodia): Frequency, development, genetics and musical background. *Annals of Human Genetics, 43*, 369–382

Koelsch, S., Gunter, T. C., van Cramon, D. Y., Zysset, S., Lohmann, G., & Friederici, A. D. (2002). Bach speaks: A cortical "language-network" serves the processing of music. *NeuroImage, 17*, 956–966.

Krumhansl, C. L. (1990). *Cognitive foundations of musical pitch*. Oxford, UK: Oxford University Press.

Krumhansl, C., & Kessler, R. (1982). Tracing the dynamic changes in perceived tonal organization in a spatial representation of musical keys. *Psychological Review, 89*, 334–368.

Laignel-Lavastine, M., & Alajouanine, T. (1921). Un cas d'agnosie auditive. *Revue Neurologique, 37*, 194–198.

Large, E. W., & Jones, M. R. (1999). The dynamics of attending: How people track time-varying events. *Psychological Review, 106*(1), 119–159.

Laskowska, I., Dalla Bella, S., Rolinska, P., Binek, M., Stachowiak, A., & Gorzelanczyk, E. J. (2006). Sensory-motor synchronization with musical and non-musical stimuli in patients with Parkinson's disase. *Journal of Cognitive Neuroscience* (Suppl.), 238–239.

Lerdahl, F., & Jackendoff, R. S. (1983). *A generative theory of tonal music*. Cambridge, MA: MIT Press.

Levitin, D. J. (1994). Absolute memory for musical pitch: Evidence from the production of learned melodies. *Perception and Psychophysics, 56,* 414–423.

Levitin, D. J., & Cook, P. R. (1996). Memory for musical tempo: Additional evidence that auditory memory is absolute. *Perception and Psychophysics, 58,* 927–935.

Liberman, A., Cooper, F., Shankweiler, D., & Studdert-Kennedy, M. (1967). Perception of the speech code. *Psychological Review, 74,* 431–461.

Lichtheim, L. (1885). On Aphasia. *Brain, 7,* 433–484.

Liégeois-Chauvel, C., Peretz, I., Babaï, M., Laguitton, V., & Chauvel, P. (1998). Contribution of different cortical areas in the temporal lobes to music processing. *Brain, 121,* 1853–1867.

Lissauer, M. (1890). Ein fall von seelenblindheit nebst einem beitrage zur theorie derselben. *Archiv für Psychiatrie und Nervenkrankheiten, 21,* 222–270 (translated from German by M. Jackson (1988). A case of visual agnosia with a contribution to theory. *Cognitive Neuropsychology, 5,* 157–192).

London, J. (2004). *Hearing in time. Psychological aspects of musical meter.* New York: Oxford University Press.

Maess, B., Koelsch, S., Gunter, T. C., & Friederici, A. D. (2001). Musical syntax is processed in Broca's area: An MEG study. *Nature Neuroscience, 4,* 540–545.

Mann, V., & Liberman, P. (1983). Some differences between phonetic and auditory modes of perception. *Cognition, 14,* 211–235.

Marin, O. S. M., & Perry, D. W. (1999). Neurological aspects of music perception. In D. Deutsch (Ed.), *The psychology of music* (2nd ed.). San Diego, CA: Academic Press.

Mavlov, L. (1980). Amusia due to rhythm agnosia in a musician with left hemisphere damage: A non auditory supramodal defect. *Cortex, 16,* 321–338.

Mendez, M. (2001). Generalized auditory agnosia with spared music recognition in a left-hander. Analysis of a case with a right temporal stroke. *Cortex, 37,* 139–150.

Mendez, M. F., & Geehan, G. R. (1988). Cortical auditory disorders: Clinical and psychoacoustic features. *Journal of Neurology, Neurosurgery and Psychiatry, 51,* 1–9.

Metz-Lutz, M.-N., & Dahl, E. (1984). Analysis of word comprehension in a case of pure worddeafness. *Brain and Language, 23,* 13–25.

Midorikawa, A., & Kawamura, M. (2000). A case of musical agraphia. *NeuroReport, 11,* 3053–3057.

Midorikawa, A., Kawamura, M., & Kezuka, M. (2003). Musical alexia for rhythm notation: A discrepancy between pitch and rhythm. *Neurocase, 9,* 232–238.

Mithen, S. (2006). *The singing Neanderthals.* Cambridge, Mass.: Harvard University Press.

Moore, B. C. J. (1997). *An introduction to the psychology of hearing* (4th ed.). San Diego, CA: Academic Press.

Motomura, N., Yamadori, A., Mori, E., & Tamaru, F. (1986). Auditory agnosia: Analysis of a case with bilateral subcortical lesions. *Brain, 109,* 379–391.

Nyberg, L., & Tulving, E. (1996). Classifying human long-term memory: Evidence from converging dissociations. *European Journal of Cognitive Psychology, 8,* 163–183.

Patel, A. D., & Peretz, I. (1997). Is music autonomous from language? A neuropsychological appraisal. In I. Deliège & J. Sloboda (Eds.), *Perception and cognition of music* (pp. 191–215). London: Erlbaum Psychology Press.

Patel, A. D., Peretz, I., Tramo, M., & Labrecque, R. (1998). Processing prosodic and musical patterns: A neuropsychological investigation. *Brain and Language, 61*(2), 123–144.

Peretz, I. (1990). Processing of local and global musical information in unilateral brain damaged patients. *Brain, 113,* 1185–1205.

Peretz, I. (1993a). Auditory agnosia: A functional analysis. In S. McAdams & E. Bigand (Eds.), *Thinking in sound: The cognitive psychology of human audition* (pp. 199–230). Oxford, UK: Oxford University Press.

Peretz, I. (1993b). Auditory atonalia for melodies. *Cognitive Neuropsychology, 10,* 21–56.

Peretz, I. (1996). Can we loose memories for music? The case of music agnosia in a nonmusician. *Journal of Cognitive Neuroscience, 8*(6), 481–496.

Peretz, I., (2001). Music perception and recognition. In B. Rapp (Ed.), *The handbook of cognitive neuropsychology* (pp. 519-540). Philadelphia: Psychology Press.

Peretz, I. (2006). The nature of music from a biological perspective. *Cognition, 100*, 1-32.

Peretz, I., Ayotte, J., Zatorre, R., Mehler, J., Ahad, P., Penhune, V., & Jutras, B. (2002). Congenital amusia: A disorder of fine-grained pitch discrimination. *Neuron, 33*, 185-191.

Peretz, I., & Babaï, M. (1992). The role of contour and intervals in the recognition of melody parts: Evidence from cerebral asymmetries in musicians. *Neuropsychologia, 30*(3), 277-292.

Peretz, I., Belleville, S., & Fontaine, F. S. (1997). Dissociations entre musique et langage après atteinte cérébrale: Un nouveau cas d'amusie sans aphasie. *Revue Canadienne de Psychologie Expérimentale, 51*(4), 354-367.

Peretz, I., Champod, S., & Hyde, K. (2003). Varieties of Musical Disorders: The Montreal Battery of Evaluation of Amusia. *Annals of the New York Academy of Sciences, 999*, 58-75.

Peretz, I., & Coltheart, M. (2003). Modularity of music processing. *Nature Neuroscience, 6*(7), 688-691.

Peretz, I., Gagnon, L., & Bouchard, B. (1998). Music and emotion: Perceptual determinants, immediacy and isolation after brain damage. *Cognition, 68*, 111-141.

Peretz, I. & Hyde, K. (2003). What is specific to music processing? Insights from congenital amusia. *Trends in Cognitive Sciences, 7*(8), 362-367.

Peretz, I., Kolinsky, R., Tramo, M., Labrecque, R., Hublet, C., Demeurisse, G., et al. (1994). Functional dissociations following bilateral lesions of auditory cortex. *Brain, 117*, 1283-1302.

Peretz, I., & Morais, J. (1988). Determinants of laterality for music: Towards an information processing account. In K. Hugdahl (Ed.), *Handbook of dichotic listening: Theory, methods and research* (pp. 284-323). New York: Wiley.

Peretz, I., & Zatorre, R. J. (2003). *The cognitive neuroscience of music*. New York: Oxford University Press.

Peretz, I., & Zatorre, R. J. (2005). Brain organization for music processing. *Annual Review of Psychology, 56*, 89-114.

Phillips-Silver, J., & Trainor, L.J. (2005). Feeling the beat: Movement influences infants' rhythm perception. *Science, 308*, 1430.

Piccirilli, M., Sciarma, T., & Luzzi, S. (2000). Modularity of music: Evidence from a case of pure amusia. *Journal of Neurology, Neurosurgery, and Psychiatry, 69*, 541-545.

Platel, H., Price, C., Baron, J. C., Wise, R., Lambert, J., Frackowiak, L.S., Lechevalier, B., & Eustache, F. (1997). The structural components of music perception. A functional anatomical study. *Brain, 120*, 229-243.

Polster, M., & Rose, S. (1998). Disorders of auditory processing: Evidence for modularity in audition. *Cortex, 34*, 47-65.

Povel, D. J., & Essens, P. (1985). Perception of temporal patterns. *Music Perception, 2*, 411-440.

Rapp, B. (2001). *The handbook of cognitive neuropsychology*. Philadelphia: Psychology Press.

Repp, B. H., & Penel, A. (2002). Auditory dominance in temporal processing: New evidence from synchronization with simultaneous visual and auditory sequences. *Journal of Experimental Psychology: Human Perception and Performance, 28*, 1085-1099.

Repp, B. H., & Penel, A. (2004). Rhythmic movement is attracted more strongly to auditory than to visual rhythms. *Psychological Research, 68*, 252-270.

Sakai, K., Hikosaka, O., Miyauchi, S., Takino, R., Tamada, T., Iwata, N. K., & Nielsen, M. (1999). Neural representation of a rhythm depends on its interval ratio. *Journal of Neuroscience, 19*, 10074-10081.

Samson, S., & Zatorre, R. (1991). Recognition for text and melody of songs after unilateral temporal lobe lesion: Evidence for dual encoding. *Journal of Experimental Psychology Learning, Memory and Cognition, 17*, 793-804.

Samson, S., & Zatorre, R.J. (1992). Learning and retention of melodic and verbal information after unilateral temporal lobectomy. *Neuropsychologia, 30*, 815-826.

Satoh, M., Takeda, K., Murakami, Y., Onouchi, K., Inoue, K., & Kuzuhara, S. (2005). A case of amusia caused by the infarction of anterior portion of bilateral temporal lobes. *Cortex*, *41*, 77–83.

Schön, D., Lorber, B., Spacal, M., & Semenza, C. (2004). A selective deficit in the production of exact musical intervals following right-hemisphere damage. *Cognitive Neuropsychology*, *21*(7), 773–784.

Serafine, M. L., Crowder, R. G., & Repp, B. (1984). Integration of melody and text in memory for song. *Cognition*, *16*, 285–303.

Serafine, M. L., Davidson, J, Crowder, R. G., & Repp, B. (1986). On the nature of melody-text integration in memory for songs. *Journal of Memory and Language*, *25*, 123–135.

Shallice, T. (1988). *From neuropsychology to mental structure*. Cambridge,UK: Cambridge University Press.

Sloboda, J. A., Wise, K. J., & Peretz, I., (2005). Quantifying tone deafness in the general population. *Annals of the New York Academy of Sciences*, *1060*, 255–261.

Snyder, B. (2000). *Music and memory. An introduction*. Cambridge, MA: MIT Press.

Spreen, O., Benton, A., & Fincham, R. (1965). Auditory agnosia without aphasia. *Archives of Neurology*, *13*, 84–92.

Steinke, W. R., Cuddy, L. L., & Jakobson, L. S. (2001). Dissociations among functional subsystems governing melody recognition after right-hemisphere damage. *Cognitive Neuropsychology*, *18*, 411–437.

Stewart, L., von Kriegstein, K., Warren, J. D., & Griffiths, T. D. (2006). Music and the brain: Disorders of musical listening. *Brain*, *129*(10), 2533–2553.

Takahashi, N., Kawamura, M., Shinotou, H., Hirayaha, K., Kalia, K., & Shindo, M. (1992). Pure-word deafness due to left-hemisphere damage. *Cortex*, *28*, 295–303.

Tanaka, Y., Yamadori, A., & Mori, E. (1987). Pure word deafness following bilateral lesions. A psychophysical analysis. *Brain*, *110*, 381–403.

Tillmann, B., Bharucha, J., & Bigand, E. (2000). Implicit learning of tonality: A self-organizing approach. *Psychological Review*, *107*, 885–913.

Tillmann, B., Janata, P., & Bharucha, J. (2003). Activation of the inferior frontal cortex in musical priming. *Cognitive Brain Research*, *16*, 145–161.

Tramo, M., Bharucha, J., & Musiek, F. (1990). Music perception and cognition following bilateral lesions of auditory cortex. *Journal of Cognitive Neuroscience*, *2*, 195–212.

Trehub, S. (2003). The developmental origins of musicality. *Nature Neuroscience*, *6*(7), 669–673.

Van Lancker, D., & Canter, G. (1982). Impairments of voice and face recognition in patients with hemispheric damage. *Brain and Cognition*, *1*, 185–192.

Van Lancker, D., & Kreiman, J. (1987). Voice discrimination and recognition are separate abilities. *Neuropsychologia*, *25*, 829–834.

Vignolo, L.A. (2003). Music agnosia and auditory agnosia. Dissociations in stroke patients. *Annals of the New York Academy of Sciences*, *999*, 50–57.

Xu, D., Liu, T., Ashe, J., & Bushara, K.O. (2006). Role of the olivo-cerebellar system in timing. *Journal of Neuroscience*, *26*(22), 5990–5995.

Yaqub, B. A., Gascon, G. G., Al-Nosha, M., & Whitaker, H. (1988). Pure word deafness (Acquired verbal auditory agnosia) in an Arabic speaking patient. *Brain*, *111*, 457–466.

Wallin, N. L., Merker, B., & Brown, S. (2000). *The origins of music*. Cambridge, MA: MIT Press.

Warren, R. M., Gardner, D. A., Brubaker, B. S., & Bashford, J. A. (1991). Melodic and non-melodic sequences of tones: Effects of duration on perception. *Music Perception*, *8*, 277–290.

Warren, J., Uppenkamp, S., Patterson, R., & Griffiths, T. (2003). Separating pitch chroma and pitch height in the human brain. *Proceedings of the National Academy of Sciences*, *100*, 10038–10042.

White, B. W. (1960). Recognition of distorted melodies. *American Journal of Psychology*, *73*, 100–107.

Wilson, S. J., Pressing, J., & Wales, R. J. (2002). Modelling rhythmic function in a musician poststroke. *Neuropsychologia*, *40*, 1494–1505.

Zatorre, R. J. (1988). Pitch perception of complex tones and human temporal-lobe function. *Journal of the Acoustical Society of America*, *84*, 566–572.

Zatorre, R. J. (2001). Neural specialization for tonal processing. *Annals of the New York Academy of Sciences, 930,* 193–210.

Zatorre, R. J., & Belin, P. (2001) Spectral and temporal processing in human auditory cortex. *Cerebral Cortex, 11,* 946–953.

Zatorre, R. J., Belin, P., & Penhune, V. B. (2002). Structure and function of auditory cortex: Music and speech. *Trends in Cognitive Sciences, 6,* 37–46

Zatorre, R. J., Halpern, A. R., Perry, D. W., Meyer, E., & Evans, A. C. (1996). Hearing in the mind's ear: A PET investigation of musical imagery and perception. *Journal of Cognitive Neuroscience, 8,* 29–46.

Zatorre, R. J., & Peretz, I. (2001). The biological foundations of music. *Annals of the New York Academy of Sciences, 930.*

CHAPTER 15

The Dynamic Brainstem: Implications for Auditory Processing Disorder

KAREN BANAI AND NINA KRAUS

From the cochlea to the auditory cortex, sound is encoded in multiple locations along the ascending auditory pathway, eventually leading to our conscious perception. Although there is no doubt that the cortex plays a major role in perception of speech, music, and other meaningful auditory signals, recent studies, reviewed in this chapter, suggest that subcortical encoding of sound is not merely a series of bottom-up processes successively transforming the acoustic signal to more complex neural code. Rather, subcortical processing dynamically interacts with cortical processing to reflect important nonsensory factors such as musical expertise (Musacchia, Sams, Skoe, & Kraus, 2007; Wong, Skoe, Russo, Dees, & Kraus, 2007), linguistic experience (Krishnan, Xu, Gandour, & Cariani, 2005), and attention (Galbraith, Bhuta, Choate, Kitahara, & Mullen, 1998; Galbraith, Olfman, & Huffman, 2003).

In this chapter, we focus on the encoding of speech-sounds at the upper brainstem/midbrain (the speech-ABR) in humans, emphasizing the fidelity of encoding within an individual, how encoding is affected by expertise, and how it is disrupted in clinical populations intersecting auditory processing disorder (APD). Because current electrophysiologic techniques provide reliable means to test subcortical, but not cortical encoding of sound at the individual listener level, we propose that these properties of subcortical auditory processing carry special relevance to the study and understanding of APD. Namely, these properties allow us to define an individual as having an APD if specific elements of their response are significantly disrupted. We can then ask whether individuals manifesting a certain physiological pattern also share similar perceptual, literacy-related, and cognitive profiles, and whether current definitions of APD, language disorders or learning problems can account for the observed profiles, or whether these physiological deficits and accompanying profiles "cut across" diagnoses.

Fidelity of Subcortical Encoding of Sound: Characteristics of Normal Subcortical Encoding of Speech Sounds

Synchronized neural activity in response to sounds can be measured noninvasively in humans by means of auditory evoked potentials. Simple (brief nonspeech) stimuli evoke an orderly pattern of responses from the auditory nuclei in low brainstem (waves I–III) and rostal (waves V–Vn, the FFR) brainstem nuclei, clinically known as the click-evoked ABR (Boston & Møller, 1985; Møller, 1999; Møller & Jannetta, 1985; Sohmer, Pratt, & Kinarti, 1977; Worden & Marsh, 1968). Slight deviations from the timing of the normal pattern are associated with hearing loss and other pathologies (Hall, 1992; Hood, 1998). Synchronized neural activity can also be measured in response to more complex sounds like synthetic vowels or consonant-vowel syllables. At low levels of the brainstem, the evoked responses to simple and complex sounds appear similar (Song, Banai, & Kraus, 2008). Here, we review work on auditory evoked responses originating at rostal brainstem/midbrain nuclei that reflect the temporal and spectral characteristics of complex stimuli with remarkable precision (Galbraith, Arbagey, Branski, Comerci, & Rector, 1995; Johnson, Nicol, & Kraus, 2005; Krishnan, 2002; Russo, Nicol, Musacchia, & Kraus, 2004; Akhoun et al, 2008).

Speech is a signal whose temporal and spectral properties change continuously. Studies in animal models indicate that many of its complex properties (formant structure, pitch, voicing, etc.) can be encoded through the firing patterns of auditory neurons (Delgutte & Kiang, 1984a, 1984b; Sachs & Young, 1979; Young & Sachs, 1979). In humans, two main classes of evoked responses (reflecting activity of large neural populations) are likely candidates to reflect these complex properties: the late waves of the auditory brainstem response (ABR), which are essentially onset responses, and the frequency following response (FFR), which reflects phase-locked activity of neural populations in the rostal brainstem, tracking the fundamental frequency of the sound and its harmonics.

Our approach to study the parallels between the acoustic properties of the speech signal and the brain evoked response is based on the source/filter model of speech production (Fant, 1970; and see Kraus & Nicol, 2005 for a detailed review of the application of the source/filter model to speech-evoked brainstem responses) and is demonstrated in Figure 15–1. In this view, the acoustic properties of the signal can be classified into one of two broad classes of responses: the source class and the filter class. The source class contains all parameters used to describe the properties of the sound source (the vocal folds in the case of speech, the strings in case of string instruments). The sound wave produced by the source is modified by the filter, that is, the shape of the vocal tract and the articulators in the case of speech or the shape of the musical instrument, and this modification produces the final acoustic structure. In the case of speech, the vocal folds produce a harmonic sound at a period determined by the rate of vibration. The filter then attenuates certain harmonics and enhances others harmonics to produce the formant structure of speech sounds.

In analyzing the physiologic response, we hypothesize that the onset and offset transient peaks of the speech-ABR reflect

Source-filter model

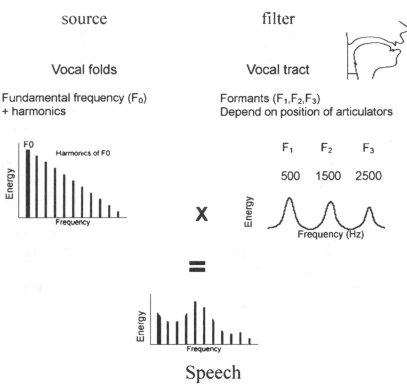

Figure 15–1. The source-filter model

mainly filter information, whereas the FFR probably reflects both source and filter properties of spectro-temporal elements and steady-state vowel-like stimuli (Kraus & Nicol, 2005; Johnson et al, in press), because the neural response shows phase-locking to the fundamental frequency of the stimulus (a source property) as well as to higher frequency formants (a filter characteristic). An examination of the evoked response to synthetic, steady-state vowels reveals a series of peaks, repeating at a rate corresponding to the fundamental frequency (F0) of the vowel—a source property. Furthermore, the spectral content of the response appears to reflect the first two formants of the vowel (Krishnan, 2002). Thus, frequency domain analyses of FFRs obtained to the synthetic vowels /u/, /ɔ/ and /a/ show that spectral peaks corresponding to the first and second formants, are increased in comparison to spectral peaks corresponding to the harmonics falling between F1 and F2 (Krishnan, 2002), thus reflecting filter properties as well.

We have been studying the brainstem response to the consonant-vowel syllable /da/ (Johnson et al., 2005; Russo et al., 2004). The brainstem response to /da/ (da-ABR) has both an onset portion occurring 6.7 ms (sd = 0.25 ms) after the stimulus onset and an FFR portion corresponding to the properties of the periodic formant transition and steady-state portion of the vowel /a/, as shown in Figure 15–2. Together, the onset and the FFR components of the da-ABR roughly reflect the acoustic parameters of the syllable /da/. The onset is a filter class response and likely repre-sents the initiation of the consonant, as it appears to be absent when a vowel is used on its own.

The speech stimulus /da/ and the response it evokes from a representative child are shown in Figure 15–2. It can be seen that the physiologic response to /da/, first reported by Cunningham, Nicol, Zecker and Kraus (2000) and described in the general population by Russo et al. (2004), includes an orderly series of peaks and troughs (peaks I through O). The initial peaks (I to A) are similar to those evoked by brief click stimuli. Waves I and III probably originate in the low brainstem, whereas peaks V and A originate in the rostal brainstem (the lateral lemniscus or inferior colliculus). Supporting the similarity between waves V and A in response to speech and clicks, Song, Banai, Russo and Kraus (2006) have reported significant correlations between the corresponding peak latencies in response to the two types of stimuli. Peak C possibly reflects the onset of voicing, whereas the later peaks (D, E, and F), comprising the FFR, occur at a rate equivalent to the fundamental frequency (F0) of the sound source and correspond to the format transition of the stimulus. Finally, peak O is likely an offset response, reflecting the end (stopping) of the sound. Figure 15–2C shows the spectra of the stimulus and the response, demonstrating how the major spectral peaks in the stimulus that fall within the phase-locking capabilities of the brainstem (F0 and F1) are represented in the response.

The feature of the speech-ABR that makes it useful in a wide array of studies and clinical applications is the high replica-bility of the response both within and across individuals. Thus, not only are the major morphologic features of the response stable over time within an individual (Russo, Nicol, Zecker, Hayes, & Kraus, 2005), the major peaks are also highly replicable between individuals (Russo et al., 2004; Akhoun et al, 2008), making deviations from the normal range easily identifiable and informative (Banai, Abrams, & Kraus, 2007; Banai & Kraus, 2006).

Supporting the separation between filter class and source class responses, significant correlations exist between latencies of the onset peaks V and A, which are considered filter class peaks. On the other hand, the latencies of the onset peaks are not correlated with the latencies of the FFR peaks or the response magnitude at the F0 (Kraus and Nicol 2005)—a source class response (Russo et al., 2004). For detailed discussions of the da-ABR, and how it is elicited and measured see Russo et al. (2004) and Johnson et al. (2005).

Because waves V and A of the speech-ABR appear to be similar to waves V and Vn of the click-evoked-ABR, it may be claimed that both reflect similar types of processing. Yet, it should be noted that whereas in the general population the latencies of wave V to click and speech are significantly correlated, this correlation breaks down in a subgroup of individuals with learning problems whose speech-ABRs are abnormal (Song et al., 2006, see below). Furthermore, different maturational patterns characterize click- and speech-evoked responses. Whereas the brainstem response to clicks is mature by 2 years of age (e.g., Salamy, 1984), the speech-evoked response only reaches adult like timing and morphology by the age of 5 (Johnson, Nicol, & Kraus, 2008). Taken together, these two lines of evidence support the idea that brainstem structures respond differently to speech- and click-sounds.

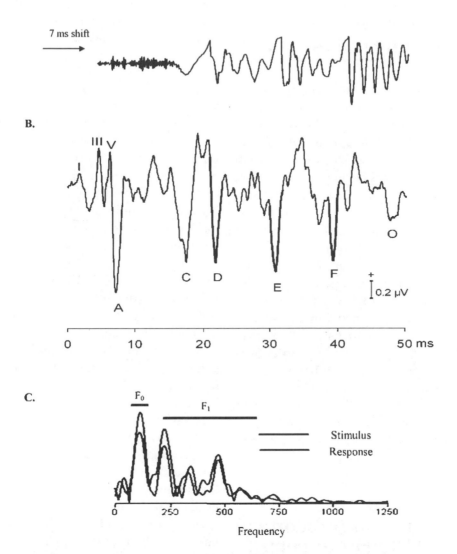

Figure 15–2. Subcortical encoding of the syllable /da/. **A.** The time/ amplitude wave form of the speech syllable /da/. **B.** The time/amplitude waveform of the brainstem response from a typical child. Labels I-O denote the characteristic peaks of the response. Waves I and III origi- nate at the low brainstem; waves V and A represent the onset of the response at the rostral brainstem. Waves D, E, and F are locked to the fundamental frequency of the /da/ stimulus. **C.** The spectra of the stim- ulus and the response from a typically developing child averaged over the entire stimulus and the last 40 ms of the response. Spectral peaks in the response correspond to F0 (103–125 Hz), and some of the higher harmonics comprising F1 (220–720 Hz). The stimulus has been filtered to mimic the phase-locking properties of the brainstem.

Malleability of Subcortical Encoding of Sound

The remarkable fidelity of subcortical encoding of speech, as measured using auditory evoked potentials, could suggest that encoding in these stations is based on automatic detection of the acoustic features of sound with no regard to higher level factors that are known to play a crucial role in perception such as expertise, attention, or context. Recent studies suggest that this is not the case, and that subcortical encoding is affected by expertise, input from other sensory modalities, and attention. Whether these influences are mediated in a top-down fashion, as predicted by the Reverse Hierarchy Theory (Hochstein & Ahissar, 2002) through the efferent, corticofugal system linking the auditory brainstem and cortex (Winer, 2006), through local mechanisms of adaptation to the acoustic properties of the input (Dean, Harper, & McAlpine, 2005), or through an interaction of afferent and efferent mechanisms is unknown.

Expertise and Subcortical Encoding of Speech

Brainstem responses to speech reflect differences in linguistic experience. The phase locking of neural activity to the pitch contour (that is the changes in F0 over time also known as pitch tracking) of Mandarin words (in which pitch provides an important cue to meaning) is stronger in native Mandarin compared to native English speakers, suggesting that the brainstems of Mandarin speakers encode Mandarin words more precisely than do the brains of English

speakers (Swaminathan et al., 2008; Krishnan et al., 2005). These findings suggest that pitch encoding mechanisms in the human brainstem are sensitive to language experience; however, they can not resolve whether this plasticity is more consistent with corticofugal modulation of the subcortical structures by language experience or with statistical learning based on the input statistics of Mandarin speech sounds.

Indeed, several recent studies on the effects of experience on subcortical encoding reached opposing conclusions. On the one hand, Xu, Krishnan, and Gandour (2006) have shown that the subcortical encoding advantage of Mandarin speakers disappears following slight manipulations to the acoustic properties of the Mandarin tokens, while still preserving their meaning and allowing Mandarin speakers to perceive them as good quality Mandarin sounds. This is more consistent with a statistical learning argument than with corticofugal modulation because it suggests that the brains of Mandarin speakers are fine tuned only to the exact contours they hear in everyday speech. In this case, knowledge of Mandarin was not sufficient to confer a brainstem encoding advantage. On the other hand, Wong et al. (2007) have shown that musical experience results in more robust encoding of linguistic pitch-patterns in the brainstem (Figure 15–3 presents more details of this study). Because the musicians in this study were native English speakers, with no prior exposure to Mandarin, it is unlikely that their more robust encoding of Mandarin sounds was the result of statistical learning of Mandarin sounds, but of a more general influence of music training on multipurpose pitch encoding mechanisms (though it could still be some other local general pitch extracting mechanism that is driven by music training but not by speaking Mandarin). The findings from the Wong et al. (2007) study suggest

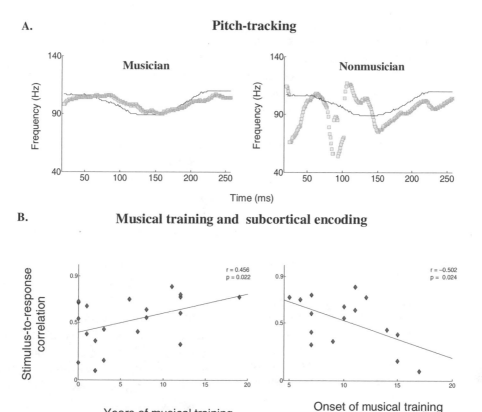

Figure 15–3. The effects of musical experience on speech encoding at the brainstem. **A.** Linguistic pitch encoding. The typical musician's brain (*left*) encodes the pitch content of Mandarin speech sounds more precisely than does the brain of the typical nonmusician (*right*). The thin line denotes the pitch contour of the stimulus, the thick line is the pitch contour extracted from the brainstem response. **B.** Musical experience and the fidelity of brainstem encoding. With increasing duration of musical training, the brainstem response more closely mimics the stimulus (indicated by increased stimulus-to-response correlation, *left*). Similarly, the age of onset of musical training is inversely correlated with the fidelity of brainstem encoding (*right*). Based on Wong, Skoe, Russo and Kraus (2007); Musacchia, Sams, Skoe and Kraus (2007).

common subcortical mechanisms for pitch processing in linguistic and nonlinguistic contexts. These findings are consistent with behavioral findings showing that Mandarin speakers use pitch information differently from native English speakers even in a nonlinguistic context when they are required to identify (but not discriminate) pitch con-

tours (Bent, Bradlow, & Wright, 2006). Similar to the Wong et al. (2007) findings, musicians also show more robust brainstem encoding of the English syllable /da/, in particular when the auditory syllable was presented together with a visual counterpart in a lip-reading condition (Musacchia et al., 2007; Musacchia, Strait, and Kraus, 2008).

Taken together, the Wong et al. (2007) and the Musacchia et al. (2007 & 2008) studies suggest that the consequences of musical experience extend across domains (e.g. language) and levels of processing in the auditory pathway (see Kraus & Banai, 2007 for further discussion of this point). Moreover, despite the well-known cortical segregation of speech and music function (Zatorre, Belin, & Penhune, 2002), a common subcortical network for speech and music is implied.

Visual Influences on Subcortical Encoding of Speech

The addition of visual input to the auditory speech stimulus, changes the way the brainstem encodes acoustic information as early as 11 ms after the onset of the acoustic stimulus (Musacchia, Sams, Nicol, & Kraus, 2006). When a visual stimulus—a face uttering a syllable or a musical instrument being played—is presented along with the acoustic stimulus (a syllable or a musical note, respectively), the brainstem response to the speech syllable is modified by the presence of the visual stimulus, and this form of auditory-visual interaction is significantly enhanced in musicians compared to non-musicians (Musacchia et al., 2007; Musacchia et al., 2008). These findings suggest sub-cortical involvement in multi-sensory integration in addition to multi-modal cortical regions typically thought to engage in this function.

Effects of Attention on Subcortical Encoding

Like visual input, attending to sound influences brainstem encoding of speech and nonspeech sounds, in addition to, and ear-

lier than the more widely documented cortical effects. Two types of attentional effects on the human FFR have been suggested. A spatial-attention (ear-related) effect and a modality effect. A spatial attention effect was observed in a dichotic listening paradigm; when two different syllables were presented simultaneously, one to each ear, and listeners were required to switch their attention between the two ears, the encoding of the fundamental frequency of the attended syllable was selectively enhanced (Galbraith et al., 1998). A small but significant effect on the FFR latency (with no effect on amplitude) was also reported with a different attentional paradigm in which listeners were required to respond to targets that occurred in the same ear as a cue ("attended") or in the contralateral ear ("unattended") (Hoormann, Falkenstein, & Hohnsbein, 2004). Frequency following response amplitudes were also found to increase when attention was directed to the auditory modality (listeners were asked to count auditory targets) compared to when attention was directed to the visual modality (listeners were asked to count visual targets while ignoring the sounds) (Galbraith et al., 2003). These findings suggest the existence of crude attentional mechanisms at the level of the auditory brainstem. These mechanisms could serve to enhance auditory encoding by direct-ing processing resources to the appropriate modality, or within the auditory modality to the appropriate ear. It is still not clear if more refined attentional, related to specific auditory features, occurs at the brainstem.

Taken together, the findings that language and musical experience, as well as inputs from the visual modality and attention affect auditory encoding of sound at subcortical levels of the auditory pathway suggest that these areas are more plastic and dynamic than was typically assumed by sensory neuroscientists, and that at least

Subcortical Encoding of Speech in Noise Can Be Improved with Training

Further evidence for the dynamic nature of subcortical auditory encoding comes from the effects of training on the speech-ABR. Russo et al. (2005) have shown that in a group of children with language-based learning disorders undergoing auditory training, the resilience of the brainstem to the degrading effects of background noise improved following training. Because the training was not specific to the syllable used to elicit the brainstem response, or to perception in noise, it is not likely that training affected local low-level mechanisms at the brainstem. This outcome therefore raises the possibility that the influences of training on the brainstem were mediated in a top-down fashion.

In addition to enhancing the brainstem response in noise, short-term training may improve pitch encoding in the brainstem in a way similar to that of long-term musical experience. Thus, when native English speakers were trained to use lexical pitch patterns to identify Mandarin words, tracking of some Mandarin pitch patterns in their brainstems became more precise (Song, Skoe, Wong, & Kraus, 2008).

Vulnerability of Subcortical Encoding of Sound

Our focus has been on children with language-based learning problems (LD). Previous work concentrated on cortical processing in this clinical group and revealed that various forms of auditory cor-

tical processing are abnormal in a substantial subgroup of this population (e.g., Baldeweg, Richardson, Watkins, Foale, & Gruzelier, 1999; Bishop & McArthur, 2004; Hari & Renvall, 2001; Heim et al., 2000; Helenius, Salmelin, Richardson, Leinonen, & Lyytinen, 2002; Kraus et al., 1996; Kujala et al., 2000; Lachmann, Berti, Kujala, & Schroger, 2005; Moisescu-Yiflach & Pratt, 2005; Nagarajan et al., 1999; Wible, Nicol, & Kraus, 2002). Our studies reveal that, in addition to cortical processing deficits, brainstem responses to speech are abnormal in about a third of children diagnosed with language-based learning problems (Banai, Nicol, Zecker, & Kraus, 2005). Compar-ed to typically developing children, in this subgroup of the LD population, waves A, C, and F were found to be delayed (King, Warrier, Hayes, & Kraus, 2002), the onset response at the upper brainstem (waves V, A) is prolonged and less synchronized (Figure 15–4), and the spectral representation of F1 (but not F0) is reduced (Wible, Nicol, & Kraus, 2004). On the other hand, the brainstem responses to click in this group are normal (Song et al., 2006) suggesting that the timing deficit in response to speech sounds does not reflect a universal deficit. A similar dissociation was reported in a group of children with specific language impairment (SLI) in which brainstem responses to pure tones were of normal latency, but responses to backward masked ones were delayed (Marler & Champlin, 2005). Finally, children on the autism spectrum have been found to have abnormal subcortical pitch-tracking, consistent with known deficits in prosody perception in this population (Russo, Bradlow, Skoe, Trommer, Nicol, Zecker and Kraus, 2008).

For a more complete discussion of our approach for determining whether speech-ABR is abnormal, as well as for normative data see Banai, Abrams, and Kraus (2007). It is of interest however to note here that the proportion and degree of speech-ABR

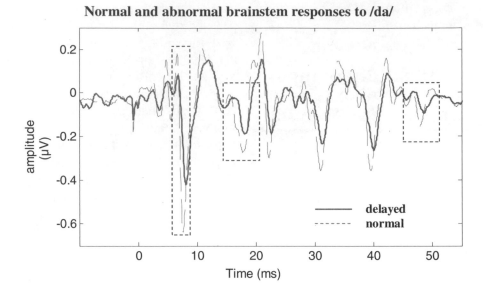

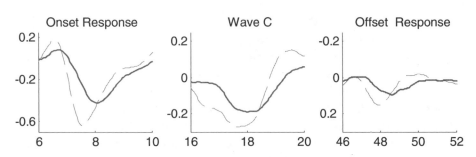

Figure 15–4. Abnormal speech ABR. *Top:* Grand averages of the time domain response in children with learning problems and abnormal responses (in *dark gray lines*) versus typically developing children (*light gray dashed line*). Dashed boxes mark the regions of the response that significantly differ between individuals with normal and abnormal responses. *Bottom:* Focus on the onset (*left*), the transition period (*middle*) and the offset (*right*) portions of the response.

deficits in all of our previous studies was unrelated to the specific diagnosis (APD, SLI, ADHD, or LD), with the exception of poor readers where the incidence is higher, suggesting that perhaps similar underlying physiological bases can cut across existing diagnostic categories. It should also be noted that, although these findings suggest an association between learning problems and abnormal processing at the level of the brainstem, they cannot be taken to indicate causality. Nonetheless, the reliability of the response within an individual makes the speech-ABR a useful marker of auditory function in the assessment of listening and learning disorders, and has led to the translation of the research to a clinically available tool—BioMAP (Biological Marker of Auditory Processing, Bio-logic Systems Corp, a Natus Company, Mundelein, IL).

The Relationships Between Cortical and Subcortical Auditory Processing

Because abnormal cortical processing of both nonspeech (Baldeweg et al., 1999; Corbera, Escera, & Artigas, 2006; Stoodley, Hill, Stein, & Bishop, 2006) and speech (Kraus et al., 1996; Schulte-Korne, Deimel, Bartling, & Remschmidt, 1998) sounds has been implicated in many cases of LD, whereas responses to acoustic clicks from structures up to the rostal brainstem were typically found to be normal in LDs (Grontved, Walter, & Gronborg, 1988; Jerger, Martin, & Jerger, 1987; Lauter & Wood, 1993; Mason & Mellor, 1984; McAnally & Stein, 1997; Purdy, Kelly, & Davies, 2002), the extent of auditory pathway deficit characterized using responses evoked by the same stimulus in the subgroup of LDs with abnormal speech-ABRs is of interest. We have examined auditory pathway encoding to the speech syllable /da/ across multiple levels of the auditory pathway.

At the lowest levels of the pathway, timing of peaks I and III in LDs with abnormal later peaks appears normal (Song, Banai et al., 2008), placing the rostal brainstem as the lowest possible source of deficit. On the other hand, when speech-ABR is abnormal, several aspects of auditory cortical processing appear abnormal as well. First, a strong correlation between brainstem timing and the resilience of the cortical response to the presence of background noise was found (Wible, Nicol, & Kraus, 2005). As shown in Figure 15–5A, noise had more detrimental effects on the cortical responses of individuals with delayed brainstem timing, compared to those with earlier timing, and this was true in both typically developing children and those with language based learning problems. Second, abnormal brainstem timing is associated with reduced cortical discrimination of fine acoustic differences (MMNs, Banai et al., 2005b). As shown in Figure 15–5B, as a group, individuals with abnormal speech-ABRs failed to show an MMN at all, suggesting that delayed timing in the brainstem and cortical discrimination are related. Third, the degree of brainstem deficit is associated with the degree of laterality of cortical processing of speech sounds (Abrams, Nicol, Zecker, & Kraus, 2006). As shown in Figure 15–5C, the normal pattern of leftward cortical asymmetry in response to speech sound is disrupted when brainstem timing is delayed. Finally, effects of musical experience are expressed in brainstem-cortical relationships (Musacchia et al., 2008).

Taken together these studies suggest strong relationships between auditory processing at the brainstem and the cortex. Because the brainstem and the cortex are linked by both ascending and descending pathways (see Winer, 2006 for review), these studies cannot resolve the direction of causality, namely, whether a subtle timing deficit at the brainstem adversely affects cortical processing or whether abnormal cortical processing exercises abnormal feedback on the brainstem, manifested by the pattern of timing deficits observed in individuals with abnormal speech-ABR. Recent studies in animal models are consistent with the top-down direction though (Ma & Suga, 2001; Palmer et al., 2006; Popelar, Nwabueze-Ogbo, & Syka, 2003). One possible route through which the descending pathway could exert its influence is by influencing selective attention, which in turn aids in gating of sensory information to the cortex. If processing in the cortex is not robust enough, it may not be able to properly "tune" the subcortical structures to relevant acoustic features.

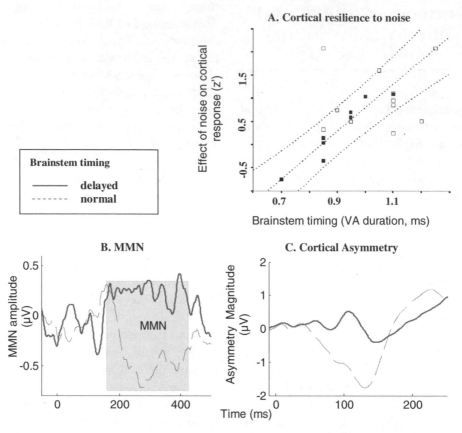

Figure 15–5. Cortical processing as a function of brainstem timing. **A.** The relationship between brainstem timing (VA duration) and the cortical suscep-tibility to noise. Filled symbols denote typically developing children; empty symbols denote children with LD showing a similar trend across both groups. z' was computed by subtracting cortical response correlations in noise from those in quiet. The larger z', the more pronounced effect noise had on response reliability. Based on Wible et al. (2004). **B.** Normally (and among individuals with early brainstem timing denoted in *light gray dashed line*) the cortical detection of rare acoustic evens among frequent ones is indexed by a negative deflection starting about 150 ms after stimulus onset (Mismatch negativity, MMN). This negative deflection is not present when brainstem tim-ing is delayed (*solid line*). Based on Banai et al. (2005). **C.** Normally, cortical processing of speech sounds is stronger in the left hemisphere of the brain, as denoted by the left asymmetry of the cortical response of individuals with early brainstem timing (*dashed line*). This pattern is disrupted when brain-stem timing is delayed (*solid line*). Based on Abrams et al. (2006).

Functional Correlates of Subcortical Encoding of Sound

How subcortical encoding of sound contributes to perception, language, and other cognitive functions is still not clear, but studies point to relationships between brainstem encoding of speech sounds and some perceptual and literacy related measures. It has been observed that more than 80% of individuals with abnormal brainstem timing are poor readers (Banai et al., 2005; Figure 15–6). This figure is higher than the proportion of poor readers typically observed in the highly heterogeneous group of individuals with LD that comprised the majority of our studies.

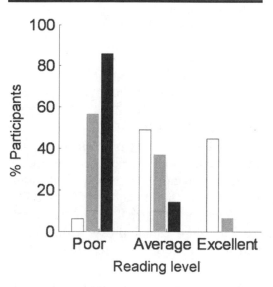

Figure 15–6. Brainstem processing and literacy. Histogram showing the distribution of reading abilities among typically developing 8- to 12-year-old children (*unfilled bars*), children with learning disabilities and normal speech-evoked ABRs (*gray bars*) and children with learning problems and abnormal speech-evoked ABRs (*black bars*). The majority of children with abnormal ABRs are poor readers. Based on Banai et al. (2005).

Regarding speech-perception, the picture is more complicated and tentative. Based on a review of unpublished data (Banai, Abrams, & Kraus, 2007), it appears that many individuals with LD and abnormal speech-ABR can have normal speech discrimination JNDs when tested behaviorally. It therefore seems that abnormal brainstem timing does not necessarily result in impaired perception of single syllables in laboratory conditions. This observation is surprising and unintuitive if one assumes that a physiologic deficit at the brainstem, with cortical correlates should have an influence on perception. However, it suggests that the link between brainstem encoding and higher level literacy related skills is not a direct outcome of abnormal speech perception at the syllable level but rather may refect a more general language deficit. Noteworthy is that in the cases where impaired perception of syllables was observed, it appears that training improves perception for individuals with abnormal brainstem timing but not for those with normal timing (C. King et al., 2002). In ongoing work, we are studying the perception of sentences presented in challenging listening conditions in individuals with abnormal speech-ABRs to investigate further the relationship between abnormal brainstem encoding and speech perception.

Poor temporal resolution, determined by elevated thresholds for the detection of backward masked tones, is characteristic of many individuals with language and learning problems (e.g., Wright et al., 1997). Although it is typically assumed that cortical processing is critical for backward masking, two studies suggest that subcortical areas of the auditory pathway may also be implicated in abnormal backward masking thresholds. In the first study, Marler and Champlin (2005) found that the auditory brainstem responses of individuals with SLI were normal when elicited with pure tones, but abnormal when the same tones were backward masked with noise. In the second study, Johnson et al. (2007) looked specifically in children with LD and poor temporal resolution (defined by performance on a backward masking task), in comparison to children with LD and normal temporal resolution. They found that as a group, children with poor temporal resolution exhibited abnormal encoding of speech at the brainstem and, furthermore, that the encoding deficit was specific to the onset and offset portion of the brainstem response, with the FFR being normal, thus linking abnormal temporal resolution with speech encoding.

Evidence for the involvement of IC (the putative neural generator of waves V and A of the speech-ABR and of the FFR) in auditory processing under challenging listening conditions, as well as in sound localization come from the few available case studies of individuals who suffered a localized lesion to the IC unilaterally or bilaterally. Whereas a bilateral lesion involving IC seems to result in auditory agnosia (Johkura, Matsumoto, Hasegawa, & Kuroiwa, 1998) or central deafness (Musiek, Charette, Morse, & Baran, 2004), unilateral lesions may result in more subtle deficits in sound localization (Champoux et al., 2007; Litovsky, Fligor, & Tramo, 2002), and in recognition of duration patterns and speech in the presence of a competing signal (Champoux et al., 2007) when the ear contralateral to the lesion is stimulated.

Implications for APD

ABRs Are Reliable in Individuals

The ABR can be recorded reliably in individuals, making it a prominent tool in the clinic (Hood, 1998). Speech-ABR is no exception (Russo et al., 2004; Akhoun et al., 2008).

The relationships among speech-ABR, literacy, and temporal resolution discussed above indicate that speech-ABRs may aid in the diagnosis and assessment of APD. Furthermore, because abnormal speech-ABRs are not characteristic of a specific type of learning disorder, but rather are found among 30% of LD individuals, irrespective of their specific diagnosis and to a greater extent in poor readers, and because APD and LD often co-occur (W. M. King, Lombardino, Crandell, & Leonard, 2003; Sharma et al., 2006), it is also likely that they characterize at least a subgroup of the individuals currently being diagnosed with APD. It could be that these individuals have a different type of disorder than those with behavioral manifestations of APD but normal speech-ABRs. Further research is required to establish the relationships between the behavioral symptoms of APD and brainstem encoding of speech.

ABRs May Be Used to Predict the Effects of Auditory Training

Auditory training is often used in remediation of both learning problems and APD, but outcomes are variable and clinicians currently do not have a way of deciding if a child is a good candidate for auditory training or not. The resilience of the speech-ABR to noise can improve with training (Russo et al., 2005). Furthermore, children with abnormal brainstem timing to speech have been shown to be more likely than those with normal brainstem timing to improve their speech perception and the resilience of their cortical responses in noise following auditory training (Hayes, Warrier, Nicol, Zecker, & Kraus, 2003; C. King et al., 2002). These findings, together with the malleability of brainstem function with long and short-term training, suggest that, in addition to objectively assessing training outcomes, clinical measurements of speech-ABRs can be used to aid in deciding on a course of therapy.

APD Research and Diagnosis Could Benefit from the Use of Objective Measures

Current diagnosis of APD is based on a battery of auditory tests, but it is often not clear how these tests relate to underlying physiologic processes that may be impaired in APD. Furthermore, it is likely that APD is not a uniform phenomenon and that individuals that are impaired on some aspects of auditory function are unimpaired on others. Subcortical encoding can be used to define subgroups that are homogeneous on a particular biological indicator (e.g. onset timing, phase-locking, noise susceptibility). Then it can be determined whether individuals within these subgroups share a similar perceptual profile. In addition to the speech-ABR discussed in detail in this chapter, another subcortical measure that has been used in research and that is sensitive to the presence of clinically diagnosed APD is the binaural interaction component (BIC) (Delb, Strauss, Hohenberg, & Plinkert, 2003; Gopal & Pierel, 1999). The BIC is a putative index of binaural processing. It is therefore possible to hypothesize that the BIC and the speech-ABRs may reveal two distinct subtypes of APD, with distinct perceptual profiles. Alternatively, they may both be impaired in the same population.

The Nature of APD

An influential current definition of APD (ASHA, 2005) suggests that the neural defi-

cits in the central nervous system that give rise to APD may be reflected by difficulties in one or more of a long list of auditory skills including sound localization and lateralization, auditory discrimination, auditory pattern recognition, multiple aspects of temporal processing, processing of competing acoustic signals, and processing of degraded acoustic signals. It also requires that these auditory deficits are not due to primarily high-order factors such as attention or memory. This heterogeneity of symptoms suggests the potential existence of distinct subtypes of APD. Attempts to define subprofiles of APD were made by Bellis and Ferre (1999) who suggested, based on case studies and clinical observations, several subtypes of APD, based on the putative underlying neurophysiology of each subtype.

1. A left hemisphere subtype characterized by deficits in auditory decoding, including deficits on auditory closure tasks, poor temporal resolution and poor performance on dichotic speech tasks (bilateral or right ear). Furthermore, individuals may have difficulties in other high-level language skills associated with left hemisphere function.

2. A right hemisphere subtype characterized by prosodic deficits including a left ear deficit on dichotic speech tasks, poor temporal patterning and poor frequency, intensity and duration discrimination. In addition, individuals may have difficulties in other high-level skills associated with the right hemisphere such as prosody perception, sight word reading, and pragmatic skills.

3. An integration deficit subtype characterized by deficits in tasks that indicate inefficient hemispheric transfer. Deficits include poor temporal patterning and left-ear deficit on dichotic speech tasks. Higher level deficits may include speech in noise and localization defi-

cits and poor performance with multi-modal cues.

This model illustrates two problems inherent in the ASHA definition of APD (ASHA, 2005). First, it suggests that a unimodal deficit confined to the auditory system alone is unlikely. Second, because individuals in each of the subgroups may have higher level deficits, the idea that the auditory deficits can not be a consequence of high-order deficits seems unlikely.

It Is Not Reasonable to Expect an Auditory-Only Disorder

The central role of the auditory modality in APD led to the suggestion that modality specificity should be incorporated into the definition and differential diagnosis of APD (Cacace & McFarland, 2005). For several reasons outlined here, we would like to claim that it is unlikely that APD is a modality specific condition. First, there is little evidence to link the general listening difficulties experienced by individuals with APD in challenging listening conditions with a *specific*, single underlying auditory physiologic deficit. In fact, the evidence from localized IC lesions discussed above are not consistent with the APD phenotype because they result in more specific deficits than those typically present in individuals diagnosed with APD. As discussed in this chapter, a specific (and subtle) timing deficit at the brainstem may be related to a general form of learning disability rather than to a specific perceptual deficit. Furthermore, the brainstem deficit is strongly linked with cortical processing abnormalities (Abrams et al., 2006; K. Banai, T. Nicol, S. Zecker, & N. Kraus, 2005a; Banai et al., 2005b; Wible et al., 2005). Second, multi-sensory processing is carried out in structures such as IC and the auditory cortex, probably influencing the subcortical auditory processes reviewed in this chapter. In addition, these processes are influenced by higher level factors such as attention and memory. These influences are not likely to be modality specific either. Indeed, in individuals with conditions overlapping APD such as developmental dyslexia, auditory perceptual deficits often co-occur with visual (Amitay, Ben-Yehudah, Banai, & Ahissar, 2002; Ramus et al., 2003) and haptic deficits (Laasonen, Service, & Virsu, 2001). Furthermore, recent studies in animal models and in humans (e.g., Alain, 2007; Brechmann et al., 2007; Moore, Palmer, Hall, & Sumner, 2007; Näätänen, Tervaniemi, Sussman, Paavilainen, & Winkler, 2001; Nelken, 2004; Scheich, Brechmann, Brosch, Budinger, & Ohl, 2007) document both high-level influence on auditory function, and the presence of multiple "cognitive" processes in the auditory cortex itself, making the idea that even performance on simple auditory tasks can be dissociated from "cognitive processes" impossible. For example, auditory processing deficits may be more dependent on cognitive factors such as working memory than on auditory encoding per se (Banai & Ahissar, 2006). It is likely that similar processes operate in individuals with APD, though to our knowledge, such a study has not been published.

Summary

Subcortical auditory processes are more dynamic than typically thought. As discussed in this chapter, they interact with other modalities and factors such as attention, visual influence, and experience. The role of subcortical auditory processes in perception and cognition is far from understood, but available data suggest that they relate to cognitive processes involved in language and music, rather than to specific aspects of fine-grained auditory perception. Taken together, the evidence challenge some of the assumptions embedded in current conceptualization of APD.

Acknowledgments. This work was supported by grants NIH/NIDCD RO1-01510, F32DC008052, NSF BCS-0544846, the National Organizaton for Hearing Research Foundation (NOHR), and by the Hugh Knowles Center, Northwestern University. We would like to thank Teri Bellis for her insightful comments on this chapter.

References

Abrams, D. A., Nicol, T., Zecker, S. G., & Kraus, N. (2006). Auditory brainstem timing predicts cerebral asymmetry for speech. *Journal of Neuroscience, 26*, 11131–11137.

Akhoun, I., Gallégo, S., Moulin, A., Ménard, M., Veuillet, E., Berger-Vachon, C., Collet, L., Thai-Van, H. (2008). The temporal relationship between speech auditory brainstem responses and the acoustic pattern of the phoneme /ba/ in normal-hearing adults. *Clincal Neurophysiology, 119*, 922–933.

Alain, C. (2007). Breaking the wave: effects of attention and learning on concurrent sound perception. *Hearing Research, 229*, 225–236.

Amitay, S., Ben-Yehudah, G., Banai, K., & Ahissar, M. (2002). Disabled readers suffer from visual and auditory impairments but not from a specific magnocellular deficit. *Brain, 125*(Pt. 10), 2272–2285.

ASHA. (2005). *(Central) Auditory Processing Disorders* American Speech-Language-Hearing Association. http://www.asha.org/members/deskref-journals/deskref/default.

Baldeweg, T., Richardson, A., Watkins, S., Foale, C., & Gruzelier, J. (1999). Impaired auditory frequency discrimination in dyslexia detected with mismatch evoked potentials. *Annals of Neurolology, 45*, 495–503.

Banai, K., Abrams, D., & Kraus, N. (2007). Sensory-based learning disability: Insights from brainstem processing of speech sounds. *International Journal of Audioliology 46*, 524–532.

Banai, K., & Ahissar, M. (2006). Auditory processing deficits in dyslexia: Task or stimulus related? *Cerebral Cortex, 16*, 1718–1728.

Banai, K., & Kraus, N. (2006). Neurobiology of (central) auditory processing disorder and language-based learning disability. In: *Handbook of Central Auditory Processing Disorder: Volume I: Auditory Neuroscience and Diagnosis*, G. D. Chermak, F. E. Musiek (eds), San Diego: Plural Publishing, pp. 89–116.

Banai, K., Nicol, T., Zecker, S. G., & Kraus, N. (2005). Brainstem timing: implications for cortical processing and literacy. *Journal of Neuroscience, 25*, 9850–9857.

Bellis, T. J., & Ferre, J. M. (1999). Multidimensional approach to the differential diagnosis of central auditory processing disorders in children. *Journal of the American Academy of Audiology, 10*, 319–328.

Bent, T., Bradlow, A. R., & Wright, B. A. (2006). The influence of linguistic experience on the cognitive processing of pitch in speech and nonspeech sounds. *Journal of Experimental Psychology and Human Perceptual Performance, 32*, 97–103.

Bishop, D. V., & McArthur, G. M. (2004). Immature cortical responses to auditory stimuli in specific language impairment: Evidence from ERPs to rapid tone sequences. *Developmental Science, 7*, F11–F18.

Boston, J. R., & Møller, A. R. (1985). Brainstem auditory-evoked potentials. *Critical Review of Biomedical Engineering, 13*, 97–123.

Brechmann, A., Gaschler-Markefski, B., Sohr, M., Yoneda, K., Kaulisch, T., & Scheich, H. (2007). Working memory-specific activity in auditory cortex: Potential correlates of sequential processing and maintenance. *Cerebral Cortex, 17*, 2544–2545.

Cacace, A. T., & McFarland, D. J. (2005). The importance of modality specificity in diagnosing central auditory processing disorder.

American Journal of Audiology, *14*, 112–123.

Champoux, F., Paiement, P., Mercier, C., Lepore, F., Lassonde, M., & Gagne, J. P. (2007). Auditory processing in a patient with a unilateral lesion of the inferior colliculus. *European Journal of Neuroscience*, *25*, 291–297.

Corbera, S., Escera, C., & Artigas, J. (2006). Impaired duration mismatch negativity in developmental dyslexia. *NeuroReport*, *17*, 1051–1055.

Cunningham, J., Nicol, T., Zecker, S., & Kraus, N. (2000). Speech-evoked neurophysiologic responses in children with learning problems: development and behavioral correlates of perception. *Ear and Hearing*, *21*, 554–568.

Dean, I., Harper, N. S., & McAlpine, D. (2005). Neural population coding of sound level adapts to stimulus statistics. *Nature Neuroscience*, *8*, 1684–1689.

Delb, W., Strauss, D. J., Hohenberg, G., & Plinkert, P. K. (2003). The binaural interaction component (BIC) in children with central auditory processing disorders (CAPD). *International Journal of Audiology*, *42*, 401–412.

Delgutte, B., & Kiang, N. Y. (1984a). Speech coding in the auditory nerve: I. Vowel-like sounds. *Journal of the Acoustical Society of America*, *75*, 866–878.

Delgutte, B., & Kiang, N. Y. (1984b). Speech coding in the auditory nerve: IV. Sounds with consonant-like dynamic characteristics. *Journal of the Acoustical Society of America*, *75*, 897–907.

Fant, G. (1970). *Acoustic theory of speech production*. The Hague: Mouton.

Galbraith, G. C., Arbagey, P. W., Branski, R., Comerci, N., & Rector, P. M. (1995). Intelligible speech encoded in the human brain stem frequency-following response. *NeuroReport*, *6*, 2363–2367.

Galbraith, G. C., Bhuta, S. M., Choate, A. K., Kitahara, J. M., & Mullen, T. A., Jr. (1998). Brain stem frequency-following response to dichotic vowels during attention. *NeuroReport*, *9*, 1889–1893.

Galbraith, G. C., Olfman, D. M., & Huffman, T. M. (2003). Selective attention affects human brain stem frequency-following response. *NeuroReport*, *14*, 735–738.

Gopal, K. V., & Pierel, K. (1999). Binaural interaction component in children at risk for central auditory processing disorders. *Scandinavian Audiology*, *28*, 77–84.

Grontved, A., Walter, B., & Gronborg, A. (1988). Auditory brain stem responses in dyslexic and normal children. A prospective clinical investigation. *Scandinavian Audiology*, *17*, 53–54.

Hall, J. W. (1992). *Handbook of auditory evoked responses*. Needham Heights, MA: Allyn & Bacon.

Hari, R., & Renvall, H. (2001). Impaired processing of rapid stimulus sequences in dyslexia. *Trends in Cognitive Sciences*, *5*, 525–532.

Hayes, E. A., Warrier, C. M., Nicol, T. G., Zecker, S. G., & Kraus, N. (2003). Neural plasticity following auditory training in children with learning problems. *Clinical Neurophysiology*, *114*, 673–684.

Heim, S., Eulitz, C., Kaufmann, J., Fuchter, I., Pantev, C., Lamprecht-Dinnesen, A., et al. (2000). Atypical organisation of the auditory cortex in dyslexia as revealed by MEG. *Neuropsychologia*, *38*, 1749–1759.

Helenius, P., Salmelin, R., Richardson, U., Leinonen, S., & Lyytinen, H. (2002). Abnormal auditory cortical activation in dyslexia 100 msec after speech onset. *Journal of Cognitive Neuroscience*, *14*, 603–617.

Hochstein, S., & Ahissar, M. (2002). View from the top: hierarchies and reverse hierarchies in the visual system. *Neuron*, *36*, 791–804.

Hood, L. J. (1998). *Clinical applications of the auditory brainstem response*. San Diego, CA: Singular.

Hoormann, J., Falkenstein, M., & Hohnsbein, J. (2004). Effects of spatial attention on the brain stem frequency-following potential. *NeuroReport*, *15*, 1539–1542.

Jerger, S., Martin, R. C., & Jerger, J. (1987). Specific auditory perceptual dysfunction in a learning disabled child. *Ear and Hearing*, *8*, 78–86.

Johkura, K., Matsumoto, S., Hasegawa, O., & Kuroiwa, Y. (1998). Defective auditory recognition after small hemorrhage in the inferior colliculi. *Journal of the Neurological Sciences, 161*, 91-96.

Johnson, K. L., Nicol, T. G., & Kraus, N. (2005). Brain stem response to speech: A biological marker of auditory processing. *Ear and Hearing, 26*, 424-434.

Johnson, K. L., Nicol T., Kraus, N. (2008). Developmental plasticity in the human auditory brainstem. *Journal of Neuroscience,* 4000-4007.

Johnson, K. L., Nicol, T. G., Zecker, S. G., & Kraus, N. (2007). Auditory brainstem correlates of perceptual timing deficits. *Journal of Cognitive Neuroscience, 19*, 376-385.

Johnson, K. L., Nicol, T. G., Zecker, S. G., Bradlow, A., Skoe, E., Kraus, N. (2008). Brainstem encoding of voiced consonant-vowel stop syllables. *Clinical Neurophysiology,* in press.

King, C., Warrier, C. M., Hayes, E., & Kraus, N. (2002). Deficits in auditory brainstem pathway encoding of speech sounds in children with learning problems. *Neuroscience Letters, 319*, 111-115.

King, W. M., Lombardino, L. J., Crandell, C. C., & Leonard, C. M. (2003). Comorbid auditory processing disorder in developmental dyslexia. *Ear and Hearing, 24*, 448-456.

Kraus, N., & Banai, K. (2007). Auditory-processing malleability: Focus on language and music. *Current Directions in Psychological Science, 16*, 105-110.

Kraus, N., McGee, T. J., Carrell, T. D., Zecker, S. G., Nicol, T. G., & Koch, D. B. (1996). Auditory neurophysiologic responses and discrimination deficits in children with learning problems. *Science, 273*, 971-973.

Kraus, N., & Nicol, T. (2005). Brainstem origins for cortical 'what' and 'where' pathways in the auditory system. *Trends in Neuroscience, 28*, 176-181.

Krishnan, A. (2002). Human frequency-following responses: Representation of steady-state synthetic vowels. *Hearing Research, 166*, 192-201.

Krishnan, A., Xu, Y., Gandour, J., & Cariani, P. (2005). Encoding of pitch in the human brainstem is sensitive to language experience. *Brain Research and Cognitive Brain Research, 25*, 161-168.

Kujala, T., Myllyviita, K., Tervaniemi, M., Alho, K., Kallio, J., & Naatanen, R. (2000). Basic auditory dysfunction in dyslexia as demonstrated by brain activity measurements. *Psychophysiology, 37*, 262-266.

Laasonen, M., Service, E., & Virsu, V. (2001). Temporal order and processing acuity of visual, auditory, and tactile perception in developmentally dyslexic young adults. *Cognitive Af-fect and Behavioral Neuroscience, 1*, 394-410.

Lachmann, T., Berti, S., Kujala, T., & Schroger, E. (2005). Diagnostic subgroups of developmental dyslexia have different deficits in neural processing of tones and phonemes. *International Journal of Psychophysiology, 56*, 105-120.

Lauter, J. L., & Wood, S. B. (1993). Auditory brainstem synchronicity in dyslexia measured using the REPs/ABR protocol. *Annals of the New York Academy of Sciences, 682*, 377-379.

Litovsky, R. Y., Fligor, B. J., & Tramo, M. J. (2002). Functional role of the human inferior colliculus in binaural hearing. *Hearing Research, 165*, 177-188.

Ma, X., & Suga, N. (2001). Plasticity of bat's central auditory system evoked by focal electric stimulation of auditory and/or somatosensory cortices. *Journal of Neurophysiology, 85*, 1078-1087.

Marler, J. A., & Champlin, C. A. (2005). Sensory processing of backward-masking signals in children with language-learning impairment as assessed with the auditory brainstem response. *Journal of Speech Language and Hearing Research, 48*, 189-203.

Mason, S. M., & Mellor, D. H. (1984). Brain-stem, middle latency and late cortical evoked potentials in children with speech and language disorders. *Electroencephalography and Clinical Neurophysiology, 59*, 297-309.

McAnally, K. I., & Stein, J. F. (1997). Scalp potentials evoked by amplitude-modulated tones in dyslexia. *Journal of Speech Language and Hearing Research, 40*, 939-945.

Moiseacu-Yiflach, T., & Pratt, H. (2005). Auditory event related potentials and source current density estimation in phonologic/auditory dyslexics. *Clinical Neurophysiology, 116*, 2632-2647.

Møller, A. R. (1999). Neural mechanisms of BAEP. *Electroencephalography and Clinical Neurophysiology Suppl, 49*, 27-35.

Møller, A. R., & Jannetta, P. (1985). Neural generators of the auditory brainstem response. In J. T. Jacobson (Ed.), *The auditory brainstem response* (pp. 13-32). San Diego, CA: College-Hill Press.

Moore, D., Palmer, A., Hall, D., & Sumner, C. (2007). Hearing research special issue "Auditory cortex 2006—The listening brain." *Hearing Research, 239*,1-2.

Musacchia, G., Sams, M., Nicol, T., & Kraus, N. (2006). Seeing speech affects acoustic information processing in the human brainstem. *Experimental Brain Research, 168*, 1-10.

Musacchia, G., Sams, M., Skoe, E., & Kraus, N. (2007). Musicians have enhanced subcortical auditory and audiovisual processing of speech and music. *Proceedings of the National Academy of Science USA, 104*, 15894-15898.

Musacchia, G., Strait, D., Kraus, N. (2008). Relationships between behavior, brainstem and cortical encoding of seen and heard speech in musicians and nonmusicians. *Hearing Research, 241,* 34-42.

Musiek, F. E., Charette, L., Morse, D., & Baran, J. A. (2004). Central deafness associated with a midbrain lesion. *Journal of the American Academy of Audiology, 15*, 133-151; quiz 172-133.

Näätänen, R., Tervaniemi, M., Sussman, E., Paavilainen, P., & Winkler, I. (2001). "Primitive intelligence" in the auditory cortex. *Trends in Neuroscience, 24*, 283-288.

Nagarajan, S., Mahncke, H., Salz, T., Tallal, P., Roberts, T., & Merzenich, M. M. (1999). Cortical auditory signal processing in poor readers. *Proceedings of the Nationall Academy of Science U S A, 96*, 6483-6488.

Nelken, I. (2004). Processing of complex stimuli and natural scenes in the auditory cortex. *Current Opinion in Neurobiology, 14*, 474-480.

Palmer, A. R., Hall, D. A., Sumner, C., Barrett, D. J., Jones, S., Nakamoto, K., et al. (2006). Some investigations into non-passive listening. *Hearing Research, 229*, 148-157.

Popelar, J., Nwabueze-Ogbo, F. C., & Syka, J. (2003). Changes in neuronal activity of the inferior colliculus in rat after temporal inactivation of the auditory cortex. *Physiological Research, 52*, 615-628.

Purdy, S. C., Kelly, A. S., & Davies, M. G. (2002). Auditory brainstem response, middle latency response, and late cortical evoked potentials in children with learning disabilities. *Journal of the American Academy of Audiology, 13*, 367-382.

Ramus, F., Rosen, S., Dakin, S. C., Day, B. L., Castellote, J. M., White, S., et al. (2003). Theories of developmental dyslexia: insights from a multiple case study of dyslexic adults. *Brain, 126*(Pt 4), 841-865.

Russo, N., Nicol, T., Musacchia, G., & Kraus, N. (2004). Brainstem responses to speech syllables. *Clinical Neurophysiology, 115*, 2021-2030.

Russo, N., Nicol, T. G., Zecker, S. G., Hayes, E. A., & Kraus, N. (2005). Auditory training improves neural timing in the human brainstem. *Behavioural Brain Research, 156*, 95-103.

Russo, N. M., Bradlow, A. R., Skoe, E., Trommer, B. L., Nicol, T., Zecker, S., Kraus, N., (2008). Deficient brainstem encoding of pitch in children with autism spectrum disorders. *Clinical Neurophysiology, 119*,1720-1731.

Sachs, M. B., & Young, E. D. (1979). Encoding of steady-state vowels in the auditory nerve: representation in terms of discharge rate. *Journal of the Acoustical Society of America, 66*, 470-479.

Salamy, A. (1984). Maturation of the auditory brainstem response from birth through early childhood. *Journal of Clinical Neurophysiology, 1*, 293-329.

Scheich, H., Brechmann, A., Brosch, M., Budinger, E., & Ohl, F. W. (2007). The cognitive auditory cortex: Task-specificity of stimulus representations. *Hearing Research, 229*, 213-214.

Schulte-Korne, G., Deimel, W., Bartling, J., & Remschmidt, H. (1998). Auditory processing and dyslexia: evidence for a specific speech processing deficit. *NeuroReport, 9*, 337-340.

Sharma, M., Purdy, S. C., Newall, P., Wheldall, K., Beaman, R., & Dillon, H. (2006). Electrophysiological and behavioral evidence of auditory processing deficits in children with reading disorder. *Clinical Neurophysiology, 117*, 1130–1144.

Sohmer, H., Pratt, H., & Kinarti, R. (1977). Sources of frequency following responses (FFR) in man. *Electroencephalography and Clinical Neurophysiology, 42*, 656–664.

Song, J. H., Banai, K., & Kraus, N. (2008). Brainstem timing deficits in children with learning impairment may result from corticofugal origins. *Audiology and Neurootology, 13*, 335–344.

Song, J. H., Banai, K., Russo, N. M., & Kraus, N. (2006). On the relationship between speech- and nonspeech-evoked auditory brainstem responses. *Audiology and Neurootology, 11*, 233–241.

Song, J. H., Skoe, E., Wong, P. C., & Kraus, N. (2008). Plasticity in the adult human auditory brainstem following short-term linguistic training. *Journal of Cognitive Neuroscience.* DOI: 10.1162/jocn.2008. 20131.

Stoodley, C. J., Hill, P. R., Stein, J. F., & Bishop, D. V. (2006). Auditory event-related potentials differ in dyslexics even when auditory psychophysical performance is normal. *Brain Research, 1121*, 190–199.

Swaminathan, J., Krishnan, A., Grandour, J. T. (2008). Pitch encoding in speech and nonspeech contexts in the human auditory brainstem. *Neuroreport, 19*, 1163–1167.

Wible, B., Nicol, T., & Kraus, N. (2002). Abnormal neural encoding of repeated speech stimuli in noise in children with learning problems. *Clinical Neurophysiology, 113*, 485–494.

Wible, B., Nicol, T., & Kraus, N. (2004). Atypical brainstem representation of onset and formant structure of speech sounds in children with language-based learning problems. *Biological Psychology, 67*, 299–317.

Wible, B., Nicol, T., & Kraus, N. (2005). Correlation between brainstem and cortical auditory processes in normal and language-impaired children. *Brain, 128*(Pt. 2), 417–423.

Winer, J. A. (2006). Decoding the auditory corticofugal systems. *Hearing Research, 212*(1–2), 1–8.

Wong, P. C., Skoe, E., Russo, N. M., Dees, T., & Kraus, N. (2007). Musical experience shapes human brainstem encoding of linguistic pitch patterns. *Nature Neuroscience, 10*, 420–422.

Worden, F. G., & Marsh, J. T. (1968). Frequency-following (microphonic-like) neural responses evoked by sound. *Electroencephalography and Clinical Neurophysiology, 25*, 42–52.

Wright, B. A., Lombardino, L. J., King, W. M., Puranik, C. S., Leonard, C. M., & Merzenich, M. M. (1997). Deficits in auditory temporal and spectral resolution in language-impaired children. *Nature, 387*, 176–178.

Xu, Y., Krishnan, A., & Gandour, J. T. (2006). Specificity of experience-dependent pitch representation in the brainstem. *NeuroReport, 17*, 1601–1605.

Young, E. D., & Sachs, M. B. (1979). Representation of steady-state vowels in the temporal aspects of the discharge patterns of populations of auditory-nerve fibers. *Journal of the Acoustical Society of America, 66*, 1381–1403.

Zatorre, R. J., Belin, P., & Penhune, V. B. (2002). Structure and function of auditory cortex: Music and speech. *Trends in Cognitive Science, 6*, 37–46.

CHAPTER 16

Tinnitus as a Central Auditory Processing Disorder

DIRK DE RIDDER, TOMAS MENOVSKY, AND
PAUL H. VAN DE HEYNING

Overview

Two parallel ascending pathways supply auditory information to auditory cortices and other parts of the brain, the classical (lemniscal) and the nonclassical (extralemniscal). Two descending pathways that may be regarded as reciprocal to the ascending pathways provide feedback from central structures to the periphery (Jones, 1998b; Møller, 2006a; Møller, 2003). Neurons in the classical pathways are sharply tuned and tonotopically organized, whereas neurons in the nonclassical pathways are broadly tuned and lack tonotopical organization. Neurons in the classical pathways predominantly fire tonically whereas many neurons in the nonclassical fire in burst or phasic mode (He & Hu, 2002; Hu, Senatorov, & Mooney, 1994).

Tinnitus is related to synchronous gamma band hyperactivity of the thalamo-cortical auditory columns (Llinas, Ribary, Jeanmonod, Kronberg, & Mitra, 1999; Weisz, Muller, Schlee, Dohrmann, Hartmann, & Elbert, 2007) and reorganization of the auditory cortex. Therefore, hypothetically, increased activation of the burst-firing nontonotopic nonclassical pathways may lead to perception of tinnitus of noise character, whereas increased activation of the tonic firing tonotopic classical system may produce pure-tone tinnitus.

Direct modulation of this hyperactivity/reorganization via transcranial magnetic stimulation or implanted electrodes can suppress tinnitus in selected patients (De Ridder, De Mulder, Verstraeten, Van der Klen, Sunaert, Smits, et al., 2006; Kleinjung, Eichhammer, Langguth, Jacob, Marienhagen, Hajek, et al., 2005; Londero, Langguth, De Ridder, Bonfils, & Lefaucheur, 2006). The stimulation design required for tinnitus with pure tone characteristics differs from the stimulation design required for noiselike tinnitus: tonic or single spike stimulation is capable of suppressing pure-tone tinnitus, but not noiselike tinnitus, whereas burst stimulation is capable of suppressing both kinds of tinnitus (De Ridder, Van der Loo, Van der Kelen, Menovsky, van de Heyning, & Møller, et al., 2007a; DeRidder, Van der Loo, Van der Kelen, Menovsky, van de Heyning, & Møller, 2007b).

It has been suggested that the burst-firing of neurons in the nonclassical system drives the tonically firing neurons in the classical system (Jones, 1998a, 2001). Burst firing is shown to be more powerful in activating the cerebral cortex than tonic firing (Lisman, 1997; Sherman, 2001a, 2001b; Swadlow & Gusev, 2001) and bursts may activate neurons that are not activated by tonic stimulations (unmasking dormant synapses) (Møller, 2006b), thus explaining how neurons in the nonclassical system drive neurons in the classical system.

Introduction

Central auditory processing disorder (CAPD) has been defined as a modality-specific perceptual dysfunction that is not due to peripheral hearing loss and that should be distinguishable from cognitive, language-based, and/or supramodal attentional problems (Cacace & McFarland, 2005). It has been argued that this definition is both too loose and too restrictive, and that any useful definition of CAPD must not only exclude supramodal causes of auditory deficits, but must be based on the notion of impaired brain function demonstrable for nonspeech sounds (Rosen, 2005). Therefore, tinnitus research, which only involves nonspeech sounds, might benefit CAPD research. The aim of this chapter is to develop a patho-physiologic hypothesis that could possibly explain differences in pure-tone tinnitus and noiselike tinnitus, but that could also be an auditory modality-specific manifestation of CAPD.

Tinnitus is an auditory phantom percept (Jastreboff, 1990; Mühlnickel, Elbert, Taub, & Flor, 1998) related to reorganization (Mühlnickel, et al., 1998) and hyperactivity (Eggermont & Roberts, 2004) of the auditory system. The auditory system consists of two main parallel pathways supplying auditory information to the cerebral cortex: the tonotopically organized classical (lemniscal) system, and the nontonotopic nonclassical (extralemniscal) system (Figure 16–1). The classical pathways use the ventral thalamus, the neurons of which project to the primary auditory cortex whereas the nonclassical pathways use the medial and dorsal thalamic nuclei that project to the secondary auditory cortex and association cortexes, thus bypassing the primary cortex (Møller, 2003). Whereas neurons in the classical pathways only respond to one modality of sensory stimulation, many neurons in the nonclassical pathway respond to more than one modality. Neurons in the ventral thalamus fire in a tonic or semitonic mode whereas neurons in the medial and dorsal thalamus fire in bursts (He & Hu, 2002; Hu, Senatorov, & Mooney, 1994). The nonclassical pathways receive their input from the classical pathways, which means that the ascending auditory pathways are a complex system of at least two main parallel systems that provide different kinds of processing and which interact with each other in a complex way. Both systems provide sensory input to the amygdala through a long cortical route, and in addition, the nonclassical pathways provide subcortical connections to the lateral nucleus of the amygdala from dorsal thalamic nuclei (LeDoux, 1993).

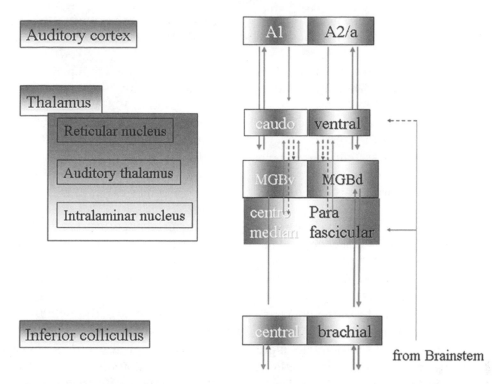

Figure 16–1. Pathways of the auditory lemniscal (*white*) and extralemniscal (*black*) system. Excitatory (*solid lines*) and inhibitory synapses (*dotted lines*) are represented.

The Nonclassical or Extralemniscal System

The nonclassical system is also known as the nonspecific system, the nontonotopic system or extralemniscal system, and has the following characteristics:

1. Phylogenetically older than the classical system (Parvizi & Damasio, 2003; Strominger, Nelson & Dougherty, 1977) (Llinas, personal communication).
2. Connects from thalamus to secondary cortex (Chiry, Tardif, Magistretti, & Clarke, 2003; Jones, 1998b, 2001, 2003; Møller, 2003).
3. More broadly tuned (less or nontonotopic) (Bordi & LeDoux, 1994; Calford, 1983; Hu et al., 1994; Jones, 2001).
4. Has a variable latency response (Bartlett & Smith, 1999; Bordi, LeDoux, Clugnet, & Pavlides, 1993; Calford, 1983).
5. Rapidly habituates to repetitive stimuli (Bartlett & Smith, 1999; Bordi & LeDoux, 1994; Calford, 1983).
6. Neurons in the medial and dorsal thalamus fire in bursts (He & Hu, 2002; Hu, et al., 1994).
7. Burst firing acts as a stimulus detector (Mooney, Zhang, Basile, Senatorov, Ngsee, Omar, et al., 2004; Sherman, 2001b).

8. Burst firing behaves in a nonlinear way (Sherman, 2001a, 2001b; Swadlow & Gusev, 2001).
9. Burst firing overrides tonic mode (Sherman, 2001a, 2001b; Swadlow & Gusev, 2001).
10. Nonclassical system drives the classical system (Jones, 1998a, 2001).
11. The nonclassical system is calbindin positive (Chiry, et al., 2003; Jones, 2001; Tardif, Chiry, Probst, Magistretti, & Clarke, 2003).
12. Calbindin increases after temporary auditory deafferentation (Caicedo, d'Aldin, Eybalin, & Puel, 1997; Forster & Illing, 2000; Garcia, Edward, Brennan, & Harlan, 2000; Syka, 2002).
13. Neurons in the nuclei of the nonclassical auditory pathways (ICX, DC, and dorsomedial MGB) respond to more than one sensory modality indicating a multimodal function (Bordi & LeDoux, 1994; Itoh, Kamiya, Mitani, Yasui, Takada, & Mizuno, 1987; Møller, 2000; Szczepaniak & Møller, 1993; Leinonen, Hyvarinen, & Sovijarvi, 1980).

4. Short latency response (Bartlett & Smith, 1999; Bordi et al., 1993; Calford, 1983).
5. Slower habituation to repetitive stimuli (Bartlett & Smith, 1999; Bordi & LeDoux, 1994; Calford, 1983).
6. Neurons in the ventral thalamus fire in a tonic or semitonic mode (He & Hu, 2002; Hu et al., 1994).
7. Tonic firing neurons are feature detectors (Mooney et al., 2004; Sherman, 2001b).
8. Tonic firing neurons behave linearly to a stimuli (Sherman, 2001a, 2001b; Swadlow & Gusev, 2001).
9. Tonic firing mode activates cortex less than burst mode (Sherman, 2001a, 2001b; Swadlow & Gusev, 2001).
10. Classical pathways are parvalbumin positive (Chiry et al., 2003; Jones, 2001; Tardif et al., 2003).
11. Parvalbumin positive cells demonstrate higher spontaneous firing rate (Kawaguchi, 2001; Kawaguchi & Kubota, 1993; Solbach & Celio, 1991).
12. Neurons respond to only one modality of sensory stimulation (Møller, 2000).

The Classical System

The classical system is also known as the specific system, the tonotopic system, or lemniscal system. It has been characterized as "slow and accurate," whereas the nonclassical system is "fast and dirty." The classical system has the following characteristics:

1. Phylogenetically more recent (Parvizi & Damasio, 2003; Strominger et al., 1977) (Llinas, personal communication).
2. Connects from thalamus to primary auditory area (Chiry, et al., 2003; Jones, 1998b, 2001, 2003; Møller, 2003).
3. (Tonotopic) (Bordi & LeDoux, 1994; Calford, 1983; Hu et al., 1994; Jones, 2001).

Hypothetical Mechanism of Central Auditory Processing

The Nonclassical System Signals That a Change in the Auditory Environment Occurs, the Classical System Transmits the Content of That Change

Sensory information is routed to the cortex via the thalamus and animals must attend selectively to stimuli that signal danger or opportunity. Sensory input must be filtered, allowing only behaviorally relevant information to capture limited attentional resources (McAlonan & Brown, 2002).

As mentioned, auditory information reaches the thalamus via two pathways: the classical tonotopic pathway transmits the content of the auditory input and the non-classical nontonotopic pathway transmits change in this auditory information (Sherman, 2001b).

From the thalamus the information reaches the primary auditory cortex (predominantly classical) and secondary auditory cortex (predominantly nonclassical) where the auditory content is compared to information contained in auditory memory. If the information is known, that is, redundant, the cortex will activate the thalamic reticular nucleus (RTN). The RTN will then shut off the classical (MGBv) and nonclassical thalamic relay nuclei (MGBv and MGBm+d) for the same information but leaving the thalamic gate open for different information. The reticular nucleus of the thalamus represents an inhibitory interface or "attentional gate," which regulates the flow of information between the thalamus and cortex (McAlonan & Brown, 2002) and the projections of cells in the auditory sector of the reticular nucleus of the thalamus to the classical thalamus (MGv) and to the nonclassical thalamus (MGd or MGm) are topographically organized, which allows for this selective information transmission (Figure 16–2).

The Arousal System Modifies the Classical System and the Nonclassical System

Auditory consciousness is probably the result of activation of the dual system, consisting of a switch on/off pathway in the posterior pons (Steriade, Contreras, Amzica, & Timofeev, 1996), specifically, the posterior mid-brain running to the intralaminar nuclei (Steriade et al., 1996; Wainer et al., 1993), most likely the cholinergic system, and a thalamocorticothalamic acceleration system driven by the intralaminar nuclei and modified by the auditory thalamus and reticular nucleus (Cotillon & Edeline, 2000). Only the nonclassical auditory pathway connects to the posterior intralaminar nuclei (PIL) (Bordi & LeDoux, 1994).

The spontaneous activity of the thalamus at rest is 5 to 15 Hz (Steriade, 2000). Recent studies of the auditory system suggest that both the auditory thalamus and the auditory sector of the reticular thalamic nucleus, but not the auditory cortex, are involved in the generation of stimulus-evoked alpha (5–15 Hz) oscillations in the thalamocortical auditory system (Cotillon & Edeline, 2000). In animals under anesthesia the oscillations were composed of both stimulus-locked (also known as evoked) and nonstimulus-locked (also known as induced) oscillations, whereas in unanesthetized animals, they were only composed of non-stimulus-locked oscillations. Thus, no evoked (i.e., stimulus-locked) oscillations are found in waking and paradoxic sleep. Both under anesthesia and in slow wave sleep (SWS), the frequency range of the oscillations is 5 to 15 Hz, and there is no frequency difference between evoked and spontaneous oscillations. The absence of oscillations in awake animals may allow each neuron to process acoustic information independently of its neighbors and may, in fact, benefit auditory perception (Cotillon-Williams & Edeline, 2003).

Low-frequency oscillations (delta and theta) depend on an increased inhibition from the reticular nucleus in the thalamus (Steriade, 2000).

Forty hertz, or greater gamma activity (30–45 Hz) might be generated by 40-Hz pacemaker cells (Steriade, 2000) in the intralaminar nuclei of the thalamus or by intra-

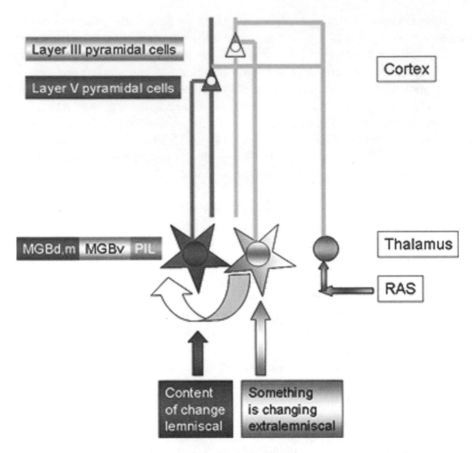

Figure 16–2. The lemniscal specific tonotopic system (*black*) and extralemniscal nonspecific nontonotopic system (*gray*) work in coherence. The arousal system (RAS) in the posterior part of the pons, via the posterior mesencephalon activates the posterior intralaminar nuclei (PIL = gray),which modulate both the extralemniscal and lemniscal system. The nontonotopic extralemniscal system tells something is changing in the auditory environment, and drives the tonotopic lemniscal system to transmit the content of this change in auditory information.

cortical feedback loss under influence of the posterior intralaminar nucleus posterior intralaminar nucleus (PIL) (Sukov & Barth, 2001). Lesions of the PIL (Barth & MacDonald, 1996) or the entire acoustic thalamus (Brett, Krishnan, & Barth, 1996) have no detectable effect on spontaneous gamma oscillations, suggesting that large intracortical networks are capable of generating and coherently synchronizing gamma oscilla-

tions independently of subcortical input. The acoustic thalamus, however, does directly modulate these oscillations, which are inhibited by stimulation of the dorsal and ventral divisions of the medial geniculate nucleus (MGd and MGv) and evoked by stimulation of the adjacent PIL (Barth & MacDonald, 1996). Burst mode stimulation of the PIL (0.5 sec of 500 Hz) induces thalamocortical 40-Hz oscillations in the auditory cortex (Brett & Barth, 1997), either via direct connections between the PIL and the cortex (Arnault & Roger, 1987, 1990) or via activation of fibers de passage (Brett & Barth, 1997). Fibers from the PIL terminate in cortical layers I (calbindin-positive nonclassical) (Chiry, et al., 2003; Hashikawa, Rausell, Molinari & Jones, 1991; Molinari et al., 1995) and VI, and at the layer III-IV (parvalbumin positive classical) (Chiry et al., 2003; Wallace, Kitzes, & Jones, 1991) border, suggesting that the same neuronal message may pass from the PIL to multiple cortical areas. Thus, the PIL may mediate a general cortical activation and may play a role in attention to auditory stimuli (Kaufman & Rosenquist, 1985) and activate both classical and nonclassical systems simultaneously via activation of an area at the border between primary and secondary cortex (Brett & Barth, 1997). Recent studies of auditory mismatch negativity, with simultaneous electroencephalographic (EEG) and magnetoencephalographic (MEG) recordings fused on functional magnetic resonance imaging (fMRI) data, demonstrate that more posteriorly located broadband-tuned neurons serve as a gating mechanism determining the extent to which unattended novel sounds enter the subject's awareness, whereas the more anteriorly located narrowly tuned neurons are more involved in subsequent attentional feature analysis (Jääskeläinen, Ahveninen, Bonmassar, Dale, Ilomoniemi, Levänen et al., 2004). In other words, the human posterior auditory cortex (most likely nonclassical), gates novel sounds to consciousness (requiring the classical primary cortex).

The intralaminar nuclei are considered the place where thalamocortical oscillations are evoked and modified (Bogen, 1995; Steriade, 2000; Steriade, Curro Dossi, & Contreras, 1993; Sukov & Barth, 2001) via interaction with the reticular nucleus of the thalamus (Cotillon & Edeline, 2000; Steri-

ade, 2000). The PIL itself is innervated by the arousal system; that is, by the adrenergic locus coeruleus, the serotoninergic dorsal raphe nucleus, and the cholinergic basal nucleus of Meynert (Arnault & Roger, 1990).

In summary, two different pathways bring auditory information to the auditory cortex and both pathways are modulated by the reticular nucleus (inhibitory) and the PIL (excitatory).

In general, the descending auditory system (Rouiller & Durif, 2004; Rouiller & Welker, 1991; Shi & Cassell, 1997) is a reciprocal system (Winer & Larue, 1987) of the ascending auditory system and consists of a descending tonotopic classical and a descending nontonotopic nonclassical system (Bartlett, Stark, Guillery, & Smith, 2000; Hazama, Kimura, Donishi, Sakoda, & Tamai, 2004).

The descending auditory pathways are connected to the auditory thalamus ipsilaterally, but to the inferior colliculus in a bilateral fashion (Winer, Chernock, Larue, & Cheung, 2002; Winer & Larue, 1987).

Separate pathways run from the primary auditory cortex to the thalamus, inferior colliculus, superior olivary complex, and cochlear nuclei in the pons, derived from different cortical cells (Weedman & Ryugo, 1996a, 1996b).

The descending pathways to the cochlea are under noradrenergic and serotoninergic influence of the arousal system by connections with the locus coeruleus and dorsal raphe nucleus (Behrens, Schofield, & Thompson, 2002; Horvath, Ribari, Repassy, Toth, Boldogkoi, & Palkovits, 2003), similarly to what is known for the ascending system (Arnault & Roger, 1990).

In summary, the interaction between the two ascending and two descending auditory systems critically depends on brainstem input and the way the nonclassical system drives the classical system.

After acute deafferentation, calbindin and parvalbumin positive cells increase in number (Caicedo, et al., 1997; Forster & Illing, 2000) and after chronic deafferentation the parvalbumin positive cells decrease in number (in the somatosensory system) (Rausell, Cusick, Taub, & Jones, 1992). This seems as if the nonclassical system is trying to compensate for the loss of activity in the tonotopic system. This also occurs in frequency-specific lesions.

Tinnitus

Studies in humans have indicated that some patients with tinnitus have an abnormal activation of the nonclassical auditory system (Møller, Møller, & Yokota, 1992). Studies of animal models of tinnitus have shown that burst firing is increased in the nonclassical system (Chen & Jastreboff, 1995; Eggermont, 2003; Eggermont & Kenmochi, 1998) and tonic firing activity is increased in the classical system (Brozoski, Bauer, & Caspary, 2002; Kaltenbach & Afman, 2000; Kaltenbach, Godfrey, Neumann, McCaslin, Afman, & Zhang, 1998; Kaltenbach, Zacharek, Zhang, & Frederick, 2004; Zacharek, Kaltenbach, Mathog, & Zhang, 2002; Zhang & Kaltenbach, 1998). Interestingly, not only tonic firing but also burst firing is increased in neurons in the primary auditory cortex in animal models of tinnitus (Ochi & Eggermont, 1997). Studies in patients with intractable tinnitus have shown that tonic electrical stimuli of the primary and secondary auditory cortex can suppress pure-tone tinnitus, but not white-noise/narrowband noise tinnitus (De Ridder et al., 2006).

Repetitive TMS is a noninvasive method capable of modulating activity of the human cortex, and by this mechanism, interfering with tinnitus perception (De Ridder et al., 2005; Eichhammer, Langguth, Marienhagen, Kleinjung, & Hajak, 2003; Kleinjung et al., 2005; Plewnia, Bartels, &

Gerloff, 2003). Repetitive TMS machines can deliver both tonic and burst stimuli. Burst stimulation is shown to be more powerful in activating the cerebral cortex than tonic stimulation (Lisman, 1997; Sherman, 2001a, 2001b; Swadlow & Gusev, 2001) and bursts may activate neurons that are not activated by tonic stimulations (unmasking dormant synapses) (Møller, 2006b).

Our recent results show that narrowband/white-noise tinnitus can only be suppressed by burst rTMS, although burst rTMS can suppress both pure-tone tinnitus and narrow-band/white-noise tinnitus. Tonic rTMS, on the other hand, can only suppress pure-tone tinnitus. As the nontonotopic (nonclassical) system provides input to the tonotopic (classical) system (Jones, 1998a, 2001), our results suggest that burst stimulation can modulate the burst firing nontonotopic nonclassical system (directly) and the tonic firing tonotopic classical system (indirectly), whereas tonic stimulation can only modulate the tonic firing tonotopic classical system (directly). A further argument supportive of this hypothesis is provided by our finding that the frequency that maximally suppresses pure-tone tinnitus is the same for tonic and burst rTMS, whereas this is not the case for narrow-band/white-noise tinnitus. Indeed, if pure-tone tinnitus is generated in the classical system and the nonclassical system drives the classical system, it is feasible that pure-tone tinnitus is equally reduced by tonic (directly) and burst (indirectly) stimulations. However, if narrowband/white-noise tinnitus is generated in the nonclassical system, it is to be expected that only burst stimulations can influence its perception because this system is not driven by another system and fires itself in bursts. Finally, recent findings (De Ridder et al., 2007b) show that lower frequencies of narrowband/white-noise tinnitus respond better to burst stimulation than higher frequencies. This could be viewed as supportive of the hypothesis, as it is known that lower pitch sounds have a wider tuning curve and thus respond more like a nontonotopic system in general.

Following these arguments, we suggest that hyperactivation of burst firings in the nontonotopic part of the auditory system could lead to white-noise tinnitus, which cannot be suppressed by tonic stimulation but only by burst stimulation, being a more powerful stimulus to modulate the cortex. Hyperactivity of the tonic firing tonotopic system would then lead to pure-tone tinnitus, which could be modified by the weaker tonic stimulation and hyperactivity of both pathways would lead to narrow-band tinnitus.

Central Auditory Processing Disorder (CAPD)

Tinnitus could be considered a CAPD resulting from highly synchronized hyperactivity of the auditory thalamocortical columns, with pure tones, white noise, and narrowband noise being generated by highly synchronous hyperactivity in the classical, nonclassical, or both systems respectively. Is this the only CAPD that results from abnormal activity of the classical or nonclassical system?

Based on studies of interaction on perceived sounds from stimulation of the somatosensory system, it has been shown that adults normally have little or no signs of involvement of the nonclassical system, whereas children normally show indications of involvement of the nonclassical system (Møller & Rollins, 2002). The perception of the strength or character of tinnitus in some individuals with tinnitus can be modulated by electrical stimulation of the median nerve (Møller, Møller, & Yokota,

1992), thus an indication of involvement of the nonclassical pathways. Median nerve stimulation can also affect the perception of sound indicating an abnormal involvement of the nonclassical pathways (Møller, Kern, & Grannemann, 2005).

In autism-related CAPD, the nonclassical system seems to persist too long. Cross-modal interaction between senses such as hearing and the somatosensory system does not occur normally in adults. As only the extralemniscal ascending auditory pathways receive somatosensory input, the presence of cross-modal interaction in autistic individuals is a sign that autism is associated with abnormal involvement of the extra-lemniscal or nonclassical auditory pathways (Møller, Kern, & Grannemann, 2005).

In order to fully explore this hypothesis, it would be very interesting to develop tests to differentially evaluate the classical and nonclassical system. Moreover, could auditory motion sensitivity testing, reduced sensitivity for low spatial and high temporal frequencies, and binaural stability testing be helpful for assessing the nonclassical system?

Conclusion

Tinnitus could possibly be considered a form of CAPD. We hypothesize that white-noise tinnitus is the result of synchronous hyperactivity of the nonclassical system, pure-tone tinnitus the result of synchronous hyperactivity of the classical system, and narrow-band noise the result of hyperactivity of both pathways. Central auditory processing disorder could be a manifestation of a loss of coherent activity between the classical and non-classical system, such as suggested for autistic CAPD. We suggest the development of tests to differentially evaluate the classical and nonclassical systems.

References

Arnault, P., & Roger, M. (1987). The connections of the peripeduncular area studied by retrograde and anterograde transport in the rat. *Journal of Comparative Neurology, 258,* 463–476.

Arnault, P., & Roger, M. (1990). Ventral temporal cortex in the rat: connections of secondary auditory areas Te2 and Te3. *Journal of Comparative Neurology, 302,* 110–123.

Barth, D. S., & MacDonald, K. D. (1996). Thalamic modulation of high-frequency oscillating potentials in auditory cortex. *Nature, 383,* 78–81.

Bartlett, E. L., & Smith, P. H. (1999). Anatomic, intrinsic, and synaptic properties of dorsal and ventral division neurons in rat medial geniculate body. *Journal of Neurophysiology, 81,* 1999–2016.

Bartlett, E. L., Stark, J. M., Guillery, R. W., & Smith, P. H. (2000). Comparison of the fine structure of cortical and collicular terminals in the rat medial geniculate body. *Neuroscience, 100,* 811–828.

Behrens, E. G., Schofield, B. R., & Thompson, A. M. (2002). Aminergic projections to cochlear nucleus via descending auditory pathways. *Brain Research, 955,* 34–44.

Bogen, J. E. (1995). On the neurophysiology of consciousness: I. An overview. *Consciousness and Cognition, 4,* 52–62.

Bordi, F., LeDoux, J., Clugnet, M. C., & Pavlides, C. (1993). Single-unit activity in the lateral nucleus of the amygdala and overlying areas of the striatum in freely behaving rats: Rates, discharge patterns, and responses to acoustic stimuli. *Behavioral Neuroscience, 107,* 757–769.

Bordi, F., & LeDoux, J. E. (1994). Response properties of single units in areas of rat auditory thalamus that project to the amygdala. I. Acoustic discharge patterns and frequency receptive fields. *Experimental Brain Research, 98,* 261–274.

Brett, B., & Barth, D. S. (1997). Subcortical modulation of high-frequency (gamma band) oscillating potentials in auditory cortex. *Journal of Neurophysiology, 78,* 573–581.

Brett, B., Krishnan, G., & Barth, D. S. (1996). The effects of subcortical lesions on evoked potentials and spontaneous high frequency (gamma-band) oscillating potentials in rat auditory cortex. *Brain Research, 721,* 155–166.

Brozoski, T. J., Bauer, C. A., & Caspary, D. M. (2002). Elevated fusiform cell activity in the dorsal cochlear nucleus of chinchillas with psychophysical evidence of tinnitus. *Journal of Neuroscience, 22,* 2383–2390.

Cacace, A. T., & McFarland, D. J. (2005). The importance of modality specificity in diagnosing central auditory processing disorder. *American Journal of Audiology, 14,* 112–123.

Caicedo, A., d'Aldin, C., Eybalin, M., & Puel, J. L. (1997). Temporary sensory deprivation changes calcium-binding proteins levels in the auditory brainstem. *Journal of Comparative Neurology, 378,* 1–15.

Calford, M. B. (1983). The parcellation of the medial geniculate body of the cat defined by the auditory response properties of single units. *Journal of Neuroscience, 3,* 2350–2364.

Chen, G. D., & Jastreboff, P. J. (1995). Salicylate-induced abnormal activity in the inferior colliculus of rats. *Hearing Research, 82,* 158–178.

Chiry, O., Tardif, E., Magistretti, P. J., & Clarke, S. (2003). Patterns of calcium-binding proteins support parallel and hierarchical organization of human auditory areas. *European Journal of Neuroscience, 17,* 397–410.

Cotillon, N., & Edeline, J. M. (2000). Tone-evoked oscillations in the rat auditory cortex result from interactions between the thalamus and reticular nucleus. *European Journal of Neuroscience, 12,* 3637–3650.

Cotillon-Williams, N., & Edeline, J. M. (2003). Evoked oscillations in the thalamo-cortical auditory system are present in anesthetized but not in unanesthetized rats. *Journal of Neurophysiology, 89,* 1968–1984.

De Ridder, D., De Mulder, G., Verstraeten, E., Van der Kelen, K., Sunaert, S., Smits, M., et al.

(2006). Primary and secondary auditory cortex stimulation for intractable tinnitus. *ORL; Journal of Oto-Rhino-Laryngology and Related Specialties, 68*, 48–54; discussion 54–45.

De Ridder, D., van der Loo, E., Van der Kelen, K., Menovsky, T., van de Heyning, P., & Møller, A. (2007a). Do tonic and burst TMS modulate the lemniscal and extralemniscal system differentially? *International Journal of Medical Sciences, 4*, 242–246.

De Ridder, D., van der Loo, E., Van der Kelen, K., Menovsky, T., van de Heyning, P., & Møller, A. (2007b). Theta, alpha and beta burst transcranial magnetic stimulation: brain modulation in tinnitus. *International Journal of Medical Sciences, 4*, 237–241.

De Ridder, D., Verstraeten, E., Van der Kelen, K., De Mulder, G., Sunaert, S., Verlooy, J., et al. (2005). Transcranial magnetic stimulation for tinnitus: influence of tinnitus duration on stimulation parameter choice and maximal tinnitus suppression *Otology and Neuro-Otology, 26*, 616–619.

Eggermont, J. J. (2003). Central tinnitus. *Auris Nasus Larynx, 30 Suppl*, S7–S12.

Eggermont, J. J., & Kenmochi, M. (1998). Salicylate and quinine selectively increase spontaneous firing rates in secondary auditory cortex. *Hearing Research, 117*, 149–160.

Eggermont, J. J., & Roberts, L. E. (2004). The neuroscience of tinnitus. *Trends in Neurosciences, 27*, 676–682.

Eichhammer, P., Langguth, B., Marienhagen, J., Kleinjung, T., & Hajak, G. (2003). Neuronavigated repetitive transcranial magnetic stimulation in patients with tinnitus: A short case series. *Biological Psychiatry, 54*, 862–865.

Forster, C. R., & Illing, R. B. (2000). Plasticity of the auditory brainstem: cochleotomy-induced changes of calbindin-D28k expression in the rat. *Journal of Comparative Neurology, 416*, 173–187.

Garcia, M. M., Edward, R., Brennan, G. B., & Harlan, R. E. (2000). Deafferentation-induced changes in protein kinase C expression in the rat cochlear nucleus. *Hearing Research, 147*, 113–124.

Hashikawa, T., Rausell, E., Molinari, M., & Jones, E. G. (1991). Parvalbumin- and calbindin-containing neurons in the monkey medial geniculate complex: differential distribution and cortical layer specific projections. *Brain Research, 544*, 335–341.

Hazama, M., Kimura, A., Donishi, T., Sakoda, T., & Tamai, Y. (2004). Topography of cortico-thalamic projections from the auditory cortex of the rat. *Journal of Neuroscience, 124*, 655–667.

He, J., & Hu, B. (2002). Differential distribution of burst and single-spike responses in auditory thalamus. *Journal of Neurophysiology, 88*, 2152–2156.

Horvath, M., Ribari, O., Repassy, G., Toth, I. E., Boldogkoi, Z., & Palkovits, M. (2003). Intracochlear injection of pseudorabies virus labels descending auditory and monoaminerg projections to olivocochlear cells in guinea pig. *European Journal of Neuroscience, 18*, 1439–1447.

Hu, B., Senatorov, V., & Mooney, D. (1994). Lemniscal and non-lemniscal synaptic transmission in rat auditory thalamus. *Journal of Physiology, 479 (Pt. 2)*, 217–231.

Itoh, K., Kamiya, H., Mitani, A., Yasui, Y., Takada, M., & Mizuno, N. (1987). Direct projections from the dorsal column nuclei and the spinal trigeminal nuclei to the cochlear nuclei in the cat. *Brain Research, 400*, 145–150.

Jääskeläinen, I. P., Ahveninen, J., Bonmassar, G., Dale, A. M., Ilmoniemi, R. J., Levänen, S., et al. (2004). Human posterior auditory cortex gates novel sounds to consciousness. *Proceedings of the National Academy of Sciences of the United States of America, 101*, 6809–6814.

Jastreboff, P. J. (1990). Phantom auditory perception (tinnitus): mechanisms of generation and perception. *Journal of Neuroscience Research, 8*, 221–254.

Jones, E. G. (1998a). A new view of specific and nonspecific thalamocortical connections. *Advances in Neurology, 77*, 49–71; discussion 72–43.

Jones, E. G. (1998b). Viewpoint: the core and matrix of thalamic organization. *Journal of Neuroscience, 85*, 331–345.

Jones, E. G. (2001). The thalamic matrix and thalamocortical synchrony. *Neurosciences, 24,* 595–601.

Jones, E. G. (2003). Chemically defined parallel pathways in the monkey auditory system. *Annals of the New York Academy of Sciences, 999,* 218–233.

Kaltenbach, J. A., & Afman, C. E. (2000). Hyperactivity in the dorsal cochlear nucleus after intense sound exposure and its resemblance to tone-evoked activity: A physiological model for tinnitus. *Hearing Research, 140,* 165–172.

Kaltenbach, J. A., Godfrey, D. A., Neumann, J. B., McCaslin, D. L., Afman, C. E., & Zhang, J. (1998). Changes in spontaneous neural activity in the dorsal cochlear nucleus following exposure to intense sound: relation to threshold shift. *Hearing Research, 124,* 78–84.

Kaltenbach, J. A., Zacharek, M. A., Zhang, J., & Frederick, S. (2004). Activity in the dorsal cochlear nucleus of hamsters previously tested for tinnitus following intense tone exposure. *Neuroscience Letters, 355,* 121–125.

Kaufman, E. F., & Rosenquist, A. C. (1985). Efferent projections of the thalamic intralaminar nuclei in the cat. *Brain Research, 335,* 257–279.

Kawaguchi, Y. (2001). Distinct firing patterns of neuronal subtypes in cortical synchronized activities. *Journal of Neuroscience, 21,* 7261–7272.

Kawaguchi, Y., & Kubota, Y. (1993). Correlation of physiological subgroupings of nonpyramidal cells with parvalbumin- and calbindin$_{D28k}$-immunoreactive neurons in layer V of rat frontal cortex. *Journal of Neurophysiology, 70,* 387–396.

Kleinjung, T., Eichhammer, P., Langguth, B., Jacob, P., Marienhagen, J., Hajak, G., et al. (2005). Long-term effects of repetitive transcranial magnetic stimulation (rTMS) in patients with chronic tinnitus. *Otolaryngology and Head and Neck Surgery, 132,* 566–569.

LeDoux, J. E. (1993). Emotional memory systems in the brain. *Behavioural Brain Research, 58,* 69–79.

Leinonen, L., Hyvarinen, J., & Sovijarvi, A. R. (1980). Functional properties of neurons in the temporo-parietal association cortex of awake monkey. *Experimental Brain Research, 39,* 203–215.

Lisman, J. E. (1997). Bursts as a unit of neural information: making unreliable synapses reliable. *Trends in Neurosciences, 20,* 38–43.

Llinas, R. R., Ribary, U., Jeanmonod, D., Kronberg, E., & Mitra, P. P. (1999). Thalamocortical dysrhythmia: A neurological and neuropsychiatric syndrome characterized by magnetoencephalography. *Proceedings of the National Academy of Sciences of the United States of America, 96,* 15222–15227.

Londero, A., Langguth, B., De Ridder, D., Bonfils, P., & Lefaucheur, J. P. (2006). Repetitive transcranial magnetic stimulation (rTMS): A new therapeutic approach in subjective tinnitus? *Clinical Neurophysiology, 36,* 145–155.

McAlonan, K., & Brown, V. J. (2002). The thalamic reticular nucleus: More than a sensory nucleus? *Neuroscientist, 8,* 302–305.

Molinari, M., Dell'Anna, M. E., Rausell, E., Leggio, M. G., Hashikawa, T., & Jones, E. G. (1995). Auditory thalamocortical pathways defined in monkeys by calcium-binding protein immunoreactivity. *The Journal of Comparative Neurology, 362,* 171–194.

Møller, A. R. (2003). *Sensory systems: Anatomy, physiology, and pathophysiology.* Amsterdam: Academic Press.

Møller, A. R. (2006a). *Hearing: Its physiology and pathophysiology* (2nd ed.). Amsterdam: Elsevier Science.

Møller, A. R. (2006b). *Neural plasticity and disorders of the nervous system.* Cambridge: Cambridge University Press.

Møller, A. R. (2000). *Hearing: Its physiology and pathophysiology* (1st ed.). San Diego, CA: Academic Press.

Møller, A. R. (2003). *Sensory systems: Anatomy and physiology.* Amsterdam: Academic Press.

Møller, A. R., Kern, J. K., & Grannemann, B. (2005). Are the non-classical auditory pathways involved in autism and PDD? *Neurological Research, 27,* 625–629.

Møller, A. R., Møller, M. B., & Yokota, M. (1992). Some forms of tinnitus may involve the extralemniscal auditory pathway. *Laryngoscope*, *102*, 1165-1171.

Møller, A. R., & Rollins, P. (2002). The non-classical auditory system is active in children but not in adults. *Neuroscience Letters*, *319*, 41-44.

Mooney, D. M., Zhang, L., Basile, C., Senatorov, V. V., Ngsee, J., Omar, A., et al. (2004). Distinct forms of cholinergic modulation in parallel thalamic sensory pathways. *Proceedings of the National Academy of Sciences*, *101*, 320-324.

Muhlnickel, W., Elbert, T., Taub, E., & Flor, H. (1998). Reorganization of auditory cortex in tinnitus. *Proceedings of the National Academy of Sciences*, *95*, 10340-10343.

Ochi, K., & Eggermont, J. J. (1997). Effects of quinine on neural activity in cat primary auditory cortex. *Hearing Research*, *105*, 105-118.

Parvizi, J., & Damasio, A. R. (2003). Differential distribution of calbindin D28k and parvalbumin among functionally distinctive sets of structures in the macaque brainstem. *Journal of Comparative Neurology*, *462*, 153-167.

Plewnia, C., Bartels, M., & Gerloff, C. (2003). Transient suppression of tinnitus by transcranial magnetic stimulation. *Annals of Neurology*, *53*, 263-266.

Rausell, E., Cusick, C. G., Taub, E., & Jones, E. G. (1992). Chronic deafferentation in monkeys differentially affects nociceptive and nonnociceptive pathways distinguished by specific calcium-binding proteins and downregulates gamma-aminobutyric acid type A receptors at thalamic levels. *Proceedings of the National Academy of Sciences*, *89*, 2571-2575.

Rosen, S. (2005). "A riddle wrapped in a mystery inside an enigma:" Defining central auditory processing disorder. *American Journal of Audiology*, *14*, 139-142; discussion 143-150.

Rouiller, E. M., & Durif, C. (2004). The dual pattern of corticothalamic projection of the primary auditory cortex in macaque monkey. *Neuroscience Letters*, *358*, 49-52.

Rouiller, E. M., & Welker, E. (1991). Morphology of corticothalamic terminals arising from the auditory cortex of the rat: A Phaseolus vulgaris-leucoagglutinin (PHA-L) tracing study. *Hearing Research*, *56*, 179-190.

Sherman, S. M. (2001a). Tonic and burst firing: dual modes of thalamocortical relay. *Trends in Neuroscience*, *24*, 122-126.

Sherman, S. M. (2001b). A wake-up call from the thalamus. *Nature Neuroscience*, *4*, 344-346.

Shi, C. J., & Cassell, M. D. (1997). Cortical, thalamic, and amygdaloid projections of rat temporal cortex. *Journal of Comparative Neurology*, *382*, 153-175.

Steriade, M. (2000). Corticothalamic resonance, states of vigilance and mentation. *Journal of Neuroscience*, *101*, 243-276.

Steriade, M., Contreras, D., Amzica, F., & Timofeev, I. (1996). Synchronization of fast (30-40 Hz) spontaneous oscillations in intrathalamic and thalamocortical networks. *Journal of Neuroscience*, *16*, 2788-2808.

Steriade, M., Curro Dossi, R., & Contreras, D. (1993). Electrophysiological properties of intralaminar thalamocortical cells discharging rhythmic (approximately 40 Hz) spike-bursts at approximately 1000 Hz during waking and rapid eye movement sleep. *Journal of Neuroscience*, *56*, 1-9.

Strominger, N. L., Nelson, L. R., & Dougherty, W. J. (1977). Second order auditory pathways in the chimpanzee. *Journal of Comparative Neurology*, *172*, 349-365.

Sukov, W., & Barth, D. S. (2001). Cellular mechanisms of thalamically evoked gamma oscillations in auditory cortex. *Journal of Neurophysiology*, *85*, 1235-1245.

Swadlow, H. A., & Gusev, A. G. (2001). The impact of 'bursting' thalamic impulses at a neocortical synapse. *Nature Neuroscience*, *4*, 402-408.

Syka, J. (2002). Plastic changes in the central auditory system after hearing loss, restoration of function, and during learning. *Physiological Reviews*, *82*, 601-636.

Szczepaniak, W. S., & Møller, A. R. (1993). Interaction between auditory and somatosensory systems: A study of evoked potentials in the inferior colliculus. *Electroencephalography and Clinical Neurophysiology*, *88*, 508-515.

Tardif, E., Chiry, O., Probst, A., Magistretti, P. J., & Clarke, S. (2003). Patterns of calcium-binding proteins in human inferior colliculus: Identification of subdivisions and evidence for putative parallel systems. *Journal of Neuroscience, 116,* 1111–1121.

Wainer, B. H., Steininger, T. L., Roback, J. D., Burke-Watson, M. A., Mufson, E. J., & Kordower, J. (1993). Ascending cholinergic pathways: Functional organization and implications for disease models. *Progress in Brain Research, 98,* 9–30.

Wallace, M. N., Kitzes, L. M., & Jones, E. G. (1991). Chemoarchitectonic organization of the cat primary auditory cortex. *Experimental Brain Research, 86,* 518–526.

Weedman, D. L., & Ryugo, D. K. (1996a). Projections from auditory cortex to the cochlear nucleus in rats: synapses on granule cell dendrites. *Journal of Comparative Neurology, 371,* 311–324.

Weedman, D. L., & Ryugo, D. K. (1996b). Pyramidal cells in primary auditory cortex project to cochlear nucleus in rat. *Brain Research, 706,* 97–102.

Weisz, N., Muller, S., Schlee, W., Dohrmann, K., Hartmann, T., & Elbert, T. (2007). The neural code of auditory phantom perception. *Journal of Neuroscience, 27,* 1479–1484.

Winer, J. A., Chernock, M. L., Larue, D. T., & Cheung, S. W. (2002). Descending projections to the inferior colliculus from the posterior thalamus and the auditory cortex in rat, cat, and monkey. *Hearing Research, 168,* 181–195.

Winer, J. A., & Larue, D. T. (1987). Patterns of reciprocity in auditory thalamocortical and corticothalamic connections: Study with horseradish peroxidase and autoradiographic methods in the rat medial geniculate body. *Journal of Comparative Neurology, 257,* 282–315.

Zacharek, M. A., Kaltenbach, J. A., Mathog, T. A., & Zhang, J. (2002). Effects of cochlear ablation on noise induced hyperactivity in the hamster dorsal cochlear nucleus: Implications for the origin of noise induced tinnitus. *Hearing Research, 172,* 137–143.

Zhang, J. S., & Kaltenbach, J. A. (1998). Increases in spontaneous activity in the dorsal cochlear nucleus of the rat following exposure to high-intensity sound. *Neuroscience Letters, 250,* 197–200.

CHAPTER 17

Auditory Neuropathy: Bridging the Gap Between Basic Science and Current Clinical Concerns

ANTHONY T. CACACE AND ROBERT F. BURKARD

As interest in the topic of auditory neuropathy increases, researchers and clinicians need to ensure the specificity of the diagnosis and be able to distinguish it from other related pathologies or sites of lesion. Controversy arises when case reports in the clinical literature or when animal models in basic science literature do not make a clear distinction between anomalies affecting sensory cells within the inner ear from those impairments that affect the structural and/or functional properties of primary auditory neurons. The issue of specificity is compounded further when the term "auditory neuropathy phenotype" is used to describe putative inner hair cell lesions where evidence for an explicit neuropathy of the auditory nerve is lacking. This practice creates confusion and puts clinicians and researchers in a virtual quandary; leaving them to wonder, *what is* and *what is not* auditory neuropathy? Other related concerns surface when studies lump inner hair cell pathology and neuropathies of the auditory nerve within the same category, using surrogate terminology like "auditory dys-synchrony" and "auditory dys-synchrony disorder." This practice is also problematic because it undermines the utility of establishing accurate genotype-phenotype relationships. Taken together, these concerns have global implications on how auditory neuropathy is being conceptualized and therefore, have direct bearing on what the clinical justification(s) should be for recommending potential treatment options. In this chapter, we provide an exposition of ideas, review pertinent human and animal models, and consider other issues relevant to this topic.

Introduction

Auditory neuropathy (AN) is a primary dysfunction of the auditory nerve which can result from a variety of conditions or circumstances (genetic, metabolic, environmental, pharmacologic, etc.). It is characterized by *normal* sensory function within the cochlea (inner hair cells, IHCs; outer hair cells; OHCs, supporting cells, electrical potentials, etc.) and *abnormal* structural and/or functional properties of primary auditory neurons. The pathophysiologic features of this distinct entity are particularly evident following transient suprathreshold acoustic stimulation where the synchronous activation of single-unit activity from the auditory nerve is disrupted. In turn, these physiologic effects alter population responses from far-field detectors recorded on the scalp (e.g., auditory brainstem responses, ABRs) (e.g., Starr, Picton, Sininger, Hood, & Berlin, 1996) or from near-field sites when recordings are made on or near the promontory of the middle ear (electrocochleography, ECoG) (e.g., Santarelli & Arslan, 2002). In this later instance, one might also expect to observe normal summating potentials (SP), normal or enhanced cochlear microphonic (CM) potentials, and similar to ABRs, distinct abnormalities in the neural components of the ECoG waveform (e.g., McMahon, Patuzzi, Gibson, & Sanli, 2008). Likewise, the presence of intact otoacoustic emissions (OAEs) is an additional criteria for establishing normal OHC function, which can then be used in combination with ABRs to help clinicians and researchers establish an appropriate diagnosis. Therefore, the signature physiologic features of AN include intact transient or distortion product OAEs (TEOAEs, DPOAEs), intact CM potentials, and poorly organized (desynchronized/absent) ABRs or neural components of the ECoG waveform.

Complicating this issue, however, is the observation that speech perception abilities, vis-á-vis monosyllabic word recognition or synthetic sentence identification, can range anywhere from normal to disproportionately poor, regardless if the speech stimuli are presented in quiet, in noise, or within ipsilateral or contralateral competing-message conditions. Also included in this domain is the rollover phenomenon for monosyllabic words, an indicator of auditory-nerve dysfunction based on the performance-intensity function (e.g., Butinar, Starr, Zidar, Koustou, & Christodoulou, 2007; Doyle, Sininger & Starr, 1998; Hood, Berlin, Bordelon, & Rose, 2003; Rance, 2005; Rance, Barker, Mok, Rincon, & Garatt, 2007; Satya-Murti, Cacace, & Hanson, 1979, 1980; Starr et al., 1996; Zeng, Oba, Garde, Sininger, & Starr, 1999). Although some researchers might argue that speech recognition ability in AN is generally poor, the empirical data supporting this proposition are mixed. In fact, Satya-Murti et al. (1979, 1980) and Butinar and colleagues (2007) have shown that individuals with documented neuropathies of the auditory nerve and evidence of desynchronized or absent ABRs can have many auditory functions that are in or near the normal range, including: pure-tone thresholds, gap-detection thresholds, measures of temporal integration, psychophysical tuning curves, OAEs, and measures of speech recognition. These observations are both noteworthy and important, as they serve to demonstrate the apparent dissociation between ABRs, speech-perception abilities, and other relevant psychoacoustic tasks. They also emphasize the functional diversity of information processing within afferent auditory pathways and the adaptive plasticity or compensatory alterations that can occur at the cortical level (Satya-Murti, Wolpaw, Cacace, & Schaeffer, 1983). Additionally, acoustic-stapedius reflex abnormalities (absent responses, elevated thresholds, or significant decay in crossed or uncrossed conditions) and efferent system dysfunction (measured by OAE suppression paradigms) can also be present (e.g., Abdala, Sininger, & Starr, 2000; Berlin, Hood, Cecola, Jackson, & Sabo, 1993; Berlin, Hood, Morlet, Wilensky, St. John, Montgomery, et al., 2005; Hood, 2007; Hood & Berlin, 2001; Satya-Murti et al., 1980; Starr, McPherson, Patterson, Don, Luxford, Shannon, et al., 1991). Moreover, AN can be unilateral or bilateral (e.g., Kothe, Fleischer, Breitfuss, & Hess, 2006; Ngo, Tan, Balakrishnan, Lim, & Lazaroo, 2006; Ohwatari, Fukuda, Chida, Matsumura, Kuroda, Kashiwamura, et al., 2001; Podwell, Podwell, Gordon, Lamendola, & Gold, 2002; Salvinelli, Firrisi, Greco, Trivelli, & D'Ascanio, 2004) and can manifest with or without frequency-dependent elevations in pure-tone thresholds.

In recent years, other descriptive terminology besides AN has been used to codify this distinctive entity, including: "auditory dys-synchrony," "auditory dys-synchrony disorder," "auditory neuropathy/dys-synchrony," "auditory neuropathy/auditory-dys-synchrony," "auditory neuropathy/auditory synaptopathy," "perisynaptic audiopathy," "synaptic audiopathy," "auditory synaptopathy/neuropathy" and/or other variations on this theme (e.g., Berlin, Hood, & Rose, 2001; Beutner, Foerst, Lang-Roth, von Wedel, & Walger, 2007; Foerst, Beutner, Lang-Roth, Huttenbrink, von Wedel, & Walger, 2006; Khimich, Nouvian, Pujol, tom Dieck, Egner, Gundelfinger, et al., 2005; Kumar & Jayaram, 2006; Lesinski-Schiedat, Frohne, Hemmaouil, Battmer, & Lenarz, 2001; Moser, Strenke, Meyer, Lesinski-Schiedat, Lenartz, Beutner, et al., 2006; Ngo, et al., 2006; Rance et al., 2007; Shallop, Jin, Driscoll, & Tibesar, 2004). The issue of contention here concerns the specificity of this nomenclature and the neuroanatomic site(s) of lesion they may or may not signify. With respect to the definition of AN, the anatomical locus implied by this term is unambiguous. However, alternative terminology like "auditory dys-synchrony," or "auditory dys-synchrony disorder," lacks specificity. Other terms like "auditory neuropathy/auditory synaptopathy," "perisynaptic audiopathy," and "synaptic audiopathy," imply *presynaptic* dysfunction and as such, are not likely to be representative of a primary neuropathy per se. Consequently, our concern centers on the fact that nonspecific nomenclature or inappropriate use of available terminology is evolving into a nebulous representation of the underlying pathophysiologic substrates involved in this disorder. Thus, as innocent as it may seem but as dubious as it is, this practice creates confusion because it distorts the distinction between primary IHC anomalies (including localized defects in pre-synaptic cellular machinery), a neuropathy of the auditory nerve, brainstem dysfunction, or a combination of factors. Indeed, this conundrum has been recognized by others (e.g., Gibson & Graham, 2008; Loundon, Marcolla, Roux, Rouillon, Denoyelle, Feldman, et al., 2005; Rapin & Gravel, 2003, 2006) and remains as an area of special interest and utmost concern.

The alternative terminology noted above seems to have arisen, in part, due to the paucity of literature documenting neuroanatomic abnormalities underlying AN, particularly, but not necessarily limited to studies in humans. As we will elaborate in subsequent sections, this scenario is gradually changing as advances in genetics, results from molecular biologic investigations, and improvements in animal models are helping to clarify the anatomic, physiologic, and psychophysical differences between sensory and neural (auditory nerve) dysfunctions. Although studies of human temporal bone histology can be viewed as an undeniable asset in documenting otopathology and in helping to delineate sensory from neural dysfunctions, these analyses are most powerful when detailed behavioral and electrophysiologic studies are available and obtained as close to death as possible. Indeed, the temporal concordance of these measures is of particular importance if correlations between anatomy, physiology, and behavior are to be considered valid. Unfortunately, this is not always possible.

Starr, Michalewski, Zeng, Fujikawa-Brooks, Linthicum, Kim, et al. (2003) describe the temporal bone of an individual with a missense mutation in the MPZ gene diagnosed with hereditary motor sensory neuropathy (Charcot-Marie-Tooth, CMT disease). Based on the histology, this individual (subject 3–2) showed a normal complement of IHCs, normal OHCs (except for loss of a few cells in the apex) and profound loss of spiral ganglion (SpG) cells (>95%). Although these neuroanatomic data and audiometric test results (elevated pure-tone thresholds and poor monosyllabic word recognition; 4% right ear, 8% left ear) would correspond to an apparent neuropathy of the auditory nerve, other relevant auditory tests such as acoustic-stapedius reflexes and ABRs were not performed. Furthermore, specific results like the *absence* of TEOAEs, in lieu of the fact that OHCs were anatomically intact over much of the cochlea's length, was discrepant with the AN phenotype. Thus, there are two important distinctions to consider here; first, in purely anatomic terms, this case would meet the criteria of AN; however, in correlating these results with available physiologic data, this diagnosis is less certain. This point is raised because the physiologic justification for diagnosis usually depends on absent/abnormal acoustic-stapedius reflexes, absent or desynchronized ABRs, and normal OAEs. Although the relationship between anatomically intact OHCs and absent TEOAEs was discrepant, no clear reason was given for this lack of agreement

between the postmortem anatomy and the pre-mortem physiology. In another study, Amatuzzi, Northrop, Liberman, Thornton, Halpin, Hermann, et al. (2001) reported on temporal bone histopathology from a group of premature infants who failed newborn hearing screenings. Using a commercially available ABR screening device as the primary test of record, this assessment tool was designed to identify wave V at a relatively low stimulation level (~35–40 dB nHL) based on a computer-automated template matching detection algorithm. Of particular interest was a subset of hearing screening failures that had selective loss of IHCs as established from their temporal bones. These data were unique but limited. They were unique in showing that IHC loss was correlated with the hearing screening failures in 5 of 6 ears tested, even in lieu of the fact that the actual degree of hearing loss was never established. The authors suggest that this pattern of otopathology can be part of the amalgam of hearing-related dysfunction found in high-risk infants; they conclude, "Data from this study documenting the unexpectedly high frequency of selective inner hair cell lesions in NICU patients suggest an alternative interpretation as a primary loss of inner hair cells rather than a primary disorder of the auditory nerve (p. 635)." However, these data were limited because follow-up diagnostic testing and no other relevant auditory-related measures like OAEs were performed to allow investigators to reach this conclusion. Nevertheless, although both reports serve to illustrate the value of human temporal bone studies, they also highlight inherent limitations of this methodology when corresponding behavioral and electrophysiologic data are either discrepant or less than optimal.

A recent report by Santarelli, Starr, Michalewski, and Arslan (2008) might shed some light on the apparent tripartite sites of lesion that might be associated with AN:

IHC loss, the IHC-auditory nerve fiber synapse, and auditory-nerve disorder. Santarelli and colleagues (2008) reported difficulty in identifying the SP and compound action potential (CAP) components in ECoG recordings of some patients with AN. Using rapid rates of stimulation, they noted modest reductions in the amplitude of the SP in control subjects, and more substantial decreases in the amplitude of the CAP. In a subset of subjects with AN, where the SP/CAP complex was prolonged at low rates of stimulation, it was observed that at high rates of stimulation, the amplitude and duration were substantially reduced. The authors suggested that the marked decrease in amplitude of the SP/CAP complex, seen in subjects with AN, is consistent with *neural adaptation*; a phenomenon which suggests that the abnormalities observed lie in the auditory nerve rather than in the IHCs. Thus, the patterns of ECoG responses they identified included: (1) A present SP with absent CAP, which in their view was consistent with IHC loss; (2) Presence of both SP and CAP, consistent with a proximal auditory-nerve disorder; and (3) Presence of a prolonged neural response (identified by a substantial decrease in the response at high stimulation rates), consistent with a presumed postsynaptic nerve-terminal abnormality. These data are of interest because they offer potential site of lesion distinctions between IHC loss and abnormalities in neural transmission.

Furthermore, it is not overtly obvious from the available literature that tests of vestibular-system function can distinguish hair-cell pathology, otolithic or saccular dysfunction from a neuropathy of the vestibular portions of the nerve. This includes bithermal caloric assessment as used in the electronystagmographic (ENG) test battery and vestibular evoked myogenic potentials (VEMPs), another paradigm gaining in stature and popularity. Moreover, there are similar concerns with respect to the genetics literature, which historically, has not been very precise in documenting auditory system site(s) of lesion. In many instances, the term "deafness" has been used without further elaboration. The negative impact of this approach is felt hardest on genotype-phenotype correlations whereby IHC pathology and auditory-nerve dysfunction are often combined into a single category. In these specific circumstances, the overall concern is that these relationships are becoming irreparably diluted at a time when molecular biologic techniques can discriminate these entities with relatively good precision. Thus, we take the position that audiologic tests of sensory and neural function should be characterized separately as independent variables and not lumped into a single nonspecific category (i.e., auditory dys-synchrony). From a statistical standpoint, this suggestion is justified so that results obtained from correlation analyses or from more complex multivariate procedures, can take on greater meaning. Lastly, misdiagnosis is another distinct matter that emerges from this list of concerns and the consequences of this effect can result in providing inaccurate prognostic information and thereby impact the direction of (re)habilitation. This issue is particularly relevant when families are involved in discussions about cochlear implants (CIs) and are confronted with making important decisions regarding their young children and their futures. As we will explicate in a later section, available but limited data suggest that individuals with putative IHC lesions perform better with CIs than those with actual neuropathies of the auditory nerve. Thus, making this distinction has intrinsic value. We also contend that this distinction will become even more crucial, if and/or when restorative therapies like use of stem cells and xenotransplants, which target the auditory nerve, become commonplace.

We now consider available human and animal models and other relevant studies that shed light on these issues. Whether or not certain points of view are accepted or rejected will ultimately depend upon the strength of evidence they provide and whether or not they can bridge the gap between what is known and what is required to advance the field.

The Primary Sensory Ganglion Model of Hereditary Neuropathies and AN

Probably the first model describing the relationship between neuropathies of the peripheral nervous system that co-occur with neuropathies of the auditory nerve was proposed by Satya-Murti and Cacace (1982). These initial observations focused on two disease entities; hereditary motor and sensory neuropathy (also known as Charcot-Marie-Tooth disease, CMT) and Friedreich's ataxia (FA). Charcot-Marie-Tooth disease is the most common form of inherited neuropathy (Suter & Scherer, 2003) and FA is the most common inherited ataxia (Beal, 2000). In both cases, the dorsal root ganglion (DRG) is the major site of neuronal loss, where large caliber neurons undergo degeneration, segmental demyelination, and remyelination. Also included as disease controls were individuals with olivopontocerebellar atrophy and hereditary spastic paraplegia, because degeneration of the DRG was not a major feature of these disorders and correspondingly, ABRs were not generally affected. The logic underlying this proposition assumed that neurodegeneration seen in DRG would co-occur in the SpG. This assumption seemed reasonable because both DRG and SpG are primary

sensory ganglia populated predominantly by large caliber myelinated neurons; even though they differ in morphology (pseudomonopolar vs. bipolar) and location (peripheral vs. cranial nerves). What distinguishes these disease entities from other conditions is the fact that a peripheral auditory system site of lesion was documented by temporal bone histopathology. In these instances, anatomic evidence of a primary neural degeneration within the SpG is shown in a setting where the sensory and supporting cells within the cochlea were intact (e.g., Hallpike, Harriman, & Wells, 1980; Spoendlin, 1974). These initial observations, which localized and solidified auditory system dysfunction to the auditory nerve, were based upon electrophysiologic investigations, detailed psychoacoustic studies, and parallel tests of peripheral-nerve physiology (Cacace, Satya-Murti, & Grimes, 1983; Satya-Murti et al., 1979, 1980). When sensory nerve conduction studies are used to ascertain the status of the peripheral nervous system, results were manifest as prolonged conduction velocities, reduced amplitudes of sensory nerve compound action potentials, and/or complete absence of these responses. Indeed, the classical distinction between demyelinating (CMT1) and axonal (CMT2) forms of the disease relies on electrophysiologic assessments for this clinical categorization (e.g., Harding & Thomas, 1980). Having similar changes in electrophysiologic measures within two homologous sensory modalities adds credence to the view that the auditory findings are consistent with a neural site of lesion, like those found in DRG. Similarly, using ABRs as the metric for defining auditory system electrophysiologic dysfunction, abnormalities ranged from reduced amplitudes, interpeak latency prolongations (particularly I–III), poorly organized waveforms of later peaks, and absence or desynchronization of the response (e.g., Butinar et al.,

2007; Fabrizi, Cavalaro, Angiari, Cabrini, Taiolo, Malerba, et al., 2007; Musiek, Weider, & Mueller, 1982; Satya-Murti et al., 1979). The results observed in CMT disease overlap with the findings in FA where ABR abnormalities were generally more severe; often being desynchronized or absent (e.g., Satya-Murti et al., 1980; Taylor, McMenamin, Andermann, & Watters, 1982). Therefore, neuronal cell loss, asynchrony of impulse conduction, and subsequent transneuronal degeneration can account for abnormalities found in both auditory and spinocerebellar pathways. When this model was initially proposed in the early 1980s, CMT disease and FA were not well understood. Since that time, there have been substantial advancements in the details, underlying mechanisms, and theory subserving these disease entities (e.g., Beal, 2000; Chen & Chan, 2005; Detmer & Chan, 2007; Dürr, Cossee, Agrid, Campuzano, Mignard, Penet, et al., 1996; Harding, 1995; Kaplan, 1999; Niemann, Berger, & Suter, 2006; Puccio & Koenig, 2002; Shy, 2004; Suter & Sherer, 2003; Young & Suter, 2003; Züchner & Vance, 2006).

In summary, it is reasonable to assume that changes in spinocerebellar and auditory pathways have many pathophysiologic processes in common. In both CMT disease and FA, the major site of neuronal dysfunction occurs in DRG where large caliber sensory neurons in afferent spinal pathways undergo degeneration. Analogous dysfunction can occur in the SpG of the cochleovestibular nerve where large-caliber Type I neurons undergo similar neuropathologic and neurophysiologic changes (Cacace et al., 1983; Hallpike et al., 1980; Satya-Murti et al., 1979, 1980, 1982; Spoendlin, 1974; Starr et al., 2003). Recent neurobiologic and genetic studies suggest that anomalies in axonal transport, intracellular protein tracking, and dysfunction in mitochondrial dynamics can be linked directly or indirectly to these neurodegenerative diseases and may represent a final common pathway underling these conditions in a substantial proportion of cases.

Pharmacologically Induced Models of AN

Ouabain

Animal models have emerged which provide logical and compelling characterizations of the AN phenotype. Most notable in this regard is one derived from the application of ouabain (e.g., Lang, Schulte, & Schmiedt, 2005; Schmiedt, Okamura, Lang, & Schulte, 2002; Wang, Cao, Yin, Yang, & Chen, 2006), a ganglioside that binds to and inhibits the action of the sodium-potassium pump in the cell membrane. Experiments indicate that applying this compound to the round window is toxic to large caliber Type I neurons in the SpG. The importance of this model centers on the fact that although pharmacologically-induced "neurotoxicity" of the auditory nerve occurs in a reliable manner, IHCs, OHCs, supporting cells, and electrical potentials within the cochlea remain intact, as do small caliber unmyelinated Type II auditory neurons, which also reside in SpG.

In addition to verifying that application of ouabain to the round window results in depopulation of large caliber myelinated SpG cells, elevations in ABR or ECoG thresholds, desynchronized ABR responses and normal CMs or OAEs, also observed is another interesting effect. Based on transtympanic ECoG recordings, Wang and colleagues (2006) show an "abnormal positive potential" (APP) in lieu of the expected CAP. The APP was evident at 96 hours post-ouabain administration and corresponded to the time frame in which ABRs were absent. The APP manifests in a frequency dependent manner; being largest at 8.0 kHz and showing a graded reduction at 4.0 kHz and 2.0 kHz. As these authors point out, the APP was initially observed over 3 decades ago; first described by Aran, Charlet de Sauvage, and Pelerin (1971) in a child with kernicterus, and subsequently reported by Wong, Gibson, and Scanli (1997) in children with histories of prematurity and hypoxia. The APP appears dependent on the severity of the hearing loss (O'Leary, Mitchell, Gibson, & Sanli, 2000) with the common denominator being its linkage to AN.

In summary, the results from ouabain administration provide a convincing phenotype and a valid animal model for AN, which is also being used in stem cell research to study restoration of auditory function. The histologic data associated with this model are supported directly by functional recordings demonstrating normal OAEs and abnormal/absent ABRs and/or the neural components of the ECoG waveform.

Doxorubicin

An alternative model of AN was presented by El-Badry, Ding, McFadden, and Eddins (2007), based on the use of the pharmaceutical doxorubicin, a cytotoxic demyelinating agent. However, even when doxorubicin was injected directly into the nerve bundle within the internal auditory canal of chinchilla, the desired cytotoxic effects were not expressed in all animals. From these experiments, two subgroups emerged: Subgroup I showed no overt effects of the drug; and subgroup II showed the desired effect, but in less than 50% of the experimental group. In 10/18 animals (55.6%), normal ABRs and intact DPOAEs were reported. Histology agreed with these findings in that no hair cell loss or gross morphologic damage to auditory nerve fibers or neurons was observed in Rosenthal's canal. Only 8 of 18 (44.4%) of the animals produced the desired result,

which were characterized by absent ABRs and intact DPOAEs. Accordingly, there was no significant hair cell loss, but sustained myelin damage was apparent. Moreover, the authors note, "there was no obvious reduction in SpG numbers, despite sustained myelin damage at 2 months postinjection" (p. 1442). Although this model was not entirely effective, it was encouraging in that the desired effect was observed in a substantial proportion of the treatment group, suggesting that further development is required before it can be applied on a more widescale basis.

Carboplatin

Several reports in the literature suggest that effects of the anticancer drug carboplatin might serve as a suitable animal model for AN (e.g., Harrison, 1998; Salvi, Wang, Stecker, & Arnold, 1999). To fully understand this proposition, the effects of carboplatin are reviewed with respect to anatomic and physiologic measures obtained from the inner ear, brainstem, and cortex. We also consider whether these changes are consistent with, or different than those found in AN. The coverage that we provide on this topic is more comprehensive than some of the others because much more experimental work has been done in this area.

Reports indicate that carboplatin affects the peripheral auditory system by differentially inducing IHC loss, while sparing OHC function. These effects are *species specific* (limited to chinchilla), dose dependent, and reproducible both within and between various laboratories (e.g., Bauer & Brozoski, 2005; Salvi et al., 1999; Wake, Takeno, Ibrahim, & Harrison, 1994; Wang, Powers, Hofstetter, Trautwein, Ding, & Salvi, 1997). Neither the mechanisms of action nor the species-specific effects are completely understood. Nevertheless, the unique pattern of auditory test findings resulting from carboplatin toxicity include modest frequency-dependent elevations in auditory thresholds, intact OAEs and/or CM potentials, and, depending on the degree of IHC loss, reduced amplitude of the auditory nerve CAP (if ECoG is used) or reduced amplitude of near-field responses from the inferior colliculus (IC).

Effects of Carboplatin on OAEs and CMs

Wake, Anderson, Takeno, Mount, and Harrison (1996) recorded TEOAEs in chinchillas before and after carboplatin administration. In the post-treatment condition, where extensive loss of IHCs and a normal complement of OHCs were documented by histologic analysis, TEOAE amplitude increased in comparison to the pretreatment condition. Other studies that evaluated DPOAEs in carboplatin-treated animals found that when OHCs were spared, DPOAE amplitudes were either unaffected or increased in amplitude (e.g., Hofstetter, Ding, Powers, & Salvi, 1997; Hofstetter, Ding, & Salvi, 1997; Jock, Hamernik, Aldrich, Ahroon, Petriello, & Johnson, 1996; Liberman, Chesney, & Kujawa, 1997; Trautwein, Hofstetter, Wang, Salvi, & Nostrant, 1996). When increases in DPOAE amplitudes were observed, the authors speculated that disruption of descending efferent input via the olivocochlear bundle might be involved. This interpretation implies that a loss of tonic inhibition leads to OAE enhancement.

In the context of selective loss IHC loss, Takeno, Harrison, Ibrahim, Wake, and Mount, (1994) reported that there was little or no effect on the threshold or amplitude of the CM when OHCs were spared. This effect was subsequently confirmed and expanded on by Trautwein et al. (1996) and Chertoff, Amani-Taleshi, Guo, and Burkard (2002) for different drug levels and IHC losses.

Effects of Carboplatin on Auditory Nerve Responses

Wang et al. (1997) evaluated single-unit responses in groups of animals following single or double-dose regimens of carboplatin that resulted in moderate-to-severe loss of IHCs. In the single-dose group, for units that responded to acoustic stimulation, normal or near-normal unit thresholds and normal tuning curves were observed. In the double-dose group, only a few single units were responsive to acoustic stimulation and these units exhibited differential behaviors. In one double-dose subgroup that represented a minority of units studied, normal tuning curves and normal or near-normal thresholds were observed. In the second subgroup that represented the majority of units, thresholds were significantly elevated. Although the tuning was not quantified in the double-dose group, their morphology was characterized as V-shaped and sharply tuned (see their Figure 10). Additionally, in the carboplatin-treated animals, spontaneous and maximum unit discharge rates were reduced.

When CAPs from the auditory nerve were evaluated, response properties depended on carboplatin dosage. For example, Takeno et al. (1994) reported elevations in CAP thresholds that were in proportion to the spatial distribution of IHC loss. In the single-dose regimen that produced moderate loss of IHCs, Trautwein et al. (1996) found that CAP amplitudes were reduced, but thresholds were within the normal range. In the double-dose regimen, where 80 to 100% loss of IHCs was reported, substantial threshold elevations and dramatic reductions in CAP amplitude were observed. Liberman et al. (1997) reported that CAP thresholds were elevated when IHC loss exceeded 50%; no CAPs were observed when the loss of IHCs was total. Qiu, Salvi, Ding, and

Burkard (2000) studied a range of carboplatin dose levels across multiple test sessions. Under these conditions, CAP amplitudes decreased in proportion to the loss in IHCs; regression analysis estimated the slope of the post-carboplatin CAP threshold shift to be 2.6 dB/10% loss of IHCs.

Effects of Carboplatin on the Central Auditory Nervous System

Auditory Brainstem Responses

Takeno and colleagues (Takeno et al., 1994; Takeno, Harrison, Mount, Wake, & Harada, 1994; Wake, Takeno, Ibrahim, Harrison, & Mount, 1993; Wake et al., 1994; Wake, Takeno, Mount, & Harrison, 1996) reported elevations in ABR thresholds following carboplatin-induced IHC loss. Greater threshold elevations were observed under intravenous versus intraperitoneal routes and this effect was paralleled by a greater loss of IHCs with intravenous administration (Takeno et al., 1994).

Inferior Colliculus (IC)

Single-Unit Responses. Wake et al. (1996) recorded single-unit activity from the IC in control and carboplatin-treated chinchillas while stimulating the contralateral ear. In this sample, the experimental group showed greater loss of IHCs at the base versus apex of the cochlea with many units exhibiting normal tuning properties and thresholds similar to those obtained in control animals. When recordings were attempted at cochlear regions with complete loss of IHCs, no single-unit responses could be measured.

Near-Field Recordings. A substantial amount of work recording near-field responses from the IC has been published.

Of particular importance to AN are the detailed experiments on stimulus-related factors which focused directly on the issue of "synchrony of neural discharge" with the intent of ascertaining whether or not IHC loss leads to "dys-synchrony" of the neural response pattern (i.e., the hallmark of AN). The importance of these manipulations is based on the notion of "response synchrony" in relation to the recording of evoked potentials. For example, if we have 10,000 neurons firing simultaneously, with an amplitude value of 1 unit (i.e., a unit response), then the recorded potential would be 10,000 unit responses, with a time lag (latency) of 0 milliseconds (ms). This, of course, cannot happen in any biologic system—as numerous factors can influence the timing of the response, such a cochlear delay, neural delays to the auditory site of interest, and neural response jitter. If we were recording from the IC, then our optimal response to a broad-band stimulus might have a latency of 5 ms, and a peak-to-peak response of 5000 units. However, we know that numerous stimulus manipulations can affect response amplitude and response latency (this could be a near-field response from a site such as the IC, or a far-field response from the surface of the scalp, like the ABR). Thus, with decreasing stimulus level, increasing stimulus rate, increasing background noise level, or increasing stimulus rise-time, peak amplitudes of the response decrease and peak latencies increase. Although it might be postulated that fewer neural elements are responding per unit time, this might explain some or all of the amplitude change, but it is unclear how this would lead to an increase in response latency. Indeed, at moderate stimulus levels, considering the narrow dynamic range of many brainstem auditory neurons, this mechanism seems unlikely. Rather, a more attractive postulation is that these various stimulation factors lead to an increase in the variability in underlying unit discharge time—leading to both a decrease in response amplitude and an increase in modal response latency; a phenomenon we refer to as "dys-synchrony" of response. In the review that follows, it is postulated that by challenging the system with stimulus manipulations that desynchronize the response, we will see the expected increase in response latency and decrease in response amplitude. Furthermore, and most importantly, if IHC loss represents an animal model for AN and if the effects of AN on ABRs is to *desynchronize* the response, then these desynchronizing stimulus manipulations will lead to an exacerbation in latency and amplitude changes in chinchillas with carboplatin-induced IHC loss.

Qiu et al. (2000) compared input-output functions pre- and postcarboplatin treatment with recordings made from the round-window, IC, and auditory cortex (AC). The near-field response from the IC also showed a decrease in response amplitude, but unlike the CAP, this amplitude reduction was only seen for moderate- and high-level stimuli. Thresholds for the near-field response increased at a rate of 1 dB/per 10% loss of IHCs which was less than half that observed for CAPs. McFadden, Kasper, Ostrowski, Ding, and Salvi (1998) reported that IHC losses as large as 90% had little impact on IC threshold. They also reported that several animals showed paradoxic responses, in that responses from the IC were actually larger in the post- versus pre-carboplatin treatment conditions. Moreover, these investigators also found that IHC loss affected the forward-masking recovery functions, especially at delays of 10 to 20 ms.

In pre- and postcarboplatin treated animals, Burkard, Trautwein, and Salvi (1997) investigated changes in click-level, rate, and background noise on recordings from the IC. With respect to parametric changes in click-level, the slope of the latency-intensity function was generally similar (Figure 17–1A).

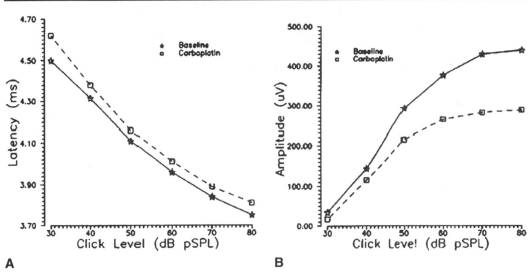

Figure 17–1. The effects of carboplatin on IC response latency (**A**) and amplitude (**B**) across click level. Reprinted with permission from Burkard, Trautwein, and Salvi. The effects of click level, click rate, and level of background masking noise on the IC potential in the normal and carboplatin-treated chinchilla. *Journal of the Acoustical Society of America, 102*(6), 3620–3627. Copyright 1997, Acoustical Society of America.

However, response amplitude decreased post-carboplatin administration (Figure 17–1B). In evaluating rate effects, Burkard and colleagues (1997) found that latency increased and amplitude decreased with increasing rate (10 to 1000 Hz). Additionally, response latencies were found to increase with rate both pre- and postcarboplatin, but again, there was only a small increase in latency at all rates post-carboplatin (Figure 17–2A).

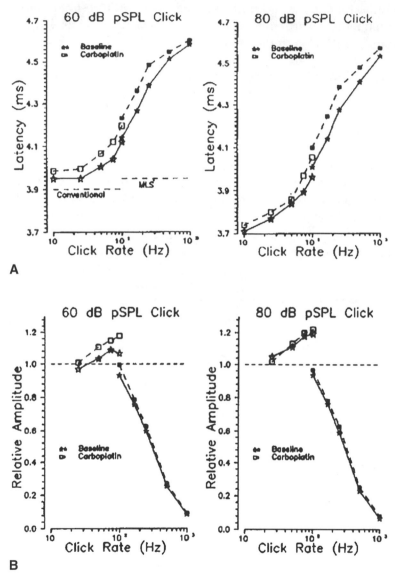

Figure 17–2. The effects of carboplatin on IC response latency (**A**) and amplitude (**B**) across click rate. Reprinted with permission from Burkard, Trautwein, and Salvi. The effects of click level, click rate, and level of background masking noise on the IC potential in the normal and carboplatin-treated chinchilla. *Journal of the Acoustical Society of America, 102*(6), 3620–3627. Copyright 1997, Acoustical Society of America.

When response amplitudes were normalized relative to the lowest rate (10 Hz condition), pre- and postcarboplatin amplitude ratios across rate were nearly identical (Figure 17–2B). When click-level was held constant and the level of a continuous broadband noise was increased in a parametric manner, response latency increased and amplitude decreased. Similar to the rate effects, latency shifts across noise level were similar pre- and postcarboplatin treatment, but again, there was a slight increase in response latency postcarboplatin administration (Figure 17–3A). When change in amplitude was plotted as a ratio of the response amplitude for the no-noise condition, pre- and postcarboplatin amplitude ratio functions were virtually identical (Figure 17–3B). Thus, based on detailed parametric studies of stimulus-related factors (input-output functions, rate, and noise-level changes), neural response behavior was similar to the precarboplatin

condition. Thus, under these conditions, there was no evidence for dys-synchrony of the neural response.

Arnold and Burkard (2002) evaluated modulation-rate transfer functions of auditory steady state responses (ASSRs) recorded from the IC and AC, pre- and postcarboplatin administration. In the precarboplatin condition, responses were largest from the IC at modulation rates of 80 and 160 Hz. Post-carboplatin responses from the IC were largest at 80 Hz. Although there were some changes in ASSR amplitude following post-carboplatin IHC loss, there was no strong evidence that selective IHC loss led to a substantial loss of neural synchrony of the response.

Probably the most pertinent study evaluating the issue of neural synchrony was performed by Phillips, Hall, Guo, and Burkard (2001). These investigators evaluated the effects of changing noise-burst rise-time on

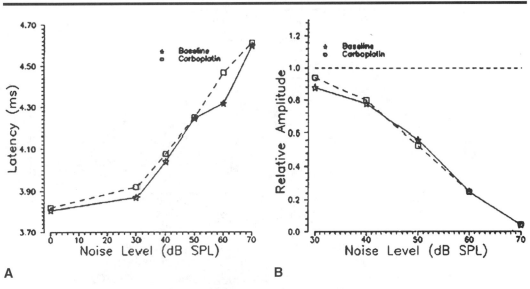

A   **B**

Figure 17–3. The effects of carboplatin on IC response latency (**A**) and amplitude (**B**) across noise level. Reprinted with permission from Burkard, Trautwein, and Salvi. The effects of click level, click rate, and level of background masking noise on the IC potential in the normal and carboplatin-treated chinchilla. *Journal of the Acoustical Society of America*, *102*(6), 3620–3627. Copyright 1997, Acoustical Society of America.

neural activity from the auditory nerve and IC, in both pre- and postcarboplatin treatment conditions. For purposes of brevity, only the results from the IC will be presented. Figure 17–4A shows response amplitudes from the IC across noise-burst level, with rise-time as the parameter. Note that with increasing rise-time and decreasing stimulus level, there is a decrease in response amplitude. These same effects occurred for CAP (data not shown). Figure 17–4C, shows response amplitude recorded from the IC

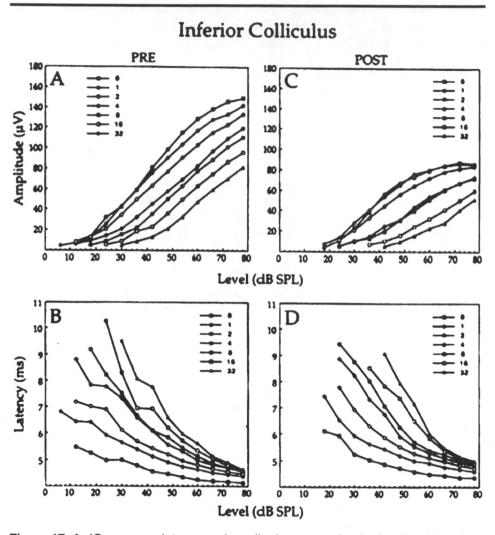

Figure 17–4. IC response latency and amplitude across stimulus level and rise-time, pre- and postcarboplatin. **A.** Response amplitude precarboplatin. **B.** Response latency precarboplatin. **C.** Response amplitude postcarboplatin. **D.** Response amplitude postcarboplatin. Reprinted from Phillips, Hall, Guo, and Burkard (2001). Sensitivity of unanaesthetized chinchilla auditory system to noise burst onset, and the effects of carboplatin. *Hearing Research, 155,* 133-142, with permission of Elsevier.

in the postcarboplatin condition. Note that like the precarboplatin data, response amplitudes decrease with decreasing noise-burst level and increasing noise-burst rise-time. This same pattern of results was seen for the CAP data. Precarboplatin IC latency data are shown in Figure 17–4B. Again, note that both stimulus level and rise-time affect response latency—specifically, that response latency increases with decreasing stimulus level and increasing stimulus rise-time. These same effects were observed in the CAP data. The effects of carboplatin on IC response latency are shown in Figure 17–4D. Note that the same basic relationship between response latency, stimulus level, and rise-time that was observed precarboplatin is seen is also seen in the postcarboplatin evaluations.

Heil (Heil, 1997a, 1997b; Heil & Irvine 1996, 1997) has shown that responses evoked from auditory nerve and cortex depend on rate of change of sound pressure (or rate of change in velocity), when one alters stimulus onset in a parametric manner. Data shown in Figure 17–4 were replotted with the abscissa scaled in terms of rate of pressure change (i.e., pascals per second; using the formula: dB SPL = $20\log_{10}$ [Pressure/20 µPa] divided by the linear rise-time in seconds) (Phillips et al., 2001). Data from the IC are shown in panels A, B, C, and D of Figure 17–5. Several points are noteworthy. First, response latency and amplitude no longer vary much with changes in stimulus rise-time. Rather, response latency decreases with increasing stimulus rate of change in pressure, while response amplitude increases with increasing rate of pressure change. Second, latency decreases and amplitude increases with increasing stimulus rate of pressure change postcarboplatin; similar effects were observed in the CAP data. These data indicate that for noise-burst stimuli gated with a linear rise-time, that

latency and amplitude of onset responses respond to the velocity of stimulus onset (in pascal/s). Most significantly, these data reveal no evidence of dys-synchrony following IHC loss.

Auditory Cortex (AC). Qiu et al. (2000) evaluated the effects of IHC loss while recording from the round window, IC and AC. For the responses obtained from AC, threshold showed a relatively small increase with increasing IHC loss (1.3 dB per 10% IHC loss), similar to that seen in the IC. In a number of instances, however, AC response amplitude actually increased postcarboplatin administration.

Arnold and Burkard (2002) investigated the modulation-rate transfer function of the ASSR recorded from the chinchilla AC pre- and postcarboplatin administration. In these experiments, multiple stimulus levels at octave modulation frequencies (ranging from 20 to 320 Hz), were used. The results showed that the ASSR peaked at 80 Hz at higher stimulus levels, both pre- and postcarboplatin administration. These data revealed little response dys-synchrony following selective IHC loss.

In summary, apart from the fact that the pattern of effects of carboplatin toxicity show some similarities to AN (elevations in auditory thresholds, intact OAEs and abnormalities on ABR tests), histopathology provides convincing and compelling evidence that carboplatin induces a selective IHC loss. By definition, this is a primary sensory cell disorder; *not* a neuropathy of the auditory nerve. However, we must temper this information with the fact that IHC lesions were typically ascertained after a time period which allowed for hair cells and neurons to degenerate. Therefore, when the temporal dynamics of hair cell and neuronal changes are taken into consideration, the sites of lesion are not clear cut (El-Badry & McFadden,

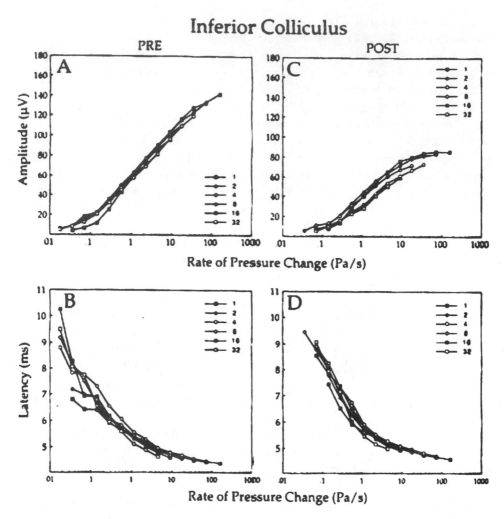

Figure 17–5. Inferior colliculus response latency and amplitude across rate of pressure change and rise-time, pre- and postcarboplatin. **A.** Response amplitude precarboplatin. **B.** Response latency precarboplatin. **C.** Response amplitude post-carboplatin. **D.** Response amplitude postcarboplatin. Reprinted from Phillips, Hall, Guo, and Burkard (2001). Sensitivity of unanesthetized chinchilla auditory system to noise burst onset, and the effects of carboplatin. *Hearing Research, 155,* 133–142, with permission of Elsevier.

2007). It is also known that Type I afferents degenerate following carboplatin adminis-tration; indeed, myelin lamellae surrounding spiral ganglion neurons and proximal nerve fibers are vacuated within hours of carbo-platin administration whereas changes to IHCs are not manifest until one or two days post-

carboplatin administration (e.g., El-Badry & McFadden, 2007; Wang, Ding, & Salvi, 2003). In contrast, Sugawara, Cortas, and Liberman (2005) demonstrate that neural degenera-tion following carboplatin administration is a secondary event, which is dependent upon whether or not supporting cells of the IHC remain intact. Clearly, these competing observations need to be reconciled before a definitive answer is available. Nevertheless, when viewed as a whole, regardless of whether eighth nerve degeneration came before or after IHC loss, it is not at all clear if or how a decrease in the number of Type I auditory neurons would lead to "dys-synchrony of response," as would be expected in a neuropathy of the auditory nerve. It is also unclear how a partial loss of IHCs could lead to such "dys-synchrony of response." Even if we speculate that dys-synchrony could emerge if a more substantial IHC lesion were induced (very near 100%), this scenario seems rather remote based on limited data that Type II afferents are responsive to sound (e.g., Robertson, 1984; Robertson, Sellick, & Patuzzi, 1999) and the fact that near-total loss of IHCs would likely result in severe-to-profound hearing loss. Viewed as a whole, available data strongly challenge the view that carbo-platin-induced IHC damage is a viable model for AN.

Diabetic Neuropathy Model

Hong and Kang (2008) proposed a mouse model of streptozotocin-induced diabetes, as a means to study AN in this disease. The development of this model is of theoretical importance and practical interest because an estimated 20% of individuals with diabetes have co-occurring or progressive peripheral neuropathies. But whether or not AN should be considered part of this complication statistic remains to be determined. In this study, streptozotocin was used as an inducing agent for diabetes, since this pharmaceutical is toxic to the insulin-producing cells of the pancreas. Four groups of animals were used ($n = 40$, 10 animals per group): controls and three experimental groups treated with 50, 100,

and 150 mg/kg of the drug. Auditory brainstem responses and middle latency potentials were used to evaluate auditory nerve, brainstem, and midbrain function. In comparison to the control group, peak latencies of wave IV and the interpeak latencies I to III and I to IV increased in the streptozotocin groups. The dominant midbrain component, labeled Pa, also increased in latency in proportion to streptozotocin dosages. However, the study had limitations. Frequency-specific assessment of auditory thresholds was not ascertained, so that any loss of peripheral hearing sensitivity was not evaluated. Additionally, the relation between blood glucose levels, ABR latencies, and interpeak latencies could not be accurately established for technical reasons. Most significantly, ABR abnormalities were subtle and no overt desynchonization of the responses were reported. Although this model is of interest, available data were both limited in scope and incomplete. Further development is necessary.

The Auditory Nerve Compression Model

Matsumoto, Sekiya, Kojima, and Ito (2008) describe a rat model of AN using direct compression of the auditory nerve as a means to induce AN. The author's rationale centers on the fact that this approach produces more targeted effects than pharmacologic treatments because it is not affected by local diffusion or systemic distribution effects. They also suggested that such results are more highly correlated with functional deficits than genetic models, which can be both subtle and variable. The effect of direct compression of the auditory nerve was tested in a sample of rats and their initial results provide the necessary validation for this model to be given consideration.

Their findings provide histologic, electro-acoustic, and electrophysiologic confirmation documenting clear neurodegeneration of the auditory nerve with preservation of cochlear hair cells, intact DPOAEs, CM potentials, and abnormal ABRs.

However, direct compression of the auditory nerve also requires unique technical skills associated with expertise in skull-base neurosurgery, knowledge of and experience with specific instrumentation (micromanipulator, pulse motor driver, and programmable controller), and use of cochlear electrophysiology for guidance and decision-making processes during experimentation. Although this method has benefits for certain highly-trained individuals, it is also inherently much more complex than pharmacologic induction of AN and has known morbidity, even for the best of surgeons. Nevertheless, direct compression of the auditory nerve is a noteworthy technique and represents a viable animal model of AN. Although limited to a subset of individuals with highly-trained surgical skills, the auditory nerve compression paradigm is summarized best by the authors, " . . . our compression model offers a unique opportunity to study the pathophysiology of AN without confounding effects induced by unspecified functional deficits in other cell types, particularly the sensory hair cells" (p. 249).

Genetic Models

The newly discovered gene mutation DFNB59 on chromosome 2q31.1-q31.3 that encodes the protein pejvakin has been implicated in producing a nonsyndromic autosomal recessive hearing loss due to a primary "neuronal" defect (Delmaghani, del Castillo, Michel, Leibovici, Aghaie, Ron, et al., 2006). Initial evidence in DFNB59 knock-in mice shows normal DPOAEs in combination with abnormalities in ABR waveforms. Although this observation is true, ABR abnormalities are less pronounced than those observed in the human phenotype (Delmaghani, del Castillo, Michel, Leibovici, Aghaie, Ron, et al., 2007). Histologic examination based on light and electron microscopy ruled out gross morphologic defects in the cochlea (i.e., IHC dysfunction), overt demyelination of the auditory nerve, and specific brainstem anomalies. It is noteworthy that pejvakin is found in cell bodies of SpG cells and in brainstem nuclei; the implication being that pejvakin is involved in auditory neuronal physiology, although in a role that is not yet completely understood. The authors speculate that pejvakin might be involved in action potential propagation or in intracellular trafficking. In those individuals with this mutation, rehabilitation options such as cochlear implants are uncertain at this time.

The Otoferlin Model and Other Issues Related to the AN Phenotype

It has been suggested that mutations in the otoferlin gene produce an "auditory neuropathy phenotype" (e.g., Rodriguez-Ballesteros, del Castillo, Martin, Moreno-Pelayo, Morera, Prieto, et al., 2003; Tekin, Akcayoz, & Incesulu, 2005; Varga, Avenarius, Kelley, Keats, Berlin, Hood, et al., 2006; Varga, Kelley, Keats, Starr, Leal, Cohn, et al., 2003). However, when this assertion is scrutinized and put in the context of newer and more detailed data, available evidence indicates that the defect characterizing this mutation is localized to the IHC and not the auditory nerve (Roux, Safieddine, Nouvian, Grati, Simmier, Bahloul, et al., 2006). The reasons for, and implications of this distinction, are expanded upon below.

The importance of these findings is evident when we consider the signaling cascade associated with transduction. Included in this enterprise are those processes involved in hair cell depolarization initiated by mechanoelectric events at the apical part of the hair cell (e.g., Hudspeth, 2005), followed by the opening of L-type voltage-gated calcium channels at the basolateral area in which glutamate-loaded synaptic vesicles fuse to the plasma membrane and are released from ribbon synapses via calcium-triggered exocitosis (e.g., Fuchs, Glowatzki, & Moser, 2003; Mammano, Bortolozzi, Ortolano, & Anselmi, 2007). Although the properties of this process are not completely understood, the roles of intrinsic calcium sensors (otoferlin), scaffolding proteins (Piccolo, Bassoon), and vesicular glutamate transporters (VGLUT1, VGLUT2, VGLUT3), are becoming appreciated as their functions are determined via specific genetic mutations (e.g., Khimich et al., 2005; Roux et al., 2006; Seal, Akil, Yi, Weber, Grant, Yoo, et al., 2008).

Indeed, ribbon synapses of the IHC are special since they produce a graded output. As such, tonic and phasic modes of transmitter release serve to transfer the frequency, intensity, and temporal fine structure of the acoustic signal to higher centers of the auditory pathway with exceptional fidelity (e.g., Fuchs, 2005; Griesinger, Richards, & Ashmore, 2005; Moser, Neef, & Khimich, 2006; von Gersdorf, 2001). The initiation of temporal coding at the level of the hair cell is of particular importance to binaural processes like sound localization, which can require microsecond resolution (e.g., Keen & Hudspeth, 2006; Nouvian, Beutner, Parsons, & Moser, 2006).

Apart from the fact that the mutation in the gene encoding otoferlin causes severe-to-profound hearing loss (e.g., Yasunaga, Grati, Cohen-Salmon, El-Amraoui, Mustapha, Salem, et al., 1999), the discovery of this protein is one of the fundamental components to understanding the release of transmitter at the ribbon synapse. In terms of its biological significance, otoferlin has six C2 domains, and as such, has been identified as the calcium ion sensor that binds with SNARE molecules (Safieddine & Wenthold, 1999) to mediate the final fusion step of pre-synaptic vesicle exocitosis; a process regulated by calcium influx (e.g., Parsons, 2006; Sterling & Mathews, 2005). Recent experiments on otoferlin and the SNARE protein syntaxin 1A have confirmed and extended these initial observations (Ramakrishnan, Drescher, & Drescher, 2008).

In accordance with human data, if otoferlin is absent from vesicles residing within the IHC, then synaptic transmission is blocked and profound hearing loss results. This is what precisely occurs in knockout mice lacking the otoferlin gene. In fact, click-evoked or tone-burst ABRs cannot be recorded, even at high levels of stimulation (~100 dB SPL). The point of emphasize here is that absence of the ABR is *not* due to dyssynchrony of neural activity (the hallmark of a neuropathy). It is attributed directly to a defect in exocitosis. Accordingly, " . . . both OHCs and the afferent auditory pathway of the adult Otof^{-1-} mice are functional, and the profound hearing impairment in these mice probably results from an IHC defect" (Roux et al., 2006, p. 281). Thus, describing the otoferlin defect as an AN is not only counterintuitive, but it is an obvious misnomer. Moreover, although it is recognized that mice with the otoferlin mutation are functionally deaf, it has also been shown that supra-threshold electrically-evoked ABRs have normal waveform morphology. This finding indicates that a substantial proportion of large-caliber auditory-nerve fibers remain intact and functional.

In summary, evidence to date indicates that the functional defect of the otoferlin mutation is presynaptic, localized to the IHCs, and results in the absence of exocytosis. When combined with histopathologic data, these effects challenge the viewpoint that mutations of the otoferlin gene represent an "auditory neuropathy phenotype." From a clinical standpoint and if the following conditions are met: (1) presence of the otoferlin mutation by genetic testing, (2) profound nonsyndromic hearing loss, (3) present OAEs, (4) absent *acoustically evoked* ABRs, and (5) present *electrically evoked* ABRs, then, in all likelihood, these factors will have prognostic value and serve as biomarkers for successful outcome via cochlear implantation (e.g., Rodriguez-Ballesteros et al., 2003; Rouillon, Marcolla, Roux, Marlin, Feldmann, Couderc, et al., 2006).

Other anomalies of the IHC that can alter the transduction process are those involving mutations of active zone scaffolding proteins like Bassoon and Piccolo (e.g., Desbach, Torres, Wittenmayer, Altrock, Zamoranet, Zuschratter et al., 2006). Scaffolding proteins can be characterized as the "molecular glue" that anchors synaptic ribbons to the plasma membrane and serves to bind, organize, and regulate active or passive forms of cellular signaling (e.g., Faux & Scott, 1996). In mice mutant for the scaffolding protein Bassoon, exocitosis is partially perturbed either because of defective attachments at the active zone or due to lack of a subset of ribbons. As a result, readily releasable pools of vesicles containing transmitter substance are diminished, synchronous synaptic transmission is reduced, and hearing sensitivity is moderately impaired (Altrock, tom Dieck, Sokolov, Meyer, Sigler, Brakebusch, et. al., 2003; Prescott & Zenisek, 2005). All of these phenomena occur in the setting where only minor reductions of calcium currents are manifest. Thus, the genetic manipulations that produce ribbon-deficient synapses are important for helping to distinguish the structural and functional relationships that can delineate IHC disturbances from those affecting primary auditory neurons (e.g., Khimich et al., 2005; Moser et al., 2006).

When ribbon synapses are defective due to the Bassoon mutation, the following characteristics are observed: an approximate 40 dB elevation in auditory thresholds, DPOAEs present over a broad bandwidth, and ABR waveforms that are morphologically intact. Indeed, the most noteworthy and distinguishing feature between Bassoon mutants, normal wild-type mice, and mice with OHC lesions, is a marked reduction in the absolute magnitude and slope of the growth function over a broad range of stimulus levels (i.e., rate of change in amplitude vs. stimulus level) using either ABRs or ASSR amplitude as the relevant metric. The reduced slope of the growth function is attributed to diminished transmitter release and therefore, reduced activation of the auditory nerve (e.g., Pauli-Mangus, Hoch, Strenzke, Anderson, Jentsch, & Moser, 2007).[1] As the Bassoon mutation is presynaptic and because it does not desynchronize the ABR, it should *not* be construed as a neuropathy. The pattern of auditory test results described above is an important observation that needs to be more fully investigated since it may be pathgnomonic of presynaptic IHC dysfunction.

Lastly, as part of the molecular machinery involved in transduction, vesicular trans-

---

[1]It is of interest to consider the fact that a reduced slope in ABR or ASSR growth function could correspond to "recruitment" a phenomenon reported in the clinical literature but thought to be associated with lesions to the auditory nerve. However, this may be a misnomer, and therefore, this topic may need to be revisited. Presynaptic IHC dysfunction, using Bassoon mutants as an example, may be a more likely scenario.

porters are necessary for loading synaptic vesicles with transmitter substance. In the IHC, the transmitter is glutamate and VGLUT1 and VGLUT2 are involved in this process. However, the function of VGLUT3 is not completely understood, but in mice mutant for this protein, profound hearing loss and nonconvulsive seizures are exhibited. In this scenario, loss of hearing is due to the absence of transmitter release from the IHC, while the organ of Corti, IHCs, OHCs, supporting cells, and its associated afferent connections are preserved; OAEs are unimpaired. Thus, in accord with otoferlin but in partial contrast to Bassoon, the mutation of VGLUT3 results in profound hearing loss due to the absence of exocitosis. To reiterate, the expression of these effects do not reflect a neuropathy of the auditory nerve and therefore, should not be represented as such. Finally, there are other parallels with respect to Bassoon and VGLUT3 mutations that are of interest; specifically, both express seizure activity as part of their phenotype. In the Bassoon mutant, recurrent seizures are accompanied by distinct changes to CNS anatomy and biochemistry as noted by manganese enhanced magnetic resonance imaging (MEMRI) and magnetic resonance spectroscopy (MRS) (Angenstein, Niessen, Goldschmidt, Lison, Altrock, Gundelfinger, et al., 2007; Angenstein, Hilfert, Zuschratter, Altrock, Niessen & Gundelfinger, 2008). In VGLUT3 mutants, seizure activity is characterized as nonconvulsive and is associated with interictal activity.

Deletion of SLC19A2, the High-Affinity Thiamine Transporter

Liberman, Tartaglini, Fleming, and Neufeld (2006) developed a mouse model of the syndrome: thiamine-responsive megaloblas-

tic anemia (TRMA), an autosomal-recessive disorder characterized by diabetes and sensorineural hearing loss. When a mutant mouse line with a targeted deletion SLC19A2 was put on a thiamine-restricted diet, loss of IHCs and to a much lesser extent OHCs was observed in the null-type mice by histologic examination; wild-type mice did not show these peripheral auditory system changes. According to Liberman and colleagues (2006), because threshold shifts for OAEs were less than the threshold shifts observed for ABRs, they assert that these effects provide evidence for an AN. However, they only show verification for selective IHC loss; the more important histologic evidence for a neuropathy of the auditory nerve was conspicuously absent. Indeed, the IHC pathology induced by the SLC19A2 deletion is unique and interesting. It supports previous work indicating that the distribution pattern of gene products that encode the high-affinity thiamine transporter is expressed more strongly in the IHCs versus OHCs (Fleming, Steinkamp, Kawatsuji, Tartaglini, Pinkus, Pinkus, et al. 2001) and supports the position that auditory dysfunction manifested by this disease is worthy of further study.

Other examples of genetic-based murine models producing selective IHC loss have been reported and are expressed with concomitant anomalies to the maculae and cristae of the vestibular system. These combined auditory and vestibular sensory system defects produce examples of hearing loss and motor-related dysfunctions that are characterized by unique circling and head-jerking behaviors (e.g., Bock, Yates, Deol, 1982; Bussoli, Kelly, & Steel, 1997). Human manifestations of this type of disturbance, although documented in the literature, are rare (e.g., Bonfils, Avan, Landero, Narcy, & Trotoux, 1991; Slack, Wright, Michaels, & Frolich, 1986).

Hypoxic/Ischemic Model

Impaired gas exchange (hypoxia) or reduced blood flow (ischemia) can be implicated in causing damage to the inner ear and central nervous system (CNS). Focusing specifically on the auditory periphery, Sawada, Mori, Mount, and Harrison (2001) developed an animal model in which long-term low-level hypoxia results in auditory dysfunction by differentially affecting IHCs versus OHCs. Based on this model and using OAEs and ABRs as physiologic monitoring tools, Sawada and colleagues found that OAEs remained intact and were generally unaffected by these manipulations, the implication being that low-level hypoxia had a primary impact on cochlear IHCs which, in turn, adversely affected ABR waveforms and thresholds. The authors suggest that secondary effects from IHC damage can induce glutamate excitotoxicity, which can cause injury to primary auditory neurons. Thus, infants exposed to similar postnatal conditions are potentially at risk for developing AN. In many different systems within the body, glutamate excitotoxicity is a well-known pathologic process that occurs following hypoxic injury; indeed, the nervous system of immature infants is particularly vulnerable to this type of insult (e.g., Khwaja & Volpe, 2008). With respect to AN, reports in the clinical and basic science literature support this correlation, particularly in premature infants (e.g., Rea & Gibson, 2003) and in animal models of hyperbilirubinemia (e.g., McDonald, Shapiro, Silverstein, & Johnston, 1998).

However, as noted above, effects of hypoxic-ischemic events are complex; they are not limited to the peripheral auditory system, and most likely, will also produce injury to the CNS along a continuum from mild to severe. In pre-term infants, hypoxic-ischemic injury is also a predisposing factor for the development of periventricular leukomalacia (PVL), a white-matter disease of the CNS observed in the watershed regions between penetrating arterial vessels from the cortex and vessels arising from deep ventricular margins. Periventricular leukomalacia also has developmental consequences correlated with impairments in sensory function, motor skills, and cognition (e.g., Hagberg, Peebles, & Mallard, 2002; Roscigno, 2002; Volpe, 2003). Models developed in experimental animals (rats) provide direct confirmation of these observations and indicate that both brain injury and impaired performance on a variety of behavioral tasks are dependent on the duration of hypoxia (Fan, Lin, Pang, Lei, Zhang, Rhodes, et al., 2005). In humans, Gadian, Aicardi, Watkins, Porter, Mishkin, and Vargha-Khadem (2000) report significant memory problems in affected individuals. These effects were attributed to damage of the hippocampus, a brain region particularly vulnerable to hypoxic-ischemic insults. Although it is generally believed that cognitive deficits do not occur in isolation from other neurologic sequelae, such as seizure disorders or cerebral palsy, Gadian and colleagues (2000) provide data that contrasts with this expectation. On the other end of the spectrum, hypoxic-ischemic injury can also result in more subtle disturbances in language and learning, which are often detected later in life and most likely manifest during early childhood educational experiences. According to the authors, these problems can be characterized as difficulty processing rapid temporal information, and can be modality specific (auditory or visually based) or polysensory in nature. According to McClure, Threldkeld, and Fitch (2007) erythropoietin administration can provide protection against this unwanted outcome and, at the same time, minimize performance deficits associated with this type of injury.

In summary, prolonged low-level hypoxia primarily and preferentially affects IHCs within the inner ear although secondary effects may induce damage to the auditory nerve through pathologic mechanisms associated with glutamate excitotoxicity (Sawada et al., 2001; Shirane & Harrison, 1987). Whereas this proposed model has more face validity than the carboplatin model, the otoferlin mutation, or the high-affinity thiamine transporter model of AN per se, it is also reasonable to say that it is much more complicated. Nevertheless, hypoxic-ischemic injury represents an important area for additional study and alerts the clinician to a complex combination of potential outcomes, particularly if this circumstance is documented early in life.

Hyperbilirubinemia

Hyperbilirubinemia is associated with AN, but the mechanism of action is not clear-cut or fully understood. Many of these reports have surfaced from the neonatal hearing-screening literature, where either anomalous outcomes were reported (e.g., Berg, Spitzer, Towers, Bartosiewicz, and Diamond, 2005; Cacace, Pinheiro, Malone, Kerwood, & Artino, 1996; Wood, Mason, Farnsworth, Davis, Curnock, & Lutman, 1998) or where diagnostic follow-up studies confirmed hearing screening failures (Katona, Buki, Farkas, Pytel, Simon-Nagy, & Hirschberg, 1993; Norton, 1993; Rhee, Park, & Jang, 1999; Sheykholeslami & Kaga, 2000). History of this insult also requires clinicians to be cognizant of the fact that hyperbilirubinemia can present as a delayed onset event and that affected individuals can recover over time (Attias & Raveh, 2007; Psarommatis, Riga, Douros, Koltsidopoulos, Douniadakis, Kapetanakis, et al., 2006; Worley, Erwin, Goldstein, Provenzale, & Ware, 1996), so that multiple assessments may be warranted.

Experimental animal models in rat, pig, and monkey have been used to evaluate the effects of hyperbilirubinemia on auditory function (e.g., Ahlfors, Shoemaker, Bennett, & Ellis, 1984; Hansen, Cashore, & Oh, 1992; Shapiro & Te Selle, 1994). Silver, Kaputulnik and Sohmer (1995) showed that asphyxia in 10-day-old versus 1-day-old jaundiced Gunn rats resulted in progressive hearing loss with absence of ABRs. According to the authors, neither asphyxia nor jaundice alone was sufficient to produce any hearing loss. Shapiro and Te Selle (1994) studied CMs and ABRs in the same animals, and showed that ABRs but not CMs were altered, indicating specific retrocochlear involvement in the Gunn rat model. Other evidence from the Gunn rat model suggests a retro-cochlear lesion; however, the results are not often severe and may require other factors to substantially desynchronize auditory nerve activity. Shaia, Shapiro, and Spencer (2005) injected sulfadimethoxine in jaundiced and nonjaundiced Gunn rats at 15 days of age; sulfa displaces bilirubin from its albumin binding sites, thus releasing it into tissue and producing pathologic effects. In this model, temporal bone histopathology using light and electron microscopy showed severely degenerated large caliber SpG neurons without abnormalities to cochlear hair cells in jaundiced but not in nonjaundiced sulfa controls. However, in a subsequent study, Rice and Shapiro (2006) noted a problem with the sulfa model in that after displacement, bilirubin levels drop to near zero and results do not correlate with neurologic dysfunction. They used single and double-dose injections of biliverdin, the precursor to bilirubin in the catabolism of hemoglobin, as an alternative method to increase bilirubin levels. This approach also produced electrophysiologic anomalies, but auditory findings were less severe than those induced with sulfadimethoxine.

Some have questioned the validity of generalizing the Gunn rat model to humans (Stern & Brodersen, 1987); Turkel (1990) offers additional criticism, "Although the possibility of reversibility of bilirubin toxicity following exchange transfusion has been raised by some studies of auditory brainstem response in newborns with hyperbilirubinemia, it is difficult to find evidence of direct toxicity of bilirubin in experimental in vivo systems, even at huge amounts (Levine, 1983). To produce kernicterus in animals, they must usually be injured first by hypoxia (Lucey, Hibbard, Behrman, et al., 1964) or hypoglycemia (Rozdilsky & Olszewski, 1961) (although the newborn kitten is an exception) (Rozdilsky & Olszewski, 1961) (p. 389)." Although this point is well taken, it may just indicate that the Gunn rat model is useful but not optimal at demonstrating these effects. As with any animal model, generalizations to humans are not always straightforward and should be made cautiously.

Thus, in humans there appears to be an association between auditory system dysfunction and hyperbilirubinemia. Although a linkage exists, we cannot establish with certainty a cause and effect relationship due to large individual differences. There can be many reasons for this; some of these reasons are not completely understood and others that may require molecular techniques to uncover. Additionally, because some presentations are life threatening, sensory evaluations are not typically considered high-priority issues at the time of presentation, which further complicates establishing cause and effect relationships. In the Gunn rat model, changes in ABRs have been interpreted to be consistent with AN, but results are often subtle and complete desynchronization of ABRs appears to be the exception and not the rule.

Restoration of Function

Having a valid animal model of AN is of particular importance to novel rehabilitation strategies, so that restoration of function can proceed on a secure footing and have the necessary translational properties that can be applied to humans. For example, when auditory neurons are significantly depopulated and IHCs, OHCs, and supporting structures remain intact, restorative approaches being studied include: xenografts (e.g., Corrales, Pan, Li, Liberman, Heller, & Edge, 2006; Hu, Ulfendahl, & Olivius, 2004; Olivius, Alexandrov, Miller, Ulfendahl, Bagger-Sjoback, & Kozlova, 2004; Olivius, Alexandrov, Miller, Ulfendahl, Bagger-Sjoback, & Kozlova, 2003) and embryonic stem-cell implants (e.g., Hu et al., 2004; Lang, Schulte, Goddard, Hedrick, Schulte, Wei, et al., 2008; Matsuoka, Kondo, Miyamoto, & Hasino, 2007; Sekiya, Kojima, Matsumoto, & Ito, 2008). Using the ouabain model of AN, Corrales et al. (2006) found that neurites (i.e., immature projections from the cell body) grew into targeted areas of the gerbil organ of Corti after embryonic stem-cell-derived mouse neural progenitor cells were injected into the trunk of the cochlear nerve. In this study, the authors report that neurons projected from the injection site through Rosenthal's canal, into the osseous spiral lamina, and into the organ of Corti, where they contacted hair cells. The authors showed distinct evidence for differentiation and regeneration, whereby stem cells showed the capacity to grow to a specific target. Matsuoka et al. (2007) transplanted a line of mesenchymal stem cells into the scala tympani and modiolar regions of the cochlea in normal and ouabain-treated gerbils. These investigators found that undifferentiated mesenchymal stem cells were only able to survive in the modiolar area. In that condition, cell counts were greater for ouabain-treated versus control animals. On the basis of enhanced stem-cell survival, the researchers were encouraged to pursue further work with this method. Additionally, after ouabain application to the round window in gerbils, Lang et al. (2008) provide evidence of differentiation and survival of embryonic stem cells in Rosenthal's canal and in perilymphatic spaces. These effects were dependent on time after injury; early implants (1 to 3 days postinjury) showed better survival than in late transplanted animals (7 days or longer).

Clinical Implications and Treatment Strategies

Based on available studies, the general consensus is that application of "conventional" hearing aids is not considered an "enabling technology" or a viable long-term rehabilitative option in cases of AN. This observation should be intuitively obvious given the reduction in channel capacity known to exist in the SpG based on the depopulation and demyelinization of large caliber auditory neurons and the secondary transneuronal degenerative effects known to occur. It is also of interest to note that limitations associated with hearing aid use is not a new revelation; this observation was made over half a century ago by an astute clinician studying nerve-deaf children secondary to *rh* incompatibility (Rosen, 1956). Nevertheless, this remains as a distinct treatment dilemma as well as a disconcerting reality for those clinicians that deal with this situation when it arises.

As we move from noninvasive to invasive procedures and consider individuals with AN and severe-to-profound hearing loss, it is less clear a priori who will benefit from CIs. Part of this uncertainty is due to limited experience based on relatively small samples sizes of individuals that have received CIs, diminished statistical power and generalizability associated with this type of information, lack of standardization of how CI data are presented in the literature, how loosely the term "benefit" is defined, and as we have emphasized throughout, the uncertainty in terms of how accurate the diagnosis of AN actually is (e.g., Buss, Labadie, Brown, Gross, Gross, & Pillsbury, 2002; Jeong, Kim, Kim, Bae, & Kim, 2007; Madden, Hilbert, Rutter, Greinwald, & Choo 2002; Mason, De Michele, Stevens, Ruth, & Hashisaki, 2003; Miyamoto, Kirk, Renshaw, & Hussain 1999; Peterson, Shallop, Driscoll, Breneman, Babb, Stoekel, et al., 2003; Runge-Samuelson, Drake, & Wackym, 2008; Shallop, Peterson, Facer, Fabry, & Driscoll 2001). For example, in those instances where investigators report that neural synchrony is "miraculously" restored following electrical stimulation at the periphery, one must seriously question whether these investigators were actually dealing with a neuropathy of the auditory nerve or putative IHC pathology that we have described herein. Clearly, this issue and those reports making such a claim remain open to interpretation and debate. Furthermore, the lack of standardization in reporting results of cochlear implantation also makes it difficult to apply data summarization techniques like meta-analysis which might prove helpful (Sinnathuray, Raut, Awa, Magee, & Toner, 2003). Based on a retrospective post hoc categorization scheme of CI use, Gibson and Sanli (2007) found that individuals with CMs that superimpose on large positive potentials (the so-called APP) and normal electrically-evoked ABRs performed better with CIs than individuals with CMs, APP, and abnormal electrically evoked ABRs. The implication being that the performance advantage for CI users with these distinctive characteristics may serve to distinguish those with IHC lesions versus those with true ANs. It is also of interest to note that the APP has *not* been reported in cases of AN when hearing loss is in the mild-to-moderate or mild-to-profound range (e.g., Santarelli et al., 2008). In retrospect, it is evident that we do not fully understand the physiology or the phenomenology of the APP, and therefore, additional efforts will be needed to validate this interesting and potentially important observation.

As we move forward in this area, there are additional points that should be emphasized. For example, it is informative to know that individuals with the otoferlin mutation and profound hearing loss due to dysfunctional IHCs reportedly perform well with CIs (e.g., Rodriguez-Ballesteros et al., 2003; Rouillon et al., 2006). These evidence-based outcome data are in contrast to other reports in the literature, such as those with Mohr-Tranebjaerg syndrome (a prototypical and histologically confirmed AN), where performance with CIs has been described as "marginal even after two years of use, with continued poor scores in standard speech, language and audiometric tests" (p. 121) (e.g., Brookes, Kanis, Tan, Tranebjaerg, Vore, & Smith, 2007). In other selected cases, such as those with CMT disease, CI performance seems to fall somewhere in between these extremes (e.g., Postelmans & Strokross, 2006; Starr et al., 2003). Other insightful information from the clinical domain provide guidance for the type of protocols that should be in place and clinical decision-making processes that are necessary when

suspected AN arises. For example, Buchman, Roush, Teagle, Brown, Zdanski, and Grose (2006) report on a sample of children ($n = 51$) with audiologic characteristics of AN where magnetic resonance imaging studies were analyzed. Significantly, in 18% (9/51) of their cohort, children with small or absent auditory nerves were identified. In those instances where auditory nerves were absent, such individuals would not be considered viable candidates for cochlear implantation. These specific circumstances require that other options need to be explored, including consideration of the auditory brainstem implant (ABI). In this context, a body of data, albeit limited in sample size and scope, is developing to suggest that in children with aplasia of the cochlear nerve, ABIs are feasible and short-term results appear encouraging (e.g., Colletti, Carner, Fiorino, Sacchetto, Miorelli, Orsi, et al., 2002). Colletti, Fiorino, Carner, Miorelli, Guida, and Colletti (2004) indicate that in two children who were unable to derive benefit from CIs, were able to detect sounds and words as early as 3 months after activation of the ABI. Furthermore, in a wide range of complex auditory and neurodevelopmental disorders, including AN, Colletti (2007) reports that children use their ABIs over 75% of the time and show continued improvement in cognitive skills. Nevertheless, evaluating long-term outcomes of this research will be necessary to judge the overall clinical utility and success of this rehabilitative option.

In cases where AN results from mitochondrial dysfunction, certain pharmacological treatments/therapies may be beneficial in stabilizing or even possibly reversing this condition, keeping in mind, however, that a downside exists with respect to this option. Most notable in this regard is the fact that multicenter double-blinded placebo-controlled clinical trials are not always available for guidance. Thus, certain words of wisdom apply, "The pursuit of an effective mitochondrial therapy remains the siren song for clinicians, luring them into unchartered areas of research" (Gillis & Kaye, 2002, p. 212). Nevertheless, when considering this option, available therapeutic mechanisms fall into three general categories of effects: electron acceptors, cofactors, and antioxidants. The most benign and perhaps most effective treatment modality that has received the majority attention in the clinical literature is the application of coenzyme Q_{10} (CoQ10; aka ubiquinone) and its analogue (e.g., idebenone). Used as an enzyme replacement therapy, CoQ10 is a potent antioxidant and free radical scavenger. Idebenone also has antioxidant properties, but in addition, stimulates oxidative phosphorylation. In instances of hearing loss secondary to hypoxia, Sato (1988) has shown in guinea pigs that CoQ10 was effective in promoting recovery from, as well as preventing metabolically related respiratory impairment to sensory hair cells in the inner ear. In diabetes mellitus associated with 3243 mitochondrial mutation, Suziki, Taniyama, Muramatsu, Atsumi, Hosokawa, Asahina, et al. (1997) found that CoQ10 may be effective in relieving neuromuscular symptoms. In maternally inherited diabetes mellitus and "neurosensory" deafness (MIDD) associated with the mitochondrial DNA 3243 (A to G) mutation, Suzuki, Hinokio, Ohtomo, Hirai, Hirai, Chiba, et al. (1998) found that CoQ10 treatment prevented progressive loss of hearing and had no overt side effects. In Kearns-Sayre syndrome, where abnormalities in somatosensory evoked potentials (SEPs) and ABRs can occur, Nakamura, Takahashi, Kitaguchi, Yorifuji, Nishikawa, Imaoka, et al. (1995) showed that long-term CoQ10 therapy preserved these evoked responses and showed improvement in SEP latencies, indicating a

beneficial effect. In an individual with bilateral optic neuropathy with chorea, Chariot, Brugieres, Eliezer-Vanerot, Geny, Binaghi, Cesaro, et al. (1999) documented improvement on MRI scans that occurred after a 1-year treatment regimen. This individual was thought to have a genetically-uncharacterized mitochondrial disorder. In mitochondrial myopathy and lactic acidosis due to cytochrome c deficiency, Jinnai, Yamada, Kanda, Masui, Tanaka, Ozawa, et al. (1990) found that CoQ10 treatment was effective in reducing both lactate and pyruvate levels and aided in the recovery from muscle atrophy. In a case of mitochondrial encephalomyopathy with sleep apnea, Tatsumi, Takahashi, Yorifuji, Nishikawa, Kitaguchi, Hashimoto, et al. (1988) found that neither ataxia nor abnormality of pyruvate metabolism was alleviated after 6 months of therapy with CoQ10. Furthermore, although inherited ataxias are incurable, oxidative stress is a core factor in disease pathogenesis. Work in this area indicates a positive response to idebenone treatment in both adult and pediatric populations, but it also suggests that age may be an important factor in the efficacy of treatment success (e.g., Pandolfo, 2008; Pineda, Arpa, Montero, Aracil, Dominguez, Galván, et al., 2008). Certainly, these results are encouraging and with medical guidance, are worthy of exploring in early-onset AN.

Lastly, some additional thoughts concerning this pharmacologic supplement are worth mentioning. Co-enzyme Q_{10} can be purchased as an over-the-counter remedy that does not require a prescription from a physician. In our view, however, and regardless how benign it may be, indiscriminant use of this compound is not recommended; a physician's input is essential and prudent, particularly when put in the context of an individuals' diagnosis and other medications he or she may be taking. Therefore, invoking the doctrine of "caveat emptor" is appropriate. The traditional implication of this principle is that consumer's should beware. However, it is of interest to consider just who is the consumer (the buyer) and who is the seller? Is it the researcher selling therapies to clinicians? Is it the clinician selling therapies to patients; or is it the advertisements of the manufacturer that are directed to all involved? Because CoQ10 is sold in health-food stores, grocery stores, large discount stores, and pharmacies, it is hard to view this supplement as a cure, but it can be viewed as a way to potentially modify the progression of the disease. It would appear that individual consumers have the ultimate responsibility in decision-making. Therefore, consumers need to be educated and understand that expectation of a positive result from a theoretically useful but unproven therapy, which often lacks double-blinded placebo-controlled trials, may not be justified. Indeed, such circumstances should be viewed with caution and skepticism.

Summary

In retrospect, several pertinent issues need to be kept in mind, particularly when dealing with children diagnosed with AN, so that known pitfalls associated with certain testing paradigms can be avoided. Most important is the fact that absence of the ABR does *not* preclude useful hearing. In fact, hearing sensitivity could be in or near the normal range under these circumstances; an observation that is not new (initial observations were made over 25 years ago), but one that is useful to reiterate (Berlin, Morlet, & Hood, 2003; Butinar et al., 2007; Satya-Murti et al, 1980, 1983). Therefore, in young children with AN, the importance of behav-

ioral assessment to cross-check the validity of electrophysiologic testing in establishing hearing sensitivity cannot be overstated. Other issues are equally important. Psarommatis et al. (2006) and Attias and Raveh (2007) provide evidence that infants diagnosed with AN at or near birth can show partial or even full recovery on retesting 5.5 to 12 months later. Under these circumstances, the decision to pursue cochlear implantation early in life should be made cautiously. When audiologic tests indicate profound hearing loss that are consistent with AN, imaging studies including MRI and/or high-resolution computed tomography examinations are imperative so that small or absent auditory nerves can be identified (e.g., Adunka, Jewells, & Buchman, 2007). As noted by Buchman and colleagues (2006), 18% of children fall into this category. Moreover, genetic studies should also be pursued rigorously, particularly in instances where nonsyndromic severe-to-profound hearing loss show a pattern of test results where ABRs are absent and OAEs are present. In this context, if the mutation of the otoferlin gene is confirmed by genetic testing and if electrically evoked ABRs can be elicited, then available evidence suggests that cochlear implantation is a viable option and has a good chance of being successful. Because the otoferlin mutation is *not* a neuropathy, this is additional good news for those affected with this condition.

Conclusion

Several human and animal models are available which can be considered suitable candidates for studying AN. The selection of appropriate models can be viewed as an evolutionary process. Clearly, not all models will be suitable, not all models will withstand scientific scrutiny, and, certainly, not all models will withstand the test of time. Therefore, by necessity, some will need to be rejected. We concur with the position taken by others that the term "auditory neuropathy" should be reserved only for those who have a disorder of the auditory nerve, and should not be applied to conditions of sensory cell loss, such as those involving putative IHC lesions (e.g., Gibson & Graham, 2008; Loundon et al., 2005; Rapin & Gravel, 2003, 2006). This is more than a matter of semantics, as one would expect differences in presenting symptoms (e.g., Santarelli et al., 2008), as well as differences in viable treatment modalities and outcomes. Moreover, we need additional postmortem anatomic data with detailed behavioral and physiologic results to help distinguish IHC abnormalities from those with true neuropathies of the auditory nerve. Of course, animal models can be very helpful but extrapolation and translation to humans requires a certain degree of caution. In our view, probably the most attractive animal models for AN are those based on ouabain administration and direct compression because they target the auditory nerve; most notably, large caliber neurons. Other presumed models of AN that have been reviewed are both unique and important in their own right. However, they are not necessarily appropriate, optimal, or sufficient to be included in this category. These include models based on: a mutation of the otoferlin gene, carboplatin administration, deletion of the high-affinity thiamine transporter SLC19A2 to simulate thiamine-responsive megaloblastic anemia, mutations in the active zone scaffolding protein Bassoon, and mutations in one of the vesicular glutamate transporters, VGLUT3. Indeed, there is strong evidence to indicate that these conditions are more closely aligned with primary IHC dysfunction rather than

with frank neuropathies of the auditory nerve. Although we recognize that some of these issues may be debatable, for the most part, this statement is true and it is supported by compelling data.

Lastly, we emphasize that specificity of the diagnosis and the ability to distinguish AN from other related pathologies or sites of lesion are essential core issues for future research to consider and therefore are key elements for strengthening this area of investigation. Such improvements will be beneficial for prospective investigations where the application of novel (re)habilitation strategies, including those where restoration of function is the ultimate goal. At this point in time, we do not have complete answers to all the relevant questions that have been posed about this condition. We also realize that this is a very challenging area. Nevertheless, it is our hope and expectation that advancements in future research will be illuminating and fruitful in solving the problems we presently face.

References

Abdala, C., Sininger, Y. S., & Starr, A. (2000). Distortion product otoacoustic emission suppression in subjects with auditory neuropathy. *Ear and Hearing, 21,* 542–553.

Adunka, O. F., Jewells, V., & Buchman, C. A. (2007). Value of computed tomography in the evaluation of children with cochlear nerve deficiency. *Otology and Neuro-Otology, 28,* 597–604.

Ahlfors, C. E., Shoemaker, C. T., Bennett, S. H., & Ellis, W. G. (1984). Bilirubin associated with abnormalities in the auditory brainstem response in an infant rhesus monkey model. *Pediatric Research, 18,* 308.

Altrock, W. D., tom Dieck, S., Sokolov, M., Meyer, A. C., Sigler, A., Brakebusch, C., et. al. (2003). Functional inactivation of a fraction of excitatory synapses in mice deficient for the active zone protein Bassoon. *Neuron, 37,* 787–800.

Amatuzzi, M., Northrop, C., Libermann, M., Thornton, A., Halpin, C., Hermann, B., et al. (2001). Selective inner hair cell loss in premature infants and cochlea pathological patterns from neonatal intensive care unit autopsies. *Archives of Otolaryngology and Head and Neck Surgery, 127,* 629–636.

Angenstein, F., Niessen, H. G., Goldschmidt, J., Lison, H., Altrock, W. D., Gundelfinger, E. D., et al. (2007). Manganese-enhanced MRI reveals structural and functional changes in the cortex of Bassoon mutant mice. *Cerebral Cortex, 17,* 28–36.

Agenstein, F., Hilfert, L., Zuschratter, W., Altrock, D., Neissen, H. G., & Gundelfinger, E. D. (2008). Morphological and metabolic changes in the cortex of mice lacking the functional presynaptic active zone protein Bassoon: A combined 1H-NMR spectroscopy and histochemical study. *Cerebral Cortex, 18,* 890–897.

Aran, J., Charlet de Sauvage, R., & Pelerin, J. (1971). Comparison of electrocochleographic and audiographic thresholds. Statistical study. *Review of Laryngology, Otology, and Rhinology, 92,* 477–491.

Arnold, S., & Burkard, R. (2002). Inner hair cell loss and steady-state evoked potentials from the inferior colliculus and auditory cortex of the chinchilla. *Journal of the Acoustical Society of America, 112,* 590–599.

Attias, J., & Raveh, E. (2007). Transient deafness in young candidates for cochlear implants. *Audiology and Neuro-Otology, 12,* 325–333.

Bauer, C., & Brozoski, T. J. (2005). Cochlear structure and function after round window application of ototoxins. *Hearing Research, 201,* 121–131.

Beal, M. F. (2000). Energetics and the pathogenesis of neurodegenerative disease. *Trends in Neuroscience, 23,* 298–304.

Berg, A. L., Spitzer, J. B., Towers, H. M., Bartosiewicz, C., & Diamond, B. E. (2005). Newborn hearing screening in the NICU: Profile of failed auditory brainstem response/passed otoacoustic emission. *Pediatrics, 116,* 933–938.

Berlin, C. I., Hood, L. J., Cecola, R. P., Jackson, D. F., & Sabo, P. (1993). Does type I afferent dysfunction reveal itself through lack of efferent suppression? *Hearing Research, 65,* 40–50.

Berlin, C. I., Hood, L. J., Morlet, T., Wilensky, D., St. John, P., Montgomery, E., et al. (2005). Absent or elevated middle ear muscle reflexes in the presence of normal otoacoustic emissions: A universal finding in 136 cases of auditory neuropathy/dys-synchrony. *Journal of the American Acadamy of Audiology, 16,* 546–553.

Berlin, C.I., Hood, L., & Rose, K. (2001). On renaming auditory neuropathy as auditory dys-synchrony: Implications for a clearer understanding of the underlying mechanisms and management options. *Audiology Today, 13,* 15–17.

Berlin, C. I., Morlet, T., & Hood, L. (2003). Auditory neuropathy/dyssynchrony: Its diagnosis and management. *Pediatric Clinics of North America, 50,* 331–340.

Beutner, D., Foerst, A., Lang-Roth, R., von Wedel, H., & Walger, M. (2007). Risk factors for auditory neuropathy/auditory synaptopathy. *Journal of Oto-Rhino-Laryngology and Related Specialties, 69,* 239–244.

Bock, G. R., Yates, G. R., & Deol, M. S. (1982). Cochlear potentials in the Bronx Waltzer mutant mouse. *Neuroscience Letters, 34,* 19–25.

Bonfils, P., Avan, P., Landero, A., Narcy, P., & Trotoux, J. (1991). Progressive hereditary deafness with predominant inner hair cell loss. *American Journal of Otology, 12,* 203–206.

Brookes, J. T., Kanis, A. B., Tan, L. Y., Tranebjaerg, L., Vore, A., & Smith, R. J. (2007). Cochlear implantation in deafness-dystonia-optic neuronopathy (DDON) syndrome. *International Journal of Pediatric Otorhinolaryngology, 72,* 121–126.

Buchman, C A., Roush, P. A., Teagle, H. F., Brown, C. J., Zdanski, C. J., & Grose, J. H. (2006). Auditory neuropathy characteristics in children with cochlear nerve deficiency. *Ear and Hearing, 27,* 399–408.

Burkard, R., Trautwein, P., & Salvi, R. (1997). The effects of click level, click rate and level of background masking noise on the inferior colliculus potential (ICP) in the normal and carboplatin-treated chinchilla. *Journal of the Acoustical Society of America, 102,* 3620-3627.

Buss, E., Labadie, R., Brown, C. J., Gross, A. J., Gross, J. H., & Pillsbury, H. C. (2002). Outcome of cochlear implantation in pediatric auditory neuropathy. *Audiology and Neuro-Otology, 23,* 328-332.

Bussoli, T., Kelly, A., & Steel, K. P. (1997). Localization of the Bronx Waltzer (bv) deafness gene to mouse chromosome 5. *Mammalian Genome, 8,* 714-717.

Butinar, D., Starr, A., Zidar, J., Koutsou, P., & Christodoulou, K. (2007). Auditory nerve is affected in one of two different point mutations of the neurofiliment light gene. *Clinical Neurophysiology, 119,* 367-375.

Cacace, A. T., Satya-Murti, S., & Grimes, C. T. (1983). Frequency selectivity and temporal processing in Friedreich ataxia: Clinical aspects in two patients. *Annals of Otology, Rhinology and Laryngology, 92,* 276-280.

Cacace, A. T., Pinheiro, J. M. B., Malone, A., Kerwood, J., & Artino, L. (1996). Cochlear deafferentation following neonatal hyperbilirubinemia. *Association for Research in Otolaryngology, 19,* 166.

Chariot, P., Brugieres, P., Eliezer-Vanerot, M. C., Geny, C., Binaghi, M., Cesaro, P., et al. (1999). Choreic movements and MRI abnormalities in the subthalamic nuclei reversible after administration of coenzyme Q10 and multiple vitamins in a patient with bilateral optic neuropathy. *Movement Disorders, 14,* 855-859.

Chen, H., & Chan, D. C. (2005). Emerging functions of mammalian mitochondrial fusion and fission. *Human Molecular Genetics, 14,* R283-R289.

Chertoff, M. E., Amani-Taleshi, D., Guo, Y., & Burkard, R. (2002). The influence of inner hair cell loss on the instantaneous frequency of the cochlear microphonic. *Hearing Research, 174,* 93-100.

Colletti, L. (2007). Beneficial auditory and cognitive effects of auditory brainstem implanta-tion in children. *Acta Otolarygologica, 127,* 943-946.

Colletti, V., Carner, M., Fiorino, F., Sacchetto, L., Miorelli, V., Orsi, A., et al. (2002). Hearing restoration with auditory brainstem implant in three children with cochlear nerve aplasia. *Otology and Neuro-Otology, 23,* 682-693.

Colletti, V., Fiorino, F. Carner, M., Miorelli, V., Guida, M., & Colletti, L. (2004). Auditory brainstem implant as a salvage treatment after unsuccessful cochlear implantation. *Otology and Neuro-Otology, 25,* 485-496.

Corrales, C. E., Pan, L., Li, H., Liberman, M. C., Heller, S., & Edge, A. S. (2006). Engraphment and differentiation of embryonic stem cell-derived neural progenitor cells in the cochlear-nerve trunk: growth of processes into the organ of Corti. *Journal of Neurobiology, 66,* 1498-1500.

Delmaghani, S., del Castillo, F. J., Michel, V., Leibovici, M., Aghaie, A., Ron, U., et al. (2006). Mutations in the gene encoding pejvakin, a newly identified protein of the afferent auditory pathway, cause DFNB59 auditory neuropathy. *Nature Genetics, 38,* 770-778.

Delmaghani, S., del Castillo, F. J., Michel, V., Leibovici, M., Aghaie, A., Ron, U., et al. (2007). Mutations in the gene encoding pejvakin, a novel protein expressed in the afferent auditory pathway, causes DFNB59 auditory neuropathy in man and mouse. *Association for Research in Otolaryngology, 30,* 170.

Detmer, S. A., & Chan, D. C. (2007). Functions and dysfunctions of mitochondrial dynamics. *Nature Reviews Molecular and Cell Biology, 8,* 870-879.

Doyle, K. J., Sininger, Y., & Starr, A. (1998). Auditory neuropathy in childhood. *Laryngoscope, 108,* 1374-1377.

Dresbach, T., Torres, V., Wittenmayer, N., Altrock, W. D., Zamorano, P., Zuschratter, W., et al. (2006). Assembly of active zone precursor vesicles: Obligatory trafficking of presynaptic cytomatrix protcins bassoon and piccolo via a trans-Golgi compartment. *Journal of Biological Chemistry, 281,* 6038-6047.

Dürr, A., Cossee, A., Agrid, Y., Campuzano, V., Mignard, C., Penet C., et al. (1996). Clinical and genetic abnormalities in patients with Friedreich's ataxia. *New England Journal of Medicine, 335,* 1169–1175.

El-Badry, M. M., Ding, D. L., McFadden, S. L., & Eddins, A. C. (2007). Physiological effects of auditory nerve myelinopathy in chinchillas. *European Journal of Neuroscience, 25,* 1437–1446.

El-Badry, M. M., & McFadden, S. L. (2007). Electrophysiological correlates of progressive sensorineural pathology in carboplatin-treated chinchillas. *Brain Research, 23,* 122–130.

Fabrizi, G. M., Cavallaro, T., Angiari, C., Cabrini, I., Taiolo, F., Malerba, G., et al. (2007). Charcot-Marie-tooth disease type 2E, a disorder of the cytoskeleton. *Brain 130,* 1–10.

Fan, L-W., Lin, S., Pang, Y., Lei, M., Zhang, F., Rhodes, P., et al. (2005). Hypoxic-ischemic induced neurological dysfunction and brain injury in the neonatal rat. *Behavioral Brain Research, 165,* 80–90.

Faux, M. C., & Scott, A. S. (1996). Molecular glue: Kinase anchoring and scaffolding proteins. *Cell, 85,* 9–12.

Fleming, J. C., Steinkamp, M. P., Kawatsuji, R., Tartaglini, E., Pinkus, J. L., Pinkus, G. S., et al. (2001). Characterization of a murine high-affinity thiamine transporter, Slc19a2. *Molecular Genetics and Metabolism, 74,* 273–280.

Foerst, A., Beutner, D., Lang-Roth, Huttenbrink, von Wedel, H., & Walger, M. (2006). Prevalence of auditory neuropathy/synaptopathy in a population of children with profound hearing loss. *International Journal of Pediatric Otorhinolaryngology, 70,* 1415–1422.

Fuchs, P. A. (2005). Time and intensity coding at the hair cell's ribbon synapse. *Journal of Physiology, 566,* 7–12.

Fuchs, P. A., Glowatzki, E., & Moser, T. (2003). The afferent synapse of cochlear hair cells. *Current Opinion in Neurobiology, 13,* 452–458.

Gadian, D. G., Aicardi, J., Watkins, K. E., Porter, D. A., Mishkin, M., & Vargha-Khadem, F. (2000). Developmental amnesia associated with early hypoxic-ischaemic injury. *Brain, 123*(Pt. 3), 499–507.

Gibson, W. P. R., & Graham, J. M. (2008). Editorial: "Auditory neuropathy" and cochlear implantation—myths and facts. *Cochlear Implants International* (published online in Wiley Interscience (www.interscience.wiley.com) DOI: 10.1002/cii.349.

Gibson, W. P. R., & Sanli, H. (2007). Auditory neuropathy: An update. *Ear and Hearing, 28,* 102S–106S.

Gillis, L., & Kaye, E. (2002). Diagnosis and management of mitochondrial diseases. *Pediatric Clinics of North America, 49,* 203–219.

Griesinger, C. B., Richards, C. D., & Ashmore, J. F. (2005). Fast vesicle replenishment allows indefatigable signaling at the first auditory synapse. *Nature, 435,* 212–215.

Hagberg, H., Peebles, D., & Mallard, C. (2002). Models of white matter injury: comparison of infectious, hypoxic-ischemic, and excitotoxic insults. *Mental Retardation Developmental Disabilities Research Review, 8,* 30–38.

Hallpike, C. S., Harriman, D. G., & Wells, C. E. (1980). A case of afferent neuropathy and deafness. *Journal of Laryngology and Otology, 94,* 945–964.

Hansen, T. W. R., Cashore, W. J., & Oh, W. (1992). Changes in piglet auditory brainstem response amplitudes without increases in serum or cerebrospinal fluid neuron-specific enolase. *Pediatric Research, 32,* 524–529.

Harding, A. E. (1995). From the syndrome of Charcot, Marie and Tooth to disorders of peripheral myelin proteins. *Brain, 118,* 809–818.

Harding, A. E., & Thomas, P. K. (1980). The clinical features of hereditary motor and sensory neuropathy I and II. *Brain, 103,* 259–280.

Harrison R. (1998). An animal model of auditory neuropathy. *Ear and Hearing, 19,* 355–361.

Heil, P. (1997a). Auditory onset responses revisited. I. First-spike timing. *Journal of Neurophysiology, 77,* 2616–2641.

Heil, P. (1997b). Auditory onset responses revisited. II. Response strength. *Journal of Neurophysiology, 77,* 2642–2660.

Heil, P., & Irvine, D. (1996). On determinants of first-spike latency in auditory cortex. *NeuroReport, 7,* 3073–3076.

Heil, P., & Irvine, D. (1997). First-spike timing of auditory-nerve fibers and comparison with auditory cortex. *Journal of Neurophysiology, 78,* 2438–2454.

Hofstetter, P., Ding, D., Powers, N. & Salvi, R. (1997). Quantitative relationship of carboplatin dose to magnitude of inner and outer hair cell loss and the reduction in distortion product otoacoustic emission amplitude in chinchillas. *Hearing Research*, *112*, 199–215.

Hofstetter, P., Ding, D., & Salvi, R. (1997). Magnitude and pattern of inner and outer hair cell loss in chinchilla as a function of carboplatin dose. *Audiology*, *36*, 301–311.

Hong, B. N., & Kang, T. H. (2008). Auditory neuropathy in streptozotocin-induced diabetic mouse. *Neuroscience Letters*, *431*, 268–272.

Hood, L. (2007). Auditory neuropathy and dys-synchrony. In R. Burkard, M. Don, & J. J. Eggermont (Eds.), *Auditory evoked potentials: Basic principles and clinical application* (pp. 275–290). Baltimore: Lippincott, Williams & Wilkins.

Hood, L. J., & Berlin, C. I. (2001). Auditory neuropathy (auditory dys-synchrony) disables efferent suppression of otoacoustic emissions. In Y. Sininger & A. Starr (Eds.), *Auditory neuropathy* (pp. 183–202). San Diego, CA: Singular.

Hood, L. J., Berlin, C. I., Bordelon, J., & Rose, K. (2003). Patients with auditory neuropathy/dys-synchrony lack efferent suppression of transient evoked otoacoustic emissions. *Journal of the American Academy of Audiology*, *14*, 302–313.

Hu, Z., Ulfendahl, M., & Olivius, N. P. (2004). Central migration of neuronal tissue and embryonic stem cells following transplantation along the adult auditory nerve. *Brain Research*, *5*, 1026, 68–73.

Hudspeth, A. J. (2005). How the ear's works work: mechanoelectrical transduction and amplification by hair cells. *C. R. Biology*, *328*, 155–162.

Jeong, S. W., Kim, L. S., Kim, B. Y., Bae, W. Y., & Kim, J. R. (2007). Cochlear implantation in children with auditory neuropathy: Outcomes and rationale. *Acta Otolaryngologica*, *558*, 36–43.

Jinnai, K., Yamada, H., Kanda, F., Masui, Y., Tanaka, M., Ozawa, T., et al. (1990). A case of mitochondrial myopathy, encephalopathy and lactic acidosis due to cytochrome c oxidase deficiency with neurogenic muscular changes. *European Neurology*, *30*, 56–60.

Jock, B., Hamernik, R., Aldrich, L., Ahroon, W., Petriello, K., & Johnson, R. (1996). Evoked-potential thresholds and cubic distortion product otoacoustic emissions in the chinchilla following carboplatin treatment and noise exposure. *Hearing Research*, *96*, 179–190.

Kaplan, J. (1999). Friedreich's ataxia is a mitochondrial disorder. *Proceedings of the National Academy of Sciences*, *28*, 10948–10949.

Katona, G., Buki, B., Farkas, Z., Pytel, J., Simon-Nagy E., & Hirschberg, J. (1993). Transitory evoked otoacoustic emission (TEOAE) in a child with profound hearing loss. *International Journal of Pediatric Otorhinolaryngology*, *26*, 263–267.

Keen, E., C., & Hudspeth, A. J. (2006). Transfer characteristics of the hair cell's afferent synapse. *Proceedings of the National Academy of Sciences*, *103*, 5537–5542.

Khimich, D., Nouvian, R., Pujol, R., tom Dieck, S., Egner, A., Gundelfinger, E. D., et al. (2005). Hair cell synaptic ribbons are essential for synchronous auditory signaling. *Nature*, *434*, 889–894.

Khwaja, O., & Volpe, J. J. (2008). Pathogenesis of cerebral white matter injury of prematurity. *Archives of Disease in Childhood Fetal Neonatal Edition*, *93*, F153–F161.

Kothe, C., Fleischer, S., Breitfuss, A., & Hess, M. (2006). Unilateral auditory neuropathy. A rare differential diagnosis of unilateral deafness. *HNO*, *54*, 215–220.

Kumar, U. A., & Jayaram, M. M. (2006). Prevalence and audiological characteristics in individuals with auditory neuropathy/auditory dys-synchrony. *International Journal of Audiology*, *45*, 360–366.

Lang, H., Schulte, B. A., & Schmiedt, R. A. (2005). Ouabain induces apoptotic cell death in type I spiral ganglion neurons, but not type II neurons. *Journal of the Association for Research in Otolaryngology*, *6*, 63–74.

Lang, H., Schulte, B. A., Goddard, J C., Hedrick, M., Schulte, J. B., Wei, L., et al. (2008). Transplantation of mouse embryonic stem cells into the cochlea of an auditory-neuropathy animal model: Effects of timing after injury. *Journal of the Association for Research in Otolaryngology, 9,* 225–240.

Liberman, M. C., Chesney, C. & Kujawa, S. (1997). Effects of selective inner hair cell loss on DPOAE and CAP in carboplatin-treated chinchillas. *Auditory Neuroscience, 3,* 255–268.

Liberman, M. C, Tartaglini, E., & Fleming, J. C., & Neufeld, E. J. (2006). Deletion of SLC19A2, the high affinity thiamine transporter, causes selective inner hair cell loss and an auditory neuropathy phenotype. *Journal of the Association for Research in Otolaryngology, 7,* 211–217.

Lesinski-Schiedat, A., Frohne, C., Hemmaouil, I., Battmer, R. D., & Lenarz, T. (2001). Subjective deafness in a case of peri-synaptic audiopathy. Isolated defects of the inner hair cells? *Laryngorhinootologie, 80,* 601–604.

Levine, R. L. (1983). The toxicity of bilirubin. In R. L. Levine & M. T. Maisels (Eds.), *Hyperbilirubinemia in the newborn, Report of the Eighty-Fifth Ross Conference on Pediatric Research* (pp. 39–46). Columbus, OH.

Loundon, N., Marcolla, A., Roux, I., Rouillon, I., Denoyelle, F., Feldman, D., et al. (2005). Auditory neuropathy or endocochlear hearing loss? *Otology and Neuro-Otology, 26,* 748–754.

Lucey, J. F., Hibbard, E., Behrman, R. E., Esquivel De Gallardo, F. O., & Windle, W. I. (1964). Kernicterus in asphyxiated newborn rhesus monkeys. *Experimental Neurology, 9,* 43.

Madden, C., Hilbert, L., Rutter, M., Greinwald, J., & Choo, D. (2002). Pediatric cochlear implantation in auditory neuropathy. *Otology and Neuro-Otology, 23,* 163–168.

Mammano, F., Bortolozzi, M., Ortolano, S., & Anselmi, F. (2007). Ca^{2+} signaling in the inner ear. *Physiology, 22,* 131–144.

Mason, J. C., De Michele, A., Stevens, C., Ruth, R. A., & Hashisaki, G. T. (2003). Cochlear implantation in patients with auditory neuropathy of varied etiologies. *Laryngoscope, 113,* 45–49.

Matsumoto, M., Sekiya, T., Kojima, K., & Ito, J. (2008). An animal experimental model of auditory neuropathy in rats by auditory nerve compression. *Experimental Neurology, 210,* 248–256.

Matsuoka, A. J., Kondo, T., Miyamoto, R. T., & Hashino, E. (2007). Enhanced survival of bone-marrow-derived pluripotent stem cells in an animal model of auditory neuropathy. *Laryngoscope, 117,* 1629–1635.

McClure, M. M., Threldkeld, S. W., & Fitch, R. H. (2007). Auditory processing and learning/memory following erythropoietin administration in neonatally hypoxic-ischemic injured rats. *Brain Research, 1132,* 203–209.

McDonald, J. W., Shapiro, S. M., Silverstein, F. S., & Johnston, M. V. (1998). Role of glutamate receptor-mediated excitotoxicity in bilirubin-induced brain injury in the Gunn rat model. *Experimental Neurology, 150,* 21–29.

McFadden, S., Kasper, C., Ostrowski, J., Ding, D., & Salvi, R. (1998). Effects of inner hair cell loss on inferior colliculus evoked potential thresholds, amplitudes and forward masking functions in chinchillas. *Hearing Research, 120,* 121–132.

McMahon, C. M., Patuzzi, R. B., Gibson, W. P. R., & Sanli, H. (2008). Frequency-specific electrochleography indicates the presynaptic and postsynaptic mechanisms of auditory neuropathy exist. *Ear and Hearing, 29,* 314–325.

Miyamoto, R. T., Kirk, K.I., Renshaw, J., & Hussain, D. (1999). Cochlear implantation in auditory neuropathy. *Laryngoscope, 109,* 181–185.

Moser, T., Neef, A., & Khimich, D. (2006). Mechanisms underlying the temporal precision of sound coding at the inner hair cell ribbon synapse. *Journal of Physiology, 576,* 55–62.

Moser, T., Strenke, N., Meyer, A., Lesinski-Schiedat, A., Lenarz, T., Beutner, D., et al. (2006). Diagnosis and therapy of auditory synaptopathy/neuropathy. *HNO 54,* 833–839.

Musiek, F. E., Weider, D. J., & Mueller, R. J. (1982). Audiologic findings in Charcot-Marie-Tooth disease. *Archives of Otolaryngology, 108,* 595–599.

Nakamura, Y., Takahashi, M., Kitaguchi, M., Yorifuji, S., Nishikawa, Y., Imaoka, H., et al. (1995). Abnormal evoked potentials of Kearns-Sayre syndrome. *Electromyography and Clinical Neurophysiology, 35,* 365–370.

Ngo, R. Y. S., Tan, H. K. K., Balakrishnan, A., Lim, S. B., & Lazaroo, D. T. (2006). Auditory neuropathy/auditory dys-synchrony detected by universal newborn hearing screening. *International Journal of Pediatric Otorhinolaryngology, 70,* 1299–1306.

Niemann, A., Berger, P., & Suter, U. (2006). Pathomechanisms of mutant proteins in Charcot-Marie-Tooth disease. *Neurology and Molecular Medicine, 8,* 217–241.

Norton, S. J. (1993). Application of transient evoked otoacoustic emissions to pediatric populations. *Ear and Hearing, 43,* 64–73.

Nouvian, R., Beutner, D., Parsons, T. D., & Moser, T. (2006). Structure and function of the hair cell ribbon synapse. *Journal of Membrane Biology, 209,* 152–165.

Ohwatari, R., Fukuda, S., Chida, E., Matsumura, M., Kuroda, T, Kashiwamura, M., et al. (2001). Preserved otoacoustic emissions in a child with a profound unilateral sensorineural hearing loss. *Auris Nasus Larynx, 28*(Suppl.), S117–S120.

O'Leary, S., Mitchell, T. E., Gibson, W. P. R., & Sanli, H. (2000). Abnormal positive potentials in round window electrocochleography. *American Journal of Otology, 21,* 813–818.

Olivius, P., Alexandrov, L., Miller, J. M., Ulfendahl, M., Bagger-Sjoback, D., & Kozlova, E. N. (2004). A model for implanting neuronal tissue into the cochlea. *Brain Research Protocols, 12,* 152–156.

Olivius, P., Threldkeld, S. W., Fitch, R. H., Alexandrov, L., Miller, J., Ulfendahl, M., et al. (2003). Allografted fetal dorsal root ganglion neuronal survival in the guinea pig cochlea. *Brain Research. 979,* 1–6.

Pandolfo, M. (2008). Drug insight: Antioxidant therapy in inherited ataxias. *Nature Clinical Practice Neurology, 4,* 86–96.

Parsons, T. D. (2006). Auditory fidelity. *Nature, 444,* 1013–1014.

Pauli-Magnus, D., Hoch, G., Strenzke, N., Anderson, S., Jentsch, T. J., & Moser, T. (2007). Detection and differentiation of sensorineural hearing loss in mice using auditory steady-state responses and transient auditory brainstem responses. *Neuroscience, 149,* 673–684.

Peterson, A., Shallop, J., Driscoll, C., Breneman, A., Babb, J., Stoekel, R., et al. (2003). Outcomes of cochlear implantation in children with auditory neuropathy. *Journal of the American Academy of Audiology, 14,* 188–201.

Phillips, D. P., Hall, S. E., Guo, Y., & Burkard. R. (2001). Sensitivity of unanaesthetized chinchilla auditory system to noise burst onset, and the effects of carboplatin. *Hearing Research, 155,* 133–42.

Pineda, M., Arpa, J., Montero, R., Aracil, A., Dominguez, F., Galván, M., et al. (2008). Idebenone treatment in pediatric and adult patients with Friedreich ataxia: Long-term follow-up. *European Journal of Pediatric Neurology,* E-pub ahead of print.

Podwell, A., Podwell, D., Gordon, T. G., Lamendola, & Gold, A. P. (2002). Unilateral auditory neuropathy: Case study. *Journal of Child Neurology, 17,* 306–309.

Postelmans, J. T., & Strokross, R. J. (2006). Cochlear implantation in a patient with deafness induced by Charcot-Marie-Tooth disease (hereditary motor and sensory neuropathies). *Journal of Laryngology and Otology, 120,* 508–510.

Prescott, E. D., & Zenisek, D. (2005). Recent progress toward understanding the synaptic ribbon. *Current Opinion in Neurobiology, 15,* 431–436.

Psarommatis, I., Riga, M., Douros, K., Koltsidopoulos, P., Douniadakis, D., Kapetanakis, I., et al. (2006). Transient infantile auditory neuropathy and its clinical implications. *International Journal of Pediatric Otorhinolaryngology, 70,* 1629–1637.

Puccio, H., & Koenig, M. (2002). Friedreich ataxia: A paradigm for mitochondrial diseases. *Current Opinions of Genetic Development, 12,* 272–277.

Qiu, C. X., Salvi, R., Ding, D. & Burkard, R. (2000). Inner hair cell loss can lead to enhancement of responses from auditory cortex in unanaesthetized chinchillas. *Hearing Research, 139,* 153–171.

Ramakrishnan, N. A., Drescher, M. J., & Drescher, D. G. (2008). Calcium-dependent interaction of otoferlin with $Ca_v1.3$ and syntaxin 1A. *Abstracts of the Association for Research in Otolaryngology, 31,* 69.

Rance, G. (2005). Auditory neuropathy/dyssynchrony and its perceptual consequences. *Trends in Amplification, 1,* 1–43.

Rance, G., Barker, E., Mok, M., Dowell, R., Rincon, A., & Garratt. R. (2007). Speech perception in noise for children with auditory neuropathy/ dys-synchrony type hearing loss. *Ear and Hearing, 28,* 351-360.

Rapin, I., & Gravel, J. S. (2003). "Auditory neuropathy": physiologic and pathologic evidence calls for more diagnostic specificity. *International Journal of Pediatric Otorhinolaryngology, 67,* 707-728.

Rapin, I., & Gravel, J. S. (2006). Auditory neuropathy: a biologically inappropriate label unless acoustic nerve involvement is documented. *Journal of the American Academy of Audiology, 17,* 147-150.

Rea , P. A., & Gibson, W. P. R. (2003). Evidence for surviving outer hair cell function in deaf ears. *Laryngoscope, 113,* 2030-2033.

Rhee, C. K., Park, H. M., & Jang, Y. J. (1999). Audiologic evaluation of neonates with severe hyperbilirubinemia using transiently evoked otoacoustic emissions and auditory brainstem responses. *Laryngoscope, 109,* 2005-2008.

Rice, A. C., & Shapiro, S. M. (2006). Biliverdin-induced brainstem auditory evoked potential abnormalities in the jaundiced Gunn rat. *Brain Research, 1107,* 215-221.

Robertson, D. (1984). Horseradish peroxidase injection of physiologically characterized afferent and efferent neurons in the guinea pig spiral ganglion. *Hearing Research, 15,* 113-121.

Robertson, D., Sellick, R. & Patuzzi, R. (1999). The continuing search for outer hair cell afferents in the guinea pig spiral ganglion. *Hearing Research, 136,* 151-158.

Rodriguez-Ballesteros, M., del Castillo, F. J., Martin, Y., Moreno-Pelayo, M. A., Morera C., Prieto F., et al. (2003). Auditory neuropathy in patients carrying mutations in the otoferlin gene (OTOF). *Human Mutatations, 22,* 451-456.

Rosen, J. (1956). Rh child: Deaf or "aphasic"? 4. Variations in the auditory disorders of the Rh child. *Journal of Speech and Hearing Disorders, 24,* 418-422.

Roscigno, C. I. (2002). Periventricular leukomalacia: pathophysiological concerns due to immature development of the brain. *Journal of Neuroscience Nursing, 34,* 296-302.

Rouillon, I., Marcolla, A., Roux, I., Marlin, S., Feldman, S., Couderc, R., et al. (2006). Results of cochlear implantation in two children with mutations in the OTOF gene. *International Journal of Pediatric Otorhinolaryngology, 70,* 689-696.

Roux, I., Safieddine, S., Nouvian, R., Grati, M., Simmier, M. C., Bahloul, A., et al. (2006). Otoferlin, defective in a human deafness form, is essential for exocytosis at the auditory ribbon synapse. *Cell, 127,* 277-289.

Rozdilsky, B., & Olszewski, J. (1961). Experimental study of the toxicity of bilirubin in newborn animals. *Journal of Neuropathology and Experimental Neurology, 20,* 193-205.

Runge-Samuelson, C. L., Drake, S., & Wackym, P. A. (2008). Quantitative analysis of electrically evoked auditory brainstem responses in implanted children with auditory neuropathy/ dyssynchrony. *Otology and Neuro-Otology, 29,* 174-178.

Safieddine, S., & Wenthold, R. J. (1999). SNARE complex at the ribbon synapses of cochlear hair cells: analysis of synaptic vesicle- and synaptic membrane-associated proteins. *European Journal of Neuroscience, 11,* 803-812.

Salvi, R. J., Wang, J., Steckler, N., & Arnold, S. (1999). Auditory deprivation of the central auditory system resulting from selective inner hair cell loss: animal model of auditory neuropathy. *Scandinavian Audiology Supplement, 51,* 1-12.

Salvinelli, F., Firrisi, L., Greco, F., Trivelli, M., & D'Ascanio, L. (2004). Preserved otoacoustic emissions in postparotitis profound unilateral hearing loss: a case report. *Annals of Oto-Rhino-Laryngology, 113,* 887-890.

Santarelli, R., & Arslan, E. (2002). Electrocochleography in auditory neuropathy. *Hearing Research, 170,* 32-47.

Santarelli, R., Starr, A, Michalewski, H. J., & Arslan, E. (2008). Neural and receptor cochlear potentials obtained by transtympanic electrocochleography in auditory neuropathy. *Clinical Neurophysiology, 119,* 1028-1041.

Sato, K. (1988). Pharmacokinetics of coenzyme Q10 in recovery of acute sensorineural hearing loss due to hypoxia. *Acta Otolaryngologica, 458,* 95–102.

Satya-Murti, S., & Cacace, A. T. (1982). Auditory evoked potentials in disorders of the primary sensory ganglion. In J. Courjon, F. Mauguiere, & M. Revol (Eds.), *Clinical Applications of Evoked Potentials in Neurology, Advances in Neurology* (Vol. 32, pp. 219–225). New York: Raven Press.

Satya-Murti, S., Cacace, A. T., & Hanson, P. (1979). Abnormal auditory evoked potentials in hereditary motor sensory neuropathy. *Annals of Neurology, 5,* 445–448.

Satya-Murti, S., Cacace, A. T., & Hanson, P. (1980). Auditory dysfunction in Friedreich ataxia: Result of spiral ganglion degeneration. *Neurology 1980, 30,* 1047–1053.

Satya-Murti, S., Wolpaw, J. R., Cacace, A. T., & Schaeffer, C. (1983). Late auditory evoked potentials can occur without brainstem potentials. *Electroencephalography and Clinical Neurophysiology, 56,* 304–308.

Sawada, S., Mori, N., Mount, R. J., & Harrison, R. V. (2001). Differential vulnerability of inner and outer hair cell systems to chronic mild hypoxia and glutamate ototoxicity: insights into the cause of auditory neuropathy. *Journal of Otolaryngology, 30,* 106–114.

Schmiedt, R. A., Okamura, H-O, Lang, H., & Schulte, B. A. (2002). Ouabain application to the round window of the gerbil cochlea: A model of auditory neuropathy and apoptosis. *Journal of the Association for Research in Otolaryngology, 3,* 223–233.

Seal, R. P., Akil, O., Yi, E., Weber, C. M., Grant, L., Yoo, J., et al. (2008). Sensorineural deafness and seizures in mice lacking vesicular glutamate transporter 3. *Neuron, 57,* 263–275.

Sekiya, T., Kojima, K., Matsumoto, M., & Ito, J. (2008). Replacement of diseased auditory neurons by cell transplantation. *Life Sciences, 1,* 2165–2176.

Shaia, W. T., Shapiro, S. M., & Spencer, R. F. (2005). The jaundiced Gunn rat model of auditory neuropathy/dyssynchrony. *Laryngoscope, 115,* 2167–2173.

Shallop, J. K., Jin, S. H., Driscoll, C. L., & Tibesar, R. J. (2004). Characteristics of electrically evoked potentials in patients with auditory neuropathy/auditory dys-synchrony. *International Journal of Audiology,* Suppl. 1, S22–S27.

Shallop, J. K., Peterson, A., Facer, G. W., Fabry, L. B., & Driscoll, C. L. (2001). Cochlear implants in five cases of auditory neuropathy: postoperative findings and progress. *Laryngoscope, 111,* 555–562.

Shapiro, S. M., & Te Selle, M. (1994). Cochlear microphonics in the jaundiced Gunn rat. *American Journal of Otolaryngology, 15,* 129–137.

Sheykholeslami, K., & Kaga, K. (2000). Otoacoustic emissions and auditory brainstem responses after neonatal hyperbilirubinemia. *International Journal of Pediatric Otorhinolaryngology, 52,* 65–73.

Shirane, M., & Harrison, R. V. (1987). The effects of deferoxamine mesylate and hypoxia on the cochlea. *Acta Otolaryngologica, 104,* 99–107.

Shy, M. E. (2004). Charcot-Marie-Tooth disease: an update. *Current Opinions in Neurology, 17,* 579–585.

Silver, S., Kaputulnik, J., & Sohmer, H. (1995). Contribution of asphyxia to the induction of hearing impairment in jaundiced Gunn rats. *Pediatrics, 95,* 579–583.

Sinnathuray, A. R., Raut, V., Awa, A., Magee, A., & Toner, J. G. (2003). A review of cochlear implantation in mitochondrial sensorineural hearing loss. *Otology and Neuro-Otology, 24,* 418–426.

Slack, R. W. T., Wright, A., Michaels, L., & Frolich, S. A. (1986). Inner hair cell loss and intracochlear clot in the preterm infant. *Clinical Otolaryngology, 11,* 443–446.

Spoendlin, H. (1974). Optic and cochleovestibular degeneration in hereditary ataxias II. Temporal bone pathology in two cases of Friedreich's ataxia with vestibulocochlear disorders. *Brain, 97,* 41–48.

Starr, A., McPherson, D., Patterson, J., Don, M., Luxford, W., Shannon, R., et al. (1991). Absence of both auditory evoked potentials and auditory percepts dependent on timing cues. *Brain, 114,* 1157-1180.

Starr, A., Michalewski, H. J., Zeng, F. G., Fujikawa-Brooks, S., Linthicum, F., Kim, C. S., et al. (2003). Pathology and physiology of auditory neuropathy with a novel mutation in the MPZ gene (Tyr145→Ser). *Brain, 126,* 1604-1619.

Starr, A., Picton, T. W., Sininger, Y., Hood, L. J., & Berlin, C. I. (1996). Auditory neuropathy. *Brain, 119,* 741-753.

Sterling, P., & Mathews, G. (2005). Structure and function of ribbon synapses. *Trends in Neurosciences, 28,* 20-29.

Stern, L., & Brodersen, R. (1987). Kernicterus research and the basic sciences: A prospect for future development. *Pediatrics, 79,* 154.

Sugawara, M., Cortas, G., & Liberman, M. C. (2005). Long-term neural survival is enhanced when supporting cells in the inner hair cell remain intact. *Association for Research in Otolaryngology, 6,* 136-147.

Suter, U., & Scherer, S. S. (2003). Disease mechanisms in inherited neuropathies. *Nature Reviews Neuroscience, 4,* 714-726.

Suziki, Y., Taniyama, M., Muramatsu, T., Atsumi, Y., Hosokawa, K., Asahina, T., et al. (1997). Diabetes mellitus associated with 3243 mitochondrial tRNA (Leu(UUR) mutation: clinical features and coenzyme Q10 treatment. *Molecular Aspects of Medicine Supplements, 18,* S181-S188.

Suzuki, S., Hinokio, Y., Ohtomo, M., Hirai, M., Hirai, A., Chiba, M., et al. (1998). (1998). The effects of coenzyme Q10 treatment on maternally inherited diabetes mellitus and deafness, and mitochondrial DNA 3243 (A to G) mutation. *Diabetologica, 41,* 584-588.

Takeno, S., Harrison, R., Mount, R., Wake, M. & Harada, Y. (1994). Induction of selective inner hair cell damage by carboplatin. *Scanning Microscopy, 8,* 97-106.

Takeno, S., Harrision, R. V., Ibrahim, D., Wake, M., & Mount, R. J. (1994). Cochlear function after selective inner hair cell degeneration induced by carboplatin. *Hearing Research, 75,* 93-102.

Tatsumi, C., Takahashi, M., Yorifuji, S., Nishikawa, Y., Kitaguchi, M., Hashimoto, S., et al. (1988).

Mitochondrial encephalomyopathy with sleep apnea. *European Neurology, 28,* 64-69.

Taylor, M. J., McMenamin, J. B., Andermann, E., & Watters, G. V. (1982). Electrophysiological investigation of the auditory system in Friedreich's ataxia. *Canadian Journal of Neurological Science, 9,* 131-135.

Tekin, M., Akcayoz, D., & Incesulu, A. (2005). A novel missense mutation in a C2 domain of OTOF results in autosomal recessive auditory neuropathy. *American Journal of Medical Genetics A, 138,* 6-10.

Trautwein, P., Hofstetter, P., Wang, J., Salvi, R., & Nostrant, A. (1996). Selective inner hair cell loss does not alter distortion product otoacoustic emissions. *Hearing Research, 96,* 71-82.

Turkel, S. B. (1990). Autopsy findings associated with neonatal hyperbilirubinemia. *Clinics in Perinatology, 17,* 381-396.

Varga, R., Avenarius, M. R., Kelley, P. M., Keats, B. J., Berlin, C. I., Hood, L. J., et al. (2006). OTOF mutations revealed by genetic analysis of hearing loss families including a potential temperature sensitive auditory neuropathy allele. *Journal of Medical Genetics, 43,* 576-581.

Varga, R., Kelley, P. M., Keats, B. J., Starr, A., Leal, S. M., Cohn, E., et al. (2003). Non-syndromic recessive auditory neuropathy is the result of mutations in the otoferlin (*OTOF*) gene. *Journal of Medical Genetics, 40,* 45-50.

Volpe, J. J. (2003). Cerebral white matter injury of the premature infant—more common than you think. *Pediatrics, 112,* 176-180.

von Gersdorff, H. (2001). Synaptic ribbons: Versatile signal transducers. *Neuron, 29,* 7-10.

Wake, M., Anderson, J., Takeno, S., Mount, R. & Harrison, R. (1996). Otoacoustic emission amplification after inner hair cell damage. *Acta Otolaryngologica, 116,* 374-381.

Wake, M., Takeno, S., Ibrahim, D., & Harrison, R. (1994). Selective inner hair cell ototoxicity induced by carboplatin. *Laryngoscope, 104,* 488-493.

Wake, M., Takeno, S., Ibrahim, D., Harrison, R., & Mount, R. (1993). Carboplatin ototoxicity: An animal model. *Journal of Laryngology and Otology, 107,* 585-589.

Wake, M., Takeno, S., Mount, R., & Harrison, R. (1996). Recording from the inferior colliculus following cochlear inner hair cell damage. *Acta Otolaryngologica, 116,* 714-720.

Wang, J., Ding, D., & Salvi, R. J. (2003). Carboplatin-induced early cochlear lesion in the chinchilla. *Hearing Research, 181,* 65-72.

Wang, L. E., Cao, K. L., Yin, S. K., Yang, Z., & Chen, Z. N. (2006). Cochlear function after selective spiral ganglion cell degeneration induced by ouabain. *Chinese Medical Journal, 119,* 974-979.

Wang, J., Powers, N. L., Hofstetter, P., Trautwein, P., Ding, D., & Salvi, R. (1997). Effects of selective inner hair cell loss on auditory nerve fiber threshold, tuning and spontaneous and driven discharge rate. *Hearing Research, 107,* 67-82.

Wong, S. H., Gibson, W. P. R., & Sanli, H. (1997). Use of transtympanic round window electrocochleography for threshold estimates in children. *American Journal of Otology, 18,* 632-636.

Wood, S., Mason, S., Farnsworth, A., Davis, A., Curnock, D. A., & Lutman, M. E. (1998). Anomalous screening outcomes from click-evoked otoacoustic emissions and auditory brainstem response tests. *British Journal of Audiology, 32,* 399-410.

Worley, G., Erwin, C. W., Goldstein, R. F., Provenzale, J. M., & Ware, R. E. (1996). Delayed development of sensorineural hearing loss after neonatal hyperbilirubinemia: A case report with brain magnetic resonance imaging. *Developmental Medicine and Child Neurology, 38,* 271-277.

Yasunaga, S., Grati, M., Cohen-Salmon, M., El-Amraoui, A., Mustapha, M., Salem, N., et al. (1999). A mutation in OTOF, encoding otoferlin, a FER-1-like protein, causes DFNB9, a nonsyndromic form of deafness. *Nature Genetics, 21,* 363-369.

Young, P., & Suter, U. (2003). The causes of Charcot-Marie-Tooth disease. *Cellular and Molecular Life Sciences, 60,* 2547-2560.

Zeng, F. G., Oba, S., Garde, S., Sininger, Y., & Starr, A. (1999). Temporal and speech processing deficits in auditory neuropathy. *NeuroReport, 10,* 3429-3435.

Züchner, S., & Vance, J. M. (2006). Mechanisms of disease: A molecular genetic update on hereditary axonal neuropathies. *Nature Clinical Practice, 2,* 45-53.

Index